I0092425

THE PRICE OF OVULATION
The Truth about Fertility Drugs
and Birth Defects – and a Solution to the Problem

Auctorem House
276 5th Ave, Ste 704-2591
New York, NY 10001
www.auctoremhouse.com
Phone: 1 888-332-7718

© 2025 Terence Mix. All rights reserved.

No part of this book may be reproduced, stored in a retrieval system, or transmitted by any means without the written permission of the author.

Published by Auctorem House: 06/02/2025

ISBN: 978-1-965687-92-5(sc)
ISBN: 978-1-965687-93-2(e)

Library of Congress Control Number: 2025912666

Any people depicted in stock imagery provided by iStock are models, and such images are being used for illustrative purposes only.

Certain stock imagery © iStock.

Because of the dynamic nature of the Internet, any web addresses or links contained in this book may have changed since publication and may no longer be valid. The views expressed in this work are solely those of the author and do not necessarily reflect the views of the publisher, and the publisher hereby disclaims any responsibility for them.

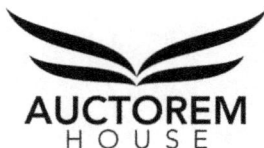

AUCTOREM
HOUSE

THE PRICE OF OVULATION
The Truth about Fertility Drugs
and Birth Defects – and a Solution to the Problem

By Terence Mix

September 30, 2007

CONTENTS

Foreword   3

Introduction   6

Chapter 1 – An Introduction to Drugs   13

Chapter 2 – Clomid on Trial: The Plaintiffs' Case   40

Chapter 3 – Clomid on Trial: The Defendant's Case   85

Chapter 4 – The Chromosome Factor   135

Chapter 5 – An Invitation to Rockville, Maryland   146

Chapter 6 – Selling the Mix Hypothesis   153

Chapter 7 – Working the System   168

Chapter 8 – Ancient Knowledge   191

Chapter 9 – Feathering the Nest   212

Chapter 10 – Controlling the Controls   219

Chapter 11 – A Homemade Study   229

Chapter 12 – The Evidence Grows   248

Chapter 13 – The Check is in the Mail   263

Chapter 14 – A Prophecy Validated   278

Chapter 15 – Back in the Saddle Again   295

Chapter 16 – Does Anyone Really Care?   309

Chapter 17 – The Federal Court of Science   338

Chapter 18 – I Rest My Case   366

Chapter 19 – Cause and Effect   400

Chapter 20 – The Epiphany   417

Chapter 21 – Where Are We Now?   444

Notes and References   475

Exhibits   493

FOREWORD

The Price of Ovulation is an extraordinary book from many perspectives. As it educates the reader in esoteric areas of law, science and medicine, the author takes us on a 35-year journey through an obstacle course imposed by a powerful pharmaceutical company, the FDA and the court system. From his groundbreaking trial and verdict, to his presentation and pleas to the U.S. Food and Drug Administration, to his multiple visits to the pharmaceutical plant and discovery of shocking and incriminating records, Terence Mix opens doors and exposes practices within the drug industry that very few outsiders ever see.

But it is when the author begins to lay out the case against clomiphene and other fertility drugs that his skills as an educator really shine. As a scientist in the field of teratology, I have participated in many studies involving clomiphene and for years have held strong suspicions about the risk presented by this drug to the human embryo. Fertility drugs have been associated with an increased incidence of birth defects in numerous epidemiology studies. Yet it was only after reviewing this incredible book that the evidence all came together. Although for over a decade, geneticists have been researching and enlightening the scientific world about the importance of cholesterol in the proper formation of embryonic organs, very few doctors are aware that clomiphene can actually impair the production of this vital lipid. That fact, along with its lengthy half-life—demonstrated by its ability to remain in the body in excess of a month, make a case against clomiphene that is hard to ignore.

The greatest value of this book, however, is an intriguing, yet credible, proposal by its author which may one day have vast and far-reaching humanitarian implications. Mix makes a persuasive case that lack of adequate cholesterol during the first 8 weeks of pregnancy is also responsible for congenital anomalies in many naturally-conceived multiple and singleton pregnancies. He points to several animal studies in which birth defects have effectively been eliminated in embryos by providing dietary supplementation of cholesterol to the pregnant mothers. If validated in appropriately-designed epidemiology studies, this book may well be a beacon of hope to one day eradicating hundreds of thousands of birth defects throughout the world.

Childlessness is a real tragedy for many couples desiring children of their own. Thus, the dramatic progress that has been made in the treatment of sterility and infertility has been one of the great successes in modern healthcare. Yet few consider that these advances in reproductive technology run counter to the body's natural selection process and don't come without risks. The Price of Ovulation not only presents both sides of this issue, it offers a compromise which allows these couples to pursue their dreams of parenthood while substantially reducing the risks.

Andrew Czeizel, M.D., Ph. D.

Professor of Genetics

World Renowned and Award-Winning Teratologist

ANDREW E. CZEIZEL, MD, PhD, is a Professor of Genetics at Eotvos Lorand University in Budapest, Hungary, and since obtaining his MD degree in 1959, has focused his education and research on the field of teratology. Along with two other scientists, he has been recognized as having discovered the protective benefits of the prenatal use of folic acid and its ability to reduce the risk of neural tube defects and other congenital malformations, for which he received the prestigious Kennedy Foundation International Award for Scientific Achievement (2000) and the United States National Council on Folic Acid award for Excellence in Research in the Field of Folic Acid and Birth Defects Prevention (2002). He is also the recipient of 11 other national and international awards and honors. Dr. Czeizel is the lead author in over 380 scientific papers published in peer-reviewed medical and scientific journals, and in excess of 40 others in which he is a co-author. Four of his published papers dealt specifically with studies evaluating the teratogenic risk of clomiphene citrate. He is a former board member of the European Teratology Society, a former president of the European Environmental Mutagen Society, one of the founders of the International

Clearinghouse for Birth Defects Monitoring Systems, and director of the World Health Organization Collaborating Centre for the Community Control of Hereditary Diseases. He is also a scientific advisor and consultant for several international committees of the World Health Organization.

INTRODUCTION

What you are about to read represents the results of a 30-plus-year investigation of the most popular fertility drug in the world. Between 1972 and 1996, I litigated eight lawsuits against the manufacturer of *Clomid*, a drug used to induce ovulation. It was contended that the drug was causing birth defects to the offspring of its users. Three of the cases went to trial. The first was tried to verdict on April 15, 1974. The other two settled before submitting the case to the jury for a decision. Four others settled before trial, and the eighth and final case was dismissed by a federal court judge after excluding my key causation witness on strongly disputed grounds. A revisit to the subject in 2004 revealed a shocking discovery and motivated the writing of this book.

You might say that Clomid and I were placed on the market for sale during the very same year. On January 4, 1967 I was admitted to the California State Bar. About four months later, Clomid was first marketed following approval by the Federal Food and Drug Administration (FDA). Destiny then stepped in and introduced the two of us in 1972. My subsequent journey over the years also took me to the FDA, where I testified in 1975, and on multiple inspection trips to the manufacturer's plant in Cincinnati. It was during these visits to Ohio that I uncovered most of my surprising evidence. Backed by the power of the judicial system, a trial attorney is in a unique position to access otherwise unavailable corporate records. Over the years, I have literally spent thousands of hours pouring through these records, looking for a "smoking gun." Not only did I find the gun, I have also found the bullets, fingerprints, names of accomplices and a long list of motives. It was the medical research, however, that provided the real inspiration for this book. As will be seen, there are a large number of incriminating studies in the published literature that have yet to be identified in the labeling on Clomid – even to this day. Many of the studies apply to other fertility drugs as well.

My principal adversary over these years was and is an old and established pharmaceutical company. The original entity began conducting business back in 1905. It later became incorporated as Vick Chemical, Inc. in 1933 and adopted the name of Richardson-Merrell, Inc. on October 21, 1960. Wm. S. Merrell Company, the Cincinnati division of Richardson-Merrell that developed, tested and marketed Clomid, changed its name to Merrell-National Laboratories in September 1971. It was under those banners that I engaged them in battle until Richardson-Merrell was purchased by Dow Chemical Company on March 10, 1981, became a subsidiary of the corporate giant, and changed its name to Merrell Dow Pharmaceuticals, Inc.

The corporate musical chairs began to pick up speed in 1990, when Merrell Dow Pharmaceuticals, Inc. merged with Marion Laboratories, Inc., and became Marion Merrell Dow, Inc. In 1995, Dow Chemical Company sold its Marion Merrell Dow stock to Hoechst AG, the world's largest chemical manufacturer, and the resulting company became Hoechst Marion Roussel, Inc. Finally, in 1999, Hoechst Marion Roussel, Inc. merged with Rhone-Poulenc Rorer Pharmaceuticals and became Aventis Pharmaceuticals, Inc. Yet throughout all of the corporate mergers, acquisitions and face lifts, there has remained a constant: product protection at any cost. The names and faces of management would change over the years, but not the corporate drive to maximize profit and the actions the company would take to achieve that ambition.

The relevant corporate history of the company is neither limited to post-1967 nor to the fertility drug that is the subject of this book. Nor is the company inexperienced in litigation. The horrific tragedy of *thalidomide* was not confined to Europe. Developed by the West German company, Chemie Grunenthal, it was reported in late 1961 that it could cause a limb reduction birth defect known as "phocomelia." Children were born with stunted limbs and other abnormalities. At the time, Richardson-Merrell had secured the license to distribute thalidomide within the United States for the treatment of insomnia. While awaiting approval for marketing from the FDA, it had distributed the drug to physician clinical investigators for the purpose of a pre-marketing study.

In June 1971 a Los Angeles jury awarded $2,200,000, including $1,100,000 in punitive damages,[1] to Margaret McCarrick and her mother, who had claimed that she received thalidomide during pregnancy only two months prior to the story breaking about its devastating effect on the human fetus.

The revelation about the cholesterol-reducing drug, *Triparanol (MER/29)*, is yet another episode in its corporate history that Merrell would prefer to forget. That story is detailed in the California appellate decision of *Toole vs. Richardson-Merrell, Inc.*[2] The plaintiff had developed cataracts in both eyes as a result of using the drug.

Between 1957 and October 1961, the Wm. S. Merrell Co. division of Richardson-Merrell conducted various animal studies on rats, monkeys and dogs to assess the potential side effects from Triparanol. During the tests by its Toxicology Department, it was discovered that all 3 species of animals began developing abnormal blood changes, then eye opacities, cataracts and in several instances blindness. One of the technicians was ordered to falsify some of the test results in her laboratory notes. Brochures to be used by physicians in human studies were also falsified. When the company filed its New Drug Application with the FDA, it submitted numerous false statements regarding the animal studies, including the falsified chart, omission of any reference to the abnormal blood changes and statements minimizing the side effects. Eye opacities were reported as mild inflammation of the eyes, and reference to blindness was eliminated from the reports. Triparanol was approved for marketing in April 1960.

When Merrell began receiving reports of human patients developing cataracts, it initially failed to report them to the FDA and withheld sending a warning to the medical profession. Finally, in April 1962, FDA officials made an unannounced visit to Merrell's laboratories and confiscated all of its records related to animal experiments. Within a month Triparanol was removed from the market. In the short time it was on sale to the general public, at least 490 people developed cataracts as a result of using Triparanol. Three employees of Merrell were indicted related to the above conduct, including Dr. Harold Werner, the vice president and director of research for the Wm. S. Merrell Co. That division and its parent, Richardson-Merrell, were both fined. The *Toole* case resulted in a verdict for the plaintiff, including an award of punitive damages, which was upheld on appeal. Dr. Werner also oversaw the early phase of testing of Clomid, and Dr. Carl Bunde, who assisted with the testing of Triparanol, was the Director of Medical Research of Merrell from 1960 to 1970, and supervised the pre-market clinical investigations of Clomid.

The anti-nausea drug, *Bendectin*, represents another chapter in Merrell's history of litigating over its pharmaceutical products. The drug was used by approximately 17.5 million women in the United States between 1957 and 1982, at which time it was voluntarily removed from the market. Principally used for the treatment of morning sickness during pregnancy, the need to assure that it posed no risk to the developing fetus was quite obvious. In large part growing out of an October 1979 story in *The National Enquirer,* relating the tragedy and lawsuit of David Mekdeci, eventually more than 1500 lawsuits nation wide were filed. It was claimed that the drug could cause a limb reduction type of birth defect similar to those caused by thalidomide.

Although the drug's potential to cause birth defects was significantly more controversial than thalidomide, the conduct of Merrell and the design of its studies to evaluate the safety of Bendectin was the subject of much criticism. It was contended by the plaintiffs that because of deficiencies in Merrell's pre-market clinical studies, they were absolutely worthless in assessing the teratogenic[3] risk of the drug. Looking also at published studies conducted by others, the plaintiffs complained that they were of little value in assessing the specific risk for limb reduction anomalies. To address the claimed deficiencies, experts were retained to reanalyze some of the published studies. The methods used in the reanalysis of these studies, as well as the use of other factors supporting the opinions of plaintiffs' experts, were challenged in various federal courts throughout the country. This eventually led to the landmark U.S. Supreme Court decision of Daubert vs. Merrell Dow Pharmaceuticals, Inc.,[4] addressing the proper method of analysis by experts.

The generic name for Clomid is *clomiphene citrate.* Beginning in 1982, the generic product was also sold under the label of Serophene, marketed by Serano Laboratories. Today, in addition to Clomid, the generic form can also be purchased under a number of different titles, including Serophene, Milophene, Clomiphene Citrate Tablets and ClomiPHENE Citrate. The package inserts for each, however, will have similar language. Although the multiple cases I have litigated only involved Clomid and its manufacturer, with some minor exceptions all product labeling will suffer from the same inadequacies and deception regardless of the product purchased. The text of this book will clearly set out the true risks of clomiphene and why not only the patients using the drug, but also most of their prescribing physicians, are being misled by labeling that continues to be approved by the FDA.

As will be seen, the criticisms that I level are not only directed at Merrell. The FDA is supposed to be our watchdog. It is to be assessing the safety and efficacy of drugs, both before and after their initial marketing. Absent the effectiveness of this federal agency, the consuming public is helpless to protect itself. Very few users of clomiphene have access to the numerous scientific studies on the drug, nor would they understand them even if they had. Other than fertility specialists, many of the prescribing physicians do little more than rely upon the package insert and the general consensus that Clomid is safe, other than the listed side effects. Many would be surprised – perhaps even shocked – at the number of published studies implicating use of clomiphene and damage to the developing embryo[5] and fetus. To a great extent, the medical profession is likewise relying upon the FDA to do its job. As will be seen, not only has the FDA dropped the ball with Clomid, it has fumbled it into the hands of Merrell and the other manufacturers of clomiphene citrate.

There have been, without question, bad apples in the bunch. Many FDA employees come from the drug industry, often previously holding important jobs with pharmaceutical companies, having developed friendships and other relationships with those now seeking approval of their company's drug products. More importantly, they frequently end up leaving their government work behind in order to enter or return to the drug industry. Many times they are hired as consultants, and sometimes end up with lucrative jobs in upper management. It does not take much imagination to see an opportunist "feathering his nest" by looking the other way or dragging his feet on a potentially damaging report.

The existence of this revolving door is an inherent problem with the whole system. Yet one must recognize that there are many ethical and devoted members of the FDA that work hard to meet their responsibilities. The FDA's file on just one drug could run up to 80,000 pages in length and more. And there are over 10,000 drugs subject to frequent review. The FDA is also another federal bureaucracy with thousands of regulations and a time-worn pecking order. It is not advisable to go above someone who has been ignoring your reports, although it is occasionally done by a staff member prepared to take the risk. Many at the FDA do an admirable job. Others, unfortunately, do not.

It is tragic, but true, that this failure is not limited to Clomid. Although this book is devoted uniquely to my experience with this fertility drug, I have had occasion over my professional life to see first hand what has gone on with other pharmaceutical products as well. Since 1972, I have tried to verdict a number of other drug product liability cases, not to mention numerous other cases that settled prior to and during trial. It is disappointing to relate that many of their histories have an all-too-familiar ring to them. Let us just say that what you are about to read is somewhat representative of what goes on between the FDA and the drug industry with most drug products, based upon one lawyer's personal observations and numerous articles and books he has read on the subject. The problems with the system will be addressed in the final chapter, along with my views of what it will take to solve them.

The subject of this book is by its very nature technical and complex. How does one present proof that a given drug causes birth defects in humans? Because this may be read by interested physicians and scientists, I have of necessity presented such evidence in medical and scientific terms. At the same time, I have attempted to reduce such terms to understandable lay language, as I would if presenting a case to a jury. The advantage of the format of a book, of course, is that we can take all of the time that is needed. I am not limited by page number and the reader can take as long as is needed to digest my presentation. Where justified, I have also presented photos of the actual documents or other evidence being discussed.

I will readily admit that I am biased and an advocate. I am a trial lawyer convinced of the position I am presenting. However, I am simply attempting to warn patients who are or will be using clomiphene and other fertility drugs. Although there will be some who will challenge the cited studies and other evidence, it is not essential that I convince the reader that the drug can cause birth defects; only that he or she appreciate the nature and level of that potential risk. The use of all drugs involves weighing its benefits against the risks. Unfortunately, clomiphene users to date have not been given that full opportunity.

Some of the events recited occurred over thirty years ago. For someone experiencing an occasional "senior moment," this might be quite challenging. Fortunately, I have preserved the records from all of my Clomid files over these many years. This includes not only correspondence, notes, memoranda, medical records, pleadings filed with the court, deposition and trial transcripts, responses to written interrogatories, and medical research, but also documents produced by Merrell and the

FDA. Whereas other closed cases with equal vintage have long since been destroyed, for some reason I was determined to preserve these documents. Perhaps, subconsciously, I sensed that one day I would be writing this book; that what I knew – and could document – about Clomid would one day be important.

Finally, some may question my motives for writing this book. Critics will say that I am after more Clomid cases, but the fact is I am near the end of my shelf life and finishing off my last couple of cases. I have no desire to jump back into the high-stress business of trial work. Others may claim that Clomid has always been an obsession of mine, and to some extent there may be a hint of truth to the charge. I have literally spent thousands of hours analyzing Clomid clinical studies and conducting medical research for no reason other than to search out the truth, and without any expectation that the work would equate to additional fees.

The fact is that in 1996 I decided to walk away from Clomid litigation. The following year, my wife and I moved to the north shore of the beautiful island of Kauai, where we spent five years until returning to California. Not long ago she approached me and encouraged that I write a book about Clomid. With my professional career near its end, she sensed that there was something unfulfilled that needed to be addressed. "You owe it to the children," she reminded, and she was right. I had knowledge that needed to be shared. I had to fulfill a commitment I had made over two decades earlier.

Little did I know that during the course of researching this book, I would happen upon a discovery that would provide me with a reward far beyond my imagination; a means of preventing thousands of birth defects throughout the world.

What follows is not for me, but for the children. A commitment fulfilled.

* * * * *

CHAPTER 1

An Introduction to Drugs

June 19, 1970 was to be a special day in the lives of Heinz and Ingrid Breimhorst. Pregnancy had not come easily. After their marriage in 1965, they had both agreed to postpone expanding their family for at least a couple of years. At that time they would be better-prepared financially for raising a child. Two years of freedom without being tied down by children would also have its benefits. So for the first couple of years Ingrid had used birth control pills.

Then in the summer of 1967 they decided that the time had arrived. Although Heinz had been born in West Germany on August 10, 1940, Ingrid's birth had been almost five years earlier on April 21, 1935, in Sweden. At 32 her biological clock was starting to tick. It was time to start working on their first little Breimhorst.

Fifteen months later they had not had any luck. Part of the problem was the irregularity of Ingrid's menstrual cycles. In sequence, she would have short, medium and long cycles. But they were never of the same duration. The short ones always varied by a couple of days, as did the medium and long ones. In a venture where timing is everything, it had been difficult to pin down the days that Ingrid had been ovulating.

So in October 1968, Ingrid went to see her OB/GYN, a Dr. Nicholas Richards.[6] After the examination and some lab tests, Dr. Richards concluded that Ingrid was in fact ovulating. However, she was "oligo-ovulatory;" that is, she ovulated every month but the timing was always irregular. He suggested some coital techniques in relation to the onset of her period, and also recommended taking her temperature every morning, using a basal body temperature (BBT) thermometer. The idea was to watch for a shift in her temperature, which would indicate the onset of ovulation. She and her husband were to have sexual intercourse on days 13 through 16 following the beginning of menstruation. Finally, the doctor urged Heinz to have a sperm test to assure that he was not contributing to the problem.

A couple of months later, Ingrid returned to report on her lack of success. They had also learned that Heinz had a low sperm count. More tests followed.

Eventually, in late spring 1969, Dr. Richards prescribed the first course of Clomid. Ingrid was to commence taking one 50 mg. tablet per day for five consecutive days, beginning the fifth day of her menstrual cycle. By now she was quite eager to get started. She was 34 and had been attempting to conceive for almost two full years.

The first course of treatment was taken in July 1969 without success. The following month they were both out of town and decided to postpone their next effort until they were back at home. But in September 1969 they hit the jackpot.

For the first 3 ½ months the pregnancy had been uneventful, and Ingrid and Heinz could not have been happier. All of their patience, perseverance and effort had paid off. Ingrid also carried her pregnancy with pride. As she began "showing," one could sense that she wanted everyone to notice. She was a mother now. And only someone who had faced the desperation of coming up empty for so long could begin to appreciate the full measure of her pride and contentment. In a little over 5 months, she would have a brand new baby – and a life-long dream would become a reality.

Then January 9, 1970 happened. Ingrid had been driving her Volkswagon bug when a Ford made a sudden left-hand turn in front of her. The resulting collision drove her abdomen into the steering wheel. Pain shot through her like a bullet, and she became instantly terrified. An effort that had extended now almost two and a half years might well have been destroyed in an instant. She was immediately rushed to an emergency room at a local hospital.

The examining physician assured Ingrid that both she and her pregnancy would be fine. A large hematoma marked the exact spot of the impact, but there had been no vaginal bleeding and the fetal heartbeat sounded normal – absolutely no sign of fetal distress. Plus, he assured the trembling mother, that baby is well-protected in the uterus. "You have absolutely nothing to be concerned about," he added. "Nothing."

And it appeared that he had been right. Right up until the first fetalgram of June 5, 1970, the pregnancy could not have gone smoother. Even then, it only demonstrated that the baby was in a transverse lie. Its position was more laterally across the uterus than down toward the cervix (uterine opening). A repeat fetalgram on June 18, 1970 disclosed the same position. A decision was made to perform a C-section, which was to take place the following morning.

On the day of delivery, Ingrid elected to have a spinal anesthesia. She was eager to be there to greet her child as he or she was brought into the world. Her special day had finally arrived. She was prepped and draped and awaiting the incision; nothing could be felt below her waist. Heinz was anxiously waiting in an adjoining room.

Dr. Richards approached and offered a reassuring smile. "This won't take long," he noted. "A couple more minutes and you'll have your baby in your arms." Ingrid responded with a tentative smile. The sooner the better, she thought. From her prone position she could not see much of what was going on.

Dr. Richards' surgical mask covered most of his face, so Ingrid could not detect his jaw go slack as he completed the incision and removed tiny Mark Breimhorst from his prenatal home. But the doctor's eyes betrayed the tragic surprise that greeted him.

The infant he had just removed had no hands.

"What's wrong?" Ingrid cried out. "What's wrong with my baby?"

Dr. Richards just shook his head as he tried to gather his thoughts. This had caught him by surprise. Nothing had been detected in either fetalgram.

"I want to see my baby!" Ingrid screamed.

Dr. Richards hesitated – then held the infant up for display. "I'm sorry," he said.

Ingrid didn't say another word as tears trickled down her face. She just extended her arms to embrace her child. He would be in need of much love and care – and it would start right now.

The Breimhorsts' initial instinct was to blame the auto accident. Neither Heinz nor Ingrid could recall any congenital anomalies in either of their family trees. Ingrid had also been religious about following every instruction given to her by Dr. Richards. The conception had been a divine event. Every precaution had been taken to insure that their precious little baby would be delivered both healthy and normal. Other than the accident, they could not recall anything that had occurred to account for this tragedy.

Five months earlier they had retained the services of an attorney, Rosalie Chapman,[7] to represent them for the accident. She had suggested that they await the outcome of the pregnancy before attempting to settle their case. That now appeared to be quite prudent advice.

But the doctors were quick to eliminate the January 9th trauma as a cause of the loss of hands. In fact, it would have been impossible for there to have been a causal connection. The hands and fingers begin forming between days 32 and 41 post-conception. Both hands were already missing when the accident occurred over a month later.

On the day of delivery, Dr.Richards had also diagnosed a left facial palsy (partial paralysis of the facial muscles), and a few weeks later Mark's pediatrician detected a limited ability to move the eyes laterally. Although they could not absolutely eliminate the auto accident as a cause of the neurological problems, all of the specialists emphasized that these anomalies had been seen together many times before. In fact, this cluster of anomalies was referred to as *Moebius syndrome*, and they were likely caused by the same event.

But what event?

If it wasn't the auto accident, then what? It could not have been Clomid. It had only been taken prior to pregnancy. How could a drug ingested several days before conception have any affect on the baby? Dr. Richards had also assured Ingrid that the only risk associated with fertility drugs was an increased possibility of multiple births.

Many times we just don't know, the doctors lamented.

The Breimhorsts, however, were not about to let the matter pass because of the uncertainty of medicine. Cause and effect; it was a basic precept of science. For every action there was a reaction. Just because science did not have an answer did not mean it was nonexistent. At one time the world did not have a clue about the devastation that thalidomide could inflict on the human embryo – a drug that deformed thousands of babies throughout Europe. They discussed the matter with their attorney. All three agreed to find out more about this clomiphene citrate.

So Ms. Chapman stopped by a local pharmacy and picked up a package insert.[8] That evening, back at her home, she read the language that set everything in motion.

"After oral administration of Clomid (clomiphene citrate) to pregnant rats during the interval of organogenesis[9] in doses of 1.6 to 200 mg./kg./day, malformations were observed in the pups from one of the five litters in the group receiving 8 mg./kg/day. Higher oral doses (40-200 mg./kg./day) inhibited fetal development and only one litter (normal) was born. Subcutaneous administration of Clomid (clomiphene citrate) to pregnant rats on one day (12th) during the period of organogenesis resulted in a dose-dependent increase in the incidence of malformations in doses of 1.6 to 1000 mg./kg. In rabbits, deformed fetuses were seen following oral doses of 20 mg./kg./day from the eighth through fifteenth day of a 32-day gestation. None was seen after the oral dose of 8 mg./kg./day."

Clomid could cause congenital malformations in the rat and rabbit. Was it merely a coincidence that Ingrid had taken a drug that could deform rats and rabbits? Why hadn't Dr. Richards informed her about these studies?

So began a series of events that would have a profound affect on my life.

"You got a couple of minutes?" The voice came from Rosalie Chapman, who was leaning through my open office door. We had shared office space for the past four months. She was also my landlord. She was the tenant of the two-office suite in the twelve-story Union Bank Tower, and the person to whom I paid my share of the monthly rent. It was early spring of 1972. At the time, my pregnant wife and I lived in Marina Del Rey, a small craft marina and adults-only apartment complex just north of LAX.

I looked up from the medical records that I had been studying for the past two hours. "No problem, Rose," I smiled. "I'll be right in." Chapman quickly disappeared and retired to her own office. I finished off the last couple of pages of the records and shoved them back into the accordion file. The review had become somewhat tedious and I welcomed the break.

I walked the short distance to her office and knocked. Whereas my office door was rarely closed, hers was never open. Like the confines of her office, Chapman was a very private person. She promptly invited me in.

I entered and dropped into one of the client chairs facing her desk. "So what's up?" I asked in my usual cheerful tone. During these early years I was always up. The enthusiasm of youth would later erode, but not now. Now I was looking forward to a bright future as a prominent trial lawyer.

"Well, Terry, I have a proposal to make. Something I think you'll be interested in." Rosalie Chapman, a brunette with a pleasant face and a quiet personality, was a few years my senior. She invariably came to the office in a suit or stylish dress, and at this stage of our relationship seemed only focused on building a successful law practice. She rarely shared information about her personal life, although I knew that she was married to a physician and lived in Palos Verdes Estates, an upscale community a short ten minutes from our Torrance, California office. "You're an experienced PI lawyer, am I right?"

I nodded my concurrence. I was a personal injury attorney, it was true. But I had been in practice for only five years and had just two jury trials under my belt, a victory and a loss. Then again I was not about to dispel any notion that magnified my skills, no matter how misguided it may have been.

"Well, I could use your help," she continued. She nodded to a five-inch thick file on her desk. "There's the biggest case in my office. Without a doubt, the most important. It's a case against a drug company, Richardson-Merrell – a birth defect case. The plaintiff is a child born without hands." She paused for a moment to observe my reaction.

I sat up a little more in my chair, unable to camouflage my interest. It was an inescapable fact that the more horrendous the injury, the bigger the case. And larger cases, if successful, translated into larger fees. This morbid interest in tragedies would continue to bother me throughout my professional life, softened only by the rationalization that they had already occurred and I was there to help alleviate the suffering. "You mean like thalidomide?"

"You might say that."

"What was the drug?" I asked.

"Clomid. It's a fertility drug, used to help women ovulate."

"And there's proof that it causes birth defects, these birth defects?"

She hesitated and looked down, as if she was looking for the right words on top of her desk. I could see that this was going to be an issue, maybe a big issue. "Well…there are animal studies. The drug has caused birth defects in animal studies. There was also a high rate of spontaneous abortions during the pre-marketing studies with women, not to mention a number of birth defects reported." She leaned forward a little. I could also see that she was doing some selling. "Look, Phil's a physician, as you know," she said, referring to her husband, "and Phil's convinced the drug is the cause. We'll get experts."

"Okay, sounds good. So Phil would be working with us, then?"

"As much as we will need."

"I'm a little confused. She took a fertility drug after she had already gotten pregnant?"

"Well, there will be some question about that, but we think the evidence will establish that she inadvertently took Clomid after she had conceived."

Another issue. Now I understood why she was talking to this "experienced" PI lawyer. Rose had no doubt shopped the case around and had come up empty. But I was an easy sell. I had never been one to shy away from difficult cases, especially only a few months after setting up my own practice. And the potential of a big lawsuit, both in fees and career advancement, would always be a strong consideration. If the case turned out to be worthless, I would dump it later. But not until every possibility had been explored. Yet I didn't want to seem too eager. We still had to negotiate the fee split.

"You know, I've never worked on one of these cases," I said. "Product liability, yeah, several of them. But not a drug case, never."

"Not many lawyers have. I've asked around. In fact, it seems very few lawyers in this state have ever tried one."

Now I was convinced. She had run it by a few big names in town and had been turned down. My presence in her office was also tempting because she could keep the case "in house." She could remain attorney of record rather than sending the clients out to another law firm for the customary referral fee.

"Terry, you're as experienced at drug cases as any other lawyer in this town," she continued. "I'd really like to see what you can do with this."

I nodded pensively. I wasn't going to make it too easy for her. "I'm interested, but what are you looking for in a fee split?"

"I was thinking 25% to you if it settles and 40% if it goes to trial. We'd be co-counsel during trial, sharing the responsibilities, of course. You can see I've already done a lot of work."

Sharing responsibilities during trial? Hardly. If we went to trial, she would be doing nothing more than sitting at the counsel table taking notes. She knew it and I knew it. Rose was primarily a transactional lawyer, with only a few court appearances to her credit. "Tell you what," I said firmly. "If it settles prior to trial, I get one third. But after trial commences, we split it 50/50, whether by settlement or jury verdict. That's my best offer. It's also subject to my review of the file, which should take no more than a day or two." I let her chew on it a moment or two then continued, "I don't expect a problem, Rose, but I'll let you know tomorrow whether I'm interested." That decision, of course, had already been made. I wasn't about ready to let this one get away, certainly not before it had been exhaustively researched.

Rose hesitated, as if she was having a problem with giving too much of the fee away. But I knew from the moment I made the proposal that it would be accepted. Not many hired guns would take a case through a jury trial without receiving 50% of the fee, no matter how much had been done in working the case up.

"Okay," she nodded with a slight smile. "We have an agreement. And if I haven't heard a rejection by tomorrow, we'll put it down in writing. Okay?"

"Sure thing, Rose."

"Oh, and one more thing. I'll be the sole contact with the clients. Interrogatories have already been answered, so there's really no reason to be seeing them right now. When it comes time for their depositions, we'll both prepare them. Same for their trial preparation. Any problem with that?"

"No problem. None at all." I knew exactly where this was coming from. In December of 1971, I had separated from a medium size law firm in Los Angeles, where I had spent my first five years in practice, the last two as a junior partner. About two dozen personal injury clients left with me and the ensuing battle wasn't pretty. The senior partners accused me of stealing their clients. I countered that I had been the only lawyer in the firm working those cases, and it was the client's decision whether to stay with the firm or go with me. My former firm would also share in the fees for the percentage of the time I spent on the lawsuits while still with the firm.

Threats were made – in both directions. One of the senior partners had even approached my bank and pressed it to cancel a credit line I had secured for starting my own practice. The effort was unsuccessful, but only added to the escalating fight. In the end, after discussions between my ex-partners and the clients, only one of them agreed to remain with the firm. But it was by far the largest of the cases. I was sure that Rose had not heard of this episode, but it was not unexpected that she would be protective of her clients. Hopefully this new case would be an ample replacement for the one I had lost.

I stood, picked up the file and said, "I'll talk to you about this tomorrow, Rose." She smiled, no doubt pleased at my decision. I quietly exited and closed the door; then entered my own office, closed its door and dropped the file on my desk. I didn't want either of our secretaries to notice as I quietly clinched my fists and uttered an exuberant, "Yeah!" under my breath.

Unlike my review of the medical records less than an hour earlier, I devoured the new file with unmitigated enthusiasm. I first viewed the pleadings to discover who I would be running up against. Richardson-Merrell was being represented by Schell & Delamer, a firm I was acquainted with that had been around forever. The partner assigned to the case was Fred Belanger. I had never met Belanger before, but was aware that he had the dubious distinction of being on the losing end of the McCarrick thalidomide trial.

I next turned my attention to the clients. Mark Breimhorst was born with the absence of both hands below the wrist, metatarsus varus (clubfoot) of the right foot and a left facial palsy, which involved a limited ability to move his eyes laterally. After their arrival from Germany and Sweden, his father and mother had met, fell in love, and eventually married on May 21, 1965. I would later learn that they were both loving and caring parents, deeply devoted to their handicapped son and helping him deal with his disabilities. At the time, the three of them lived in Redondo Beach, part of the greater South Bay area of Los Angeles County.

I learned that Heinz had a low sperm count, which may have accounted for a good part of their difficulty. But Richards still decided that use of a fertility drug would be beneficial and prescribed Clomid. Per prescriptions from Dr. Richards, Ingrid used the drug on two occasions. Based solely upon the sequence of Ingrid's short, medium and long menstrual periods, a theory was posed in a file memorandum that she may have taken two tablets after conception. Even with my limited knowledge at the time, this seemed to be a stretch.

Based upon their recorded dates of sexual intercourse, ovulation and conception probably occurred on September 20 or 21, 1969, four or five days *after* last consuming the drug. How could a drug taken prior to conception cause birth defects to the subsequent embryo or fetus? As initially suspected, this was going to be a big issue.

From file notes I learned that Ingrid had never been warned by Richards that there had been studies with animals in which birth defects had been caused by administering Clomid during pregnancy, nor had she been warned that there was any risk of causing birth defects if she inadvertently took Clomid during pregnancy. Ingrid was adamant during her initial interview that if she had been so warned, she never would have taken the drug, and certainly never would have engaged in sexual intercourse during the five days she was ingesting the tablets.

Inside the file I found a color photograph of Mark. He was sitting on the floor, surrounded by a large number of toys. No doubt induced by one or both of his parents, he was looking up at the camera with a bright smile. For all intents and purposes he looked like any other twenty-month old child, except at the end of both arms there were no hands. For several moments I studied the photograph. The client was now more than a name.

I also reviewed the Clomid package insert that had been picked up by Rose. It was illuminating for a number of reasons. One interesting statement was that Clomid was for use by *anovulatory* patients. Under the heading "Indications and Selection of Patient" it further stated, "Clomid is indicated for the treatment of *ovulatory failure* in patients desiring pregnancy...." [Emphasis added.] Ingrid definitely was not anovulatory (without ovulation) nor in "ovulatory failure." Her cycles may have been irregular but she was ovulating every month. Richards thus did not follow the package insert's instructions on selection of patient.

Nor did he require Ingrid to use BBT charts while using the drug, as mandated by Richardson-Merrell "to avoid inadvertent Clomid administration during early pregnancy." When a woman ovulates, there is a slight dip, then a rise, in her body temperature. By using a highly sensitive thermometer and recording the temperature readings on a chart, one can usually determine the time of ovulation. Not only does this become a signal when to engage in sexual intercourse, it can also represent a caution to cease taking the Clomid tablets after it takes place.

Dr. Richards had never been named as a defendant in the lawsuit. Subject to running it by Rose's husband, it seemed to me that failure to follow specific instructions set out in the package insert would be in violation of the standard of care for a prescribing physician. I would recommend that we amend the lawsuit to add Richards as a defendant.

As mentioned, the package insert cited the animal studies with rats and rabbits during which Clomid caused congenital malformations when administered during the period of organogenesis. But a very significant representation was also made by Richardson-Merrell in this context: "Although *no causative evidence of a deleterious effect of Clomid therapy on the human fetus has been seen,* such evidence in regard to the rat and the rabbit has been presented (see Pharmacology)." [Emphasis added.] There it was, boldly stated. There was absolutely no evidence that Clomid therapy could have a harmful effect on the human fetus. This went beyond a failure to warn; it was an absolute assurance of safety. If it was true, of course, we didn't have a case, unless the animal studies could be extrapolated to humans. But if it was untrue, if there was just one valid study out there that presented evidence that clomiphene citrate could have a teratogenic effect on the human embryo or fetus, it was an outright misrepresentation.

There was another important finding in the package insert, which appeared to answer my major concern about conception occurring after use of the drug. Clomid had a half-life of approximately five days. This meant that five days after Ingrid's last tablet of Clomid – perhaps the day of conception – 50% of the Clomid in that tablet and/or its metabolites still remained circulating in her body. This would be added to some remnants of the first four tablets as well.

Finally, I noticed one little problem that Rose had failed to mention. Ingrid had been in an auto accident on January 9, 1970, three and a half months into her pregnancy. Her pregnant abdomen had impacted the steering wheel as a result of the collision, and the trauma was evidenced by a nasty-looking hematoma at the point of contact. The driver of the other car had even been named as a defendant in the lawsuit.

I called Philip Chapman[10] that evening. We had met once when he stopped by the office to have lunch with Rose, and I had immediately liked him. He had a warm smile and a congenial nature that no doubt worked well for him as a family practitioner. Phil seemed very cooperative and was quite willing to answer all of my questions. He agreed that Richards' failure to follow the instructions in the package insert fell below the standard of care. He also provided some useful information about half-life, warming up to my idea regarding the pre-conception treatment. He explained that the elimination of clomiphene from Ingrid's body would not have been linear; that all of the remaining drug would not have been excreted over the next five days. Typical of half-life studies, in theory over the succeeding five days only fifty percent of the remaining 50% would be excreted, then a half of a half every five days and so on. During the half-life studies with Clomid, per the package insert, markers of the drug/metabolites "appeared in the feces 6 weeks after administration."

Rather than attempt to sell the notion that Ingrid took a couple of Clomid tablets after conception, our contention at trial would be that she did in fact conceive on September 20 or 21, 1969, but that the drug, last taken before conception, remained in the maternal and embryonic circulation up until the time that Mark's hands would have formed.

Phil also dispelled any notion that the auto accident could have been responsible for the birth defects. The hands begin to develop in the human embryo well before the trauma from the accident at 3½ months. It was remotely possible that the impact from the steering wheel could have produced the clubfoot or facial palsy, but it was highly unlikely. These three congenital anomalies had previously been reported together as a group in the medical literature and had in fact been described as Moebius syndrome.[11] Whatever had caused Mark to be born without hands no doubt produced the other anomalies as well. The driver of the other car had been joined as a defendant as a precautionary measure, in case Richardson-Merrell contended he was a cause of some of the defects.

I asked to speak to Rose on the phone. She seemed quite excited about my observations and quickly agreed to add Richards as a defendant. She expressed her pleasure that I would be joining her on the case, although I am sure that a more accurate description would have been one of relief. She reminded me that she would be preparing our agreement in the morning.

The remainder of 1972 and all of 1973 seemed to fly by. Discovery[12] continued on the case by both sides. Interrogatories were served upon us by Thelen, Marrin,

Johnson & Bridges, the law firm representing the new defendant, Richards. The depositions of Heinz and Ingrid were also taken, which provided me with the first opportunity to meet my clients. Rose and I spent several hours preparing both of them for their testimony. At the time, I also assessed how they would come across to a jury. They were foreign born, which sometimes can be a handicap, depending upon the country of origin. They were both attractive, with light hair and complexion. Their accents were only slight, which I thought might be an asset rather than a handicap. American juries tend to like Europeans. They also seemed quite honest in relating the relevant events. They were friendly and likable, which instinct told me would likely be how they would be perceived by a jury. They both did quite well during their depositions.

An extensive set of interrogatories was served upon Richardson-Merrell. The responses provided a wealth of important information: how the company was organizationally structured, the names of the various departments that studied Clomid, the names and titles of the heads of those departments, the specific date and identity of all animal studies, the names and locations of all the physician clinical investigators that conducted the company-sponsored pre-marketing investigations, the identity of all package inserts, physician brochures and other labeling materials for Clomid, the identity of all published articles on the drug, and a list describing all reported birth defects following use of the drug. Yet there was little information upon which to build our case against Merrell. That could and would only happen by looking at the actual records maintained by the company in Cincinnati, and taking the depositions of the key employees overseeing the research, testing and evaluation of the drug. Since the entire file for Clomid purportedly numbered in excess of 80,000 pages, the inspection would of necessity entail a trip to Ohio.

On December 13, 1973, I attended a trial-setting conference, during which a trial date was selected for March 11, 1974. A settlement conference was also scheduled at the courthouse for February 7, 1974. The jury trial would take place in the Southwest District branch of the Los Angeles Superior Court, located in Torrance, California. The close proximity of the trial date reminded me that there was still a major amount of preparation to be done, including rounding up our expert witnesses for testimony and my long-put-off trip to Cincinnati.

By this time my practice had grown to in excess of 50 cases and had been consuming a large part of my time. Since January 1972, I had also donated extra hours to multiple speaking engagements, part of my responsibilities as a newly-elected member of the Board of Governors of the Los Angeles Trial Lawyers Association. And I had concluded five more jury trials during the past year and a half, one of which included my first six-figure verdict. This would turn out to be a big confidence builder as I entered the home stretch on Breimhorst. But because of the time spent on that and other legal activities, I found myself facing a major challenge, with little time to pull it off.

I had left Rose's suite months earlier and opened my own office on the ninth floor of the same building. Following the depositions of Ingrid and Heinz, Rose and I had seen little of one another, but now was the time to call in the chips. Phil and Rose needed to start working on pulling together a set of expert witnesses for the trial, while I concentrated on completing the discovery against Richardson-Merrell. Defense counsel on the case would insure that this would not be an easy task.

The first thing to hit me was a motion for summary judgment brought by Richards' attorneys. Such a motion seeks to have a judgment entered in favor of the party filing the motion, based upon the contention that the responding party lacks sufficient evidence to allow a jury to decide the case. It was filed and served only 55 days before trial. It was also 43 pages long. To gather all of my evidence in defense of the motion required the use of valuable time and eliminated any possibility of flying to Cincinnati in January.

I thus initiated efforts to schedule a document inspection and depositions in Cincinnati for February 5, 1974. By the end of January I had filed my opposition papers to the motion for summary judgment. But then I was hit by a second motion, this one brought by Merrell to quash my notice to produce records at the scheduled depositions of its employees. The following day I filed my opposition to the motion to quash.

Due to some pressure from the judge at the hearing, Merrell's attorney agreed in open court to make available the requested records and took its motion off calendar. I returned to my office, scheduled my flight and reservations at a hotel near Merrell-

National Laboratories, and started prepping for the employee depositions. At this point I felt like I was stumbling, sliding back one step for every two I took forward. I was making progress, but I feared not fast enough to be ready on March 11, 1974.

A Long Overdue Trip to Cincinnati

It was February 5, 1974, and a cold, gray, overcast day in Cincinnati. Carl Bunde, M.D., Merrell's former Director of Medical Research, was unavailable. He had supervised the Clomid pre-marketing clinical studies, but would not be produced. He had been number-one on my hit list. A second choice was Mark Hoekenga, M.D. He had also participated in the Clomid clinical investigations. Merrell had agreed to produce Hoekenga, as well as Dorsey Holtkamp, Ph.D., who had been the Head of the Department of Endocrinology, and oversaw the animal teratology studies.

I entered the rented conference room at the Sheraton-Gibson Hotel, just a mile from the Merrell-National plant. My court reporter was waiting for me and took the needed information about the case. I spread my documents and notes in front of me on the conference table and waited. No more than ten minutes later the full entourage entered the room: Charles Swanson, Belanger's second in command; Frederic Lamb and John Chewning, from Merrell's in-house legal staff; Wendell Mortimer, from the Thelen, Marrin firm; and Albert Holzhauer, a senior partner in the firm representing the defendant driver. The last to arrive was the witness, Mark Hoekenga. After introductions all around the table, the court reporter administered the oath and we started what turned out to be a somewhat fruitless deposition. Before I could launch into my standard admonition to the witness, Swanson rose to his feet and made an announcement that would set the tone for the rest of the day.

"Counsel, I would like to read a statement into the record, if I may at this point." He held a note in his hand so as to avoid any misstatement. "Pursuant to a stipulation entered into between the defendant Richardson-Merrell and the plaintiff, the defendant stipulated that, subject to all appropriate objections in the premises, they would have 12 individual project reports entitled 'Reproduction' or 'Teratology' *available*." The word "available" was given some emphasis, as to forewarn that a point was about to be made.

"Subject to this stipulation," he continued, "the defendant Richardson-Merrell will not make all of the project reports available upon the grounds that they are not relevant to the subject matter of the lawsuit and not calculated to lead to the discovery of admissible evidence. Discovery so far has disclosed that the defendant's product was prescribed prior to conception."

I was perplexed. Even with his notes, he had just acknowledged making an agreement in open court that all of these key animal studies would be made "available" at this deposition, yet then announced that they would *not* be made "available." I sensed that the second "available" had inadvertently been dropped into his rehearsed statement. If you're going to play a game of semantics, you can't get careless with the words. He essentially admitted that they were not going to do what he had assured a judge would in fact take place at this deposition. Swanson then attempted to justify their position. Evidence had established that Ingrid had taken Clomid only prior to conception, he assured, and all but two of the studies involved administering the drug to animals post-conception. The two reports involving preconception treatment would be produced, but none of the teratology studies. Merrell also produced their records related to the 58 infants born with birth defects during the clinical investigations, as well as copies of the Clomid Drug Experience Reports (DERs) of congenital malformations voluntarily reported by the medical profession after marketing had commenced.

I began to boil inside, but kept telling myself to maintain control. Unleashing my anger on Merrell's three legal representatives would only send me off on a journey to nowhere. I had to make the best of a bad situation.

After identifying with specificity all of the non-produced studies, I methodically proceeded to interrogate the witness about his entire career up to the present, including his education, training, employment and a full description of all jobs held with Merrell over the years, including his responsibilities.

I then began my education on how a drug goes through the process of acquiring FDA approval for marketing. After preliminary animal and laboratory studies, an Investigational New Drug (IND) application is filed with the FDA. This is for the purpose of obtaining approval to commence studies in humans termed "clinical investigations." The two primary objectives of the clinical investigations are to determine safety and efficacy. What are its side effects and does it work? The actual physicians that conduct the studies (clinical investigators) are generally outside specialists, treating patients for the problem addressed by the drug, who have been retained by the pharmaceutical company. In the case of Clomid, these were physicians who specialized in female fertility problems. The clinical investigation is customarily designed, monitored, analyzed, summarized and then reported to the FDA by the drug manufacturer. It was not lost on me that such a system could lead to abuses by the company. The FDA was relying upon studies and reports supplied by an entity with a vested interest in the results. Objectivity was not part of this picture.

After the company has sufficient data from the clinical studies, it files a New Drug Application (NDA) with the FDA. This is to start the process toward marketing the drug. The Clomid NDA was filed on February 23, 1965, approximately two years prior to its formal approval for marketing. Following marketing, the pharmaceutical company supplies the FDA with updated data and summaries called "Periodic Reports." These are filed once every three months during the first year, then semi-annually during the second year, and annually thereafter.

Every time I posed a question related to assessing the drug's teratological potential when ingested during pregnancy, it was met with an objection and an instruction not to answer. Persistent questioning, however, produced some interesting responses.

"Let me ask you this, relative to the half-life factor I referred to: Were any clinical investigations performed to determine whether or not if conception occurred during the half-life period – whether there could be in fact a teratogenic effect from the drug?"

"No specific studies were set up to determine that. As I said before, all pregnancies were followed to determine the outcome whenever Clomid was ingested, including if it was ingested during pregnancy."

"Were any statistics compiled specifically to make an evaluation as to any possible teratogenic effect during the half-life period?" I asked.

"Only in the sense that I referred to earlier."

"Well, relative to the clinical investigations and all the investigative reports, was any analysis made or any conclusion formulated as to the possible teratogenic effect of Clomid when conception actually occurred during the half-life period?"

"Not a specific analysis relating to half-life."

No specific study was designed to assess the risk to the embryo when conception occurred after last treatment, at a time when the drug and/or its metabolites still remained in the maternal circulation. Again, another suggestion that all Merrell was doing was tabulating the outcome of pregnancies without specifically investigating potential risks to the developing embryo.

Finally, Hoekenga recited his opinion that Clomid did not cause birth defects in humans. This was based upon two factors gleaned from the clinical investigations. First, the incidence of birth defects following use of Clomid was no greater than the incidence seen in the general population; and, second, there was no specific pattern of defects following use of the drug.

The deposition of Holtkamp was even less productive. After reviewing his education, training and employment history, and various positions with Merrell, I moved into his work history with Clomid, which was primarily limited to animal studies conducted in his Endocrinology Department. Endocrinology involves the study of the glands and hormones of the body and their related disorders. Since fertility drugs have both a direct and indirect effect on the endocrine system, Clomid fell into Holtkamp's area of expertise.

Consistent with their refusal to produce any of the teratology studies, Merrell's counsel also prohibited any questions related to those studies. Only two project reports were provided, neither of which were of any value. There was, however, one small item that hit me for the first time: Almost all of the animal teratology studies were conducted during 1962, two years *after* the clinical investigations in humans had been initiated. No doubt prompted by the thalidomide tragedy, revealed to the world in November 1961, I wondered whether the results of such studies had ever been communicated to the clinical investigators. If so, when? Holtkamp held no knowledge about such communications. One more thing to learn, and it wasn't going to happen this trip. I quickly packed up my file and the records and left for the airport.

It was not difficult to appreciate what had just taken place. I had been led in the wrong direction, sent on a goose chase going nowhere. The whole trip was almost a complete waste of time, which was exactly what defense counsel was after. I was losing days while the trial date was closing in on me. The biggest trial in my life was only five weeks away and I had absolutely no idea how I would prove our case. Was I going down in flames? I wasn't sure, but I wasn't going to make it easy for them. It was time to go back to the courthouse.

On February 13, 1974, I filed a motion to compel production of the denied records, a motion to compel answers to questions posed at the depositions, and a motion to compel answers to an earlier set of interrogatories. I also requested an award of sanctions, which included reimbursement of the costs for my trip to Cincinnati and attorney fees for my time. Sanctions may be awarded in California when a party denies discovery "without substantial justification."

Schell & Delamer filed its opposition to the motions. As expected, their principal objection was based upon the argument that the sought records and questions related to studies during which Clomid was administered *during* pregnancy, whereas Mrs. Breimhorst only ingested the drug *prior* to conception. The questions and records were thus irrelevant. To explain away the earlier agreement made in open court, Merrell's counsel argued that they had agreed to make the records "available" at the depositions, not to "produce" them. They were "available" at the depositions of February 5, 1974, they just weren't "produced." This was the word that Swanson had apparently misplaced at the deposition. The Thelen, Marrin firm filed its opposition to my motion related to similar interrogatories served on Richards.

The discovery motions were argued and submitted on February 21, 1974, in front of the Honorable William A. Ross. It was a total victory. Judge Ross ordered Merrell to produce all of the requested records, answer all of the deposition questions at a second round in Cincinnati, and to answer 29 of the 34 interrogatories that were the subject of the motion. He also ordered Merrell to reimburse all of my travel costs for my last trip to Cincinnati and to pay me attorney fees for my lost time. Richards was also ordered to answer interrogatories as well. I had won the battle, but was I losing the war? Still more time had passed, and I had yet to see the key documents and thoroughly examine Drs. Hoekenga and Holtkamp. Trial was now only 18 days away.

It was March 1, 1974, and here I was again at a hotel in Cincinnati. The skies were again gray and overcast and the temperature again cold – at least for a California boy. And in front of me again sat Hoekenga. This time, however, I drew Belanger along with Swanson. Fred Lamb was absent, but Chewning showed up again to observe and report to corporate office. Worrell also made the second trip on behalf of Richards. Everything else seemed the same, except that this time the overly-protected records were produced and I came armed with a court order. After a few preliminary matters, I began my examination.

I initially touched on the Drug Experience Reports. Since my last trip, I had spent some time reviewing the DERs previously produced. Between the date of initial marketing on May 15, 1967 and the end of 1973, there had been a total of 34 reports of Clomid-related congenital malformations reported by the medical profession. Such reports are totally voluntary. Federal law did not require members of the medical community to report suspected adverse reactions to a drug.

I had observed at least three cases with abnormal chromosomes, a few with congenital heart defects, one with the absence of fingers on one hand and a myriad of other anomalies. But what really caught my attention were *eight reports of anencephaly*. Anencephaly literally means absence of a brain, although there is usually some small remnant and a reduced spinal cord with non-closure of the skull. I had assumed that this abnormality was a somewhat rare occurrence, and that eight[13] out of 34 reports (23.5%) might be indicative of that pattern Hoekenga had previously mentioned. But how was I going to play this out with the witness? Was I going to review the anencephalic DERs with him, in hopes of extracting some concessions, or hit Merrell's witnesses with it for the first time during trial? I opted for a surprise attack. I asked for descriptions of a few of the defects, and then moved to an old subject.

"Was Clomid ever investigated as to any possible teratogenic effects, in the clinical investigation?"

"No, Clomid was not specifically evaluated to see if it would have a teratogenic effect. The outcome of every pregnancy that was temporally related with Clomid was assiduously searched for and tabulated and evaluated."

I was uncertain whether Hoekenga heard the question correctly, so I attempted to phrase it differently. "Well, in drafting the prescribed protocols was any effort made to set forth information, which you desired, that might later assist you in making a determination as to whether or not Clomid had a teratogenic effect?"

"The answer to the question is that we instructed the investigators repeatedly to advise us of the outcome of every pregnancy."

What I was beginning to increasingly appreciate was that the study was never designed to evaluate the risk of birth defects beyond simply recording and tabulating the outcome of each pregnancy produced by Clomid. With further questioning I learned that the investigators were never requested to make an ascertainment of the cause of any of the delivered birth defects. Having by now reviewed the records of the reported anomalies from the clinical investigations, I made a determination to explore this question a little deeper, to test what could or could not be concluded from the outcomes that were "tabulated and evaluated." I first called his attention to the submitted records for case number 028-183.[14]

"Can you determine by looking at these records the date of conception?" I asked, handing him the documents.

Hoekenga examined them a few moments then responded, "I cannot determine from this particular record."

"Can you determine from looking at these records whether or not the conception occurred during a treatment cycle?"

"No."

Clomid is taken for five days beginning the fifth day of the menstrual cycle. If ovulation and conception occur shortly after the last tablet, conception is considered to have occurred during a "treatment cycle." I handed him the records for case number 028-249.

"Can you determine the exact dates that Clomid was taken during the month of May, which would have been the concluding month, I believe?"

"I would not be able to determine the precise starting and stopping date," he answered, after examining the documents.

Nor could he ascertain the exact date of conception, other than it had occurred during the same month. There would be no way of knowing whether any of the drug was taken after conception, and thus during pregnancy. We next looked at Clinical Report number 028-429.

"Can you determine by looking at that, Doctor, the exact days she would have taken the drug?"

"I cannot determine the exact days."

"Does it indicate in any part of the record the date of conception?"

"The precise date is not stated."

Similar testimony was elicited from Hoekenga after reviewing Clinical Report number 028-430. From patient 065-021 it could be determined that Clomid was taken during pregnancy, but lacking a date of conception one could not ascertain how far into the pregnancy the drug was given. Clinical Report numbers 066-233, 100-116 and 100-175 failed to reveal dates of conception. Number 263-001 did not even report the year of treatment; only that it occurred during a treatment cycle, without mentioning the date of conception. Similar uncertainty also existed for 305-044 and 346-021.

I had just reviewed 11 case histories with Hoekenga from the records pertaining to the 58 birth defects reported from the clinical investigations. The others appeared to relate accurate information on the dates of Clomid treatment and the dates of conception. But twenty percent failed to reveal what I thought would be critical information. Then there were all of the other records I had never seen. According to the current package insert, there were a total of 2,369 pregnancies that occurred during the clinical investigations from which the outcome was purportedly known. What would those records reveal? Would there be similar uncertainties or even worse? Questions to which I had no answers. There was only one certainty: I would never see those records before a trial that was only 11 days away. All I could do was attempt to exploit what I had.

It was time to talk to Dr. Holtkamp about the elusive teratology studies.

After a few preliminary matters, I began my examination of Holtkamp with project report number E-62-10; then continued with numbers E-62-29, E-62-34, E-62-47, E-62-48, E-62-49, E-62-50, E-62-51, E-65-18, E-61-61, E-62-32, E-62-46 and E-71-01.

The "E" referred to the Endocrinology Department; the next two digits represented the year of the study; and the last two digits the specific report number.

I focused my questioning on the reported anomalies. In the rats, the reports described elongated snouts, hydrocephalus (fluid accumulation on brain with enlargement of skull), "head malformations" and "abnormal hind limbs." When asked to describe the limb abnormalities, Holtkamp only offered that they were non-skeletal and involved abnormal soft tissue. He had no further description of the "head malformations." In another study some had elongated snouts and "altered limbs," but he could not tell me how they were "altered" or even whether it involved the front or hind limbs. That was fine. I would play the vagueness up during trial as a possible effort at concealment. The rabbit offspring had a form of "turning under" of the hind feet or paws. Kind of like Mark's clubfoot, I would argue. Maybe the limb abnormalities did not involve limb reduction defects, but it appeared that Clomid was attacking the limbs. I would use any weapon at my disposal. I concluded on what I anticipated would be a sensitive subject – thalidomide. After a barrage of objections, I was able to pursue some questioning.

"Were any animal studies conducted in your department on thalidomide, as to its potential teratogenic effect?"

"Yes."

"Were there any findings in your studies of birth defects caused by that particular drug?"

"There were malformed fetuses of treated mothers."

"Do you have any recollection as to a description of the malformed fetuses?"

"There were limb deformities."

"You recall the nature of the limb deformities?"

"Skeletal changes were present."

"Do you recall whether or not there was a similarity in the defects that you observed in the animal studies on thalidomide as compared to the defects generally attributed to thalidomide in humans?"

"Yes."

"What were the similarities, if you recall?"

"There were some skeletal ones."

So there you are. There was a correlation between animal studies and humans, at least with this known human teratogen; another piece of useful information in my growing, though somewhat meager, arsenal. It was time to head back to California.

The Big Day Arrives

Monday, March 11, 1974. It was "D" day, or should I say "T" day? In any case, zero hour was at hand and it was time to answer ready in Department "A," the master calendar department in Torrance. From here we would be assigned out for trial to one of the half dozen trial judges hearing civil cases that had an open court. Rosalie Chapman was sitting next to me in the courtroom behind the railing, waiting for our case to be called. The room was packed with lawyers, clients and a handful of witnesses on a few short cause matters – almost standing room only. We were waiting for the judge to take the bench. Everyone seemed to be talking, except at a subdued level. I leaned over to Rose's ear.

"As I said earlier, I'm going to make a motion to continue. Got no choice. I haven't even talked to our experts. Our exhibits aren't in order, we have no trial brief, I don't even have my questions laid out for our own clients…"

"Terry, I understand, I agree. You should make the motion."

"…and I just got the deposition transcripts from Cincinnati last night."

Rose looked at me as if to say, who are you trying to convince? I got the message and nodded. I was terrified of going to trial unprepared. It was my first drug case and the biggest lawsuit in my seven-year career and I didn't want to blow it. But was I making the motion because it was the right thing to do for the case or because I was inexperienced and not up to the task? Maybe I *was* trying to convince myself.

"All rise." The voice of the courtroom bailiff was loud and clear as the Honorable Stephen R. Stothers burst through the door to the left of the bench. Immediately the room went silent. He quickly ascended to his throne, sat down, reviewed a few papers on his desk, and then directed to his clerk, "Call the trial calendar, Alex."

Alex Dugally stood and called the first case on the calendar. We were number six down the list. The cases were prioritized based upon their age, with the oldest filed cases going first. It was my hope that any open courtrooms would quickly fill up with lengthy trials. If we couldn't get into a courtroom by the end of the week, the judge would continue us over for at least three months. The first two lawyers came from the back of the room and stood in front of Judge Stothers. "We have a settlement," one announced, and the other nodded his agreement. Within five minutes they had put the settlement on the record with the court reporter and were gone.

The next two cases were short-cause matters (half a day or less) and were promptly assigned out to the same judge. By trial or settlement they would both be concluded by the end of the day and the judge again available. Stothers was now down to number four. Alex called the case and five lawyers stood up and paraded in front of the bench. This is a long one, I tried to convince myself; should last at least a month. The first four lawyers answered ready, but the fifth indicated that she needed to move for a continuance. Her client had just been in a serious auto accident and was hospitalized. She had a report from his treating doctor, if necessary.

"Hand it to the clerk," Stothers instructed.

He was not about to take her word on the matter. In turn the clerk handed the report to Stothers, who analyzed it for a minute and with an unhappy face said, "I'm going to reluctantly grant your motion."

He then preached his usual sermon for the benefit of all present that continuances were disfavored in his courtroom, and that when you come to Torrance for trial, you'd better be prepared to go out. An open courtroom was the only way to dispense justice, and as long as he was presiding judge, he would be doing what he could to cut down the backlog of cases. Didn't sound too promising, I thought.

Number five on the list was of little help either. The three lawyers all agreed that they were very close to settlement, but could use the assistance of a judge to put a few loose ends together. Stothers told them to hang around, and he would see them in chambers after he cleared the calendar. We were next up.

"Breimhorst vs. Richardson-Merrell," Alex announced.

My heart sank as we both stood and entered through the gate. We were followed by Belanger and Swanson, and Robert Worrell from the Thelen, Marrin firm. He did not look too pleased. His motion for summary judgment had been denied only a week earlier. We had also let the driver out of the case for $5,000, after counsel for Merrell and Richards both conceded, in their court-ordered answers to interrogatories, that they would not contend the auto accident was the cause of the malformations – any of them. After we stated our appearances for the record, I reluctantly said, "Plaintiffs will be making a motion for continuance, your honor."

Stothers stared down at me like he couldn't believe I hadn't heard his lecture. Steve Stothers was a former attorney who had defended cases for insurance companies. He was also ultra-conservative and his rulings from the bench reflected his conservative views, as did the close butch cut of his silver-white hair. His features were sharp and stern, although he was actually quite pleasant when in chambers or away from the courtroom. I had previously been in front of him on several occasions, but fortunately never for trial.

"What are your grounds, Counsel?"

I proceeded to lay out the whole experience, including the two trips to Cincinnati, the award of sanctions and the clear obstreperous actions on the part of defense counsel for Merrell. To deny the motion for continuance would be to condone the very conduct for which defendant was sanctioned. Belanger, of course, had a different point of view of the whole matter. Every objection that they made was proper and meritorious, and just because Judge Ross saw it differently didn't mean they lacked the right to assert those objections. Then he pounded in the final nail.

"Maybe Mr. Mix should not have waited so long to make his trip back to Ohio."

In addition to being a contemporary of Judge Stothers, Belanger no doubt knew him as a fellow member of the defense bar before he was appointed to the bench. I was convinced they were probably even drinking buddies. In any event, I knew I was dead.

"Motion denied," said Stothers, without giving it much thought.

"Well, your honor, then we would move to take the matter off calendar, to remove it from the civil active list."

"Motion denied," he repeated. He turned to his clerk. "Alex, send them to department 'D,' Judge Fredricks."

Suddenly a light went on at the end of this very long tunnel. It was a small one, but it was definitely there. So it was going to be Judge Fredricks. Thomas W. Fredricks had been our settlement judge only a few weeks earlier. We had settled only the auto case, but he seemed very interested and saw it as an important lawsuit.[15] He had also been the trial judge on a slip-and-fall case I had successfully tried the prior fall, with the resulting six-figure verdict. I had been very pleased with his judicial performance at the time. Judge Fredricks was a pleasant man with an engaging smile, a judge with the ideal temperament. He had an open mind on virtually all legal issues, and would listen carefully to both sides before making a ruling. He was as fair a judge as there was in Torrance at the time. If we had to go to trial on this date, I felt that we would receive even-handed treatment from him, and be given every opportunity to put on our best case. Maybe things weren't so bad after all. Alex Dugally[16] handed me the court's official file on the case and the five of us paraded out of the courtroom and down the hall to Department "D."

* * * * *

CHAPTER 2

Clomid on Trial:

The Plaintiffs' Case

After a few quick phone calls to clients, we all entered Department "D" and checked in with the clerk. Elma Ota had been Judge Fredricks' clerk on my earlier jury trial. We exchanged greetings and I handed her the file.

Elma digested my recent addition for a moment – a mustache. She had seen it just briefly a couple of weeks earlier, but obviously had not adjusted to the change. Due to my blonde hair and blue eyes, and somewhat youthful appearance, I decided that a little hair under my nose might add a touch of maturity. She smiled and said, "So I guess we're gonna be busy with another one of your trials."

"You know me," I said. "I'm here to entertain."

"Well, you can go entertain Judge Fredricks. He's ready to see you, so go right on in."

The five of us went through the door next to the bench and entered the back hallway. I knocked on the door to Fredricks' chambers, heard the invitation and entered. Judge Fredricks immediately rose, rounded his desk with his usual smile and extended his hand. "Nice to see everyone again," he offered. We all shook his hand and sat down. "Well, you don't have to tell me about the case. Any progress on negotiations?"

Bob Worrell was the first to react. "We do have some money, your honor. But first we'd like to chat with you privately." Worrell didn't seem to be too pleased. He was still shell-shocked at losing the motion for summary judgment. He no doubt was acting on marching orders from the insurance carrier to settle the case.

The judge looked at senior counsel for Merrell. "How about you, Mr. Belanger?"

"We're still at $75,000. We think it's very generous. I doubt the company will go a dollar more."

"Mr. Mix?" The judge was now looking at me.

"And we're still at $400,000, Judge. For both defendants, of course. But we do have some movement if they want to talk." You bet we had some movement. We didn't want to give the case away, but it was bargain basement time. I felt absolutely unprepared, not even sure what I would say in my opening statement.

"Okay," said the judge. "Why don't you and Mrs. Chapman step outside and let me hear what they have to say."

Rose and I quickly exited and returned to the courtroom. By this time, Ingrid had arrived and was anxiously waiting to hear an update on what was happening. Rose and I filled her in and waited. About a half hour later we were called back inside and spent some time alone with the judge as well. After going through this process a couple more times, we eventually settled with Richards for $65,000. Ingrid had approved without hesitation. With the driver's settlement, this gave us $70,000[17] in the bank.

We also eventually reduced our settlement demand for Merrell to $130,000, but Belanger was not about to move. "Not even a dollar," he assured. The $75,000 was still there if we wanted it. "But if you're not interested, let's have a jury decide the case." This was no doubt an effort at intimidation. The message was quite clear. They had absolutely no concern about the outcome.

Fifty-five thousand dollars was all that separated us, but it might as well have been an ocean.[18] Lines were being drawn in the sand by both sides. In my desperation, I was tempted to recommend that we drop our number even further, but I likewise began to dig in my heels. I sensed arrogance on the part of Belanger. The glove had been thrown at my feet. Needed adrenalin began pumping through me for the first time. The hell with it, I thought. Without my customary level of preparation, I started to develop a take-it-as-it-comes attitude. Damn the torpedoes, full speed ahead! We had seventy grand in the bank. Our costs were covered, so what the hell, why not?

"Okay," I said. "Let's let a jury decide the case."

Tom Fredricks did not seem the least bit upset by this decision. He told us to take a fifteen minute break and be prepared to argue any motions *in limine*[19] on the record when we got back. On the way out of chambers, Swanson handed me an 18-page trial brief and several written motions. He would be earning his stripes riding shotgun for the veteran. The originals were given to Elma back in the courtroom. Rose conferred with Ingrid while I sat down at the counsel table and began reviewing my handwritten notes. Unlike Belanger's well-drafted written motions, setting out all of the supporting legal authorities that Judge Fredricks would ever want to read, my motions would be delivered orally in open court.

Fifteen minutes later I was arguing my five motions. Belanger gave his usual eloquent opposition to each, except for my last motion to preclude anyone from mentioning the settlements to the jury. By stipulation, the amounts would be deducted from any judgment for the plaintiff. I didn't want the jury to know about receipt of the $70,000, because on a close question of whether we had proven our case, it would be easier for the jury to turn down the infant plaintiff knowing he would still be receiving some money. Conversely, Belanger no doubt didn't want the jury hearing the number because it was sufficiently high enough as to prompt a jury to infer that someone on Richards' team felt the drug might be the cause of the defects.

After we finished arguing my motions, the judge told us that they were deemed submitted and he would give us the decisions the following morning. He would also spend the afternoon reading Belanger's trial brief and written motions, and hear any argument to be made on them first thing in the morning. He told us to be prepared to start picking a jury by 10:00 AM.

By early afternoon I was back in my office, scripting out questions to ask the prospective jurors. I also structured an outline for my opening statement, sufficient enough to get by a motion for nonsuit.[20] There would have to be enough facts stated to meet all of the legal elements for establishing our case. I would also need to give the jury enough to hold their interest, yet without too much detail to avoid cornering myself on something I couldn't later prove. To a great extent, I still needed to hear how far our own expert witnesses would go. I was also hoping to score a number of points when cross-examining the defendant's witnesses, but that wouldn't occur for a couple more weeks. Do enough to hold off the wolves, I encouraged myself. Belanger would be looking to leap on every mistake and I knew there would be many. Yet I had this intuitive sense that if we survived until I could get to the defendant's experts, our case would actually get stronger with Merrell's own witnesses.

At 3:00 PM I met with Rose at her office. I needed a full list of witnesses to give to the judge in the morning. Their names would have to be read to the prospective jurors. Ingrid and Heinz and Richards were a given. We also had one of Mark's treating doctors. But who were our experts and what would they say? I was still in the dark. Just like that first day, I was again sitting across from Rosalie Chapman in one of her client chairs.

"Okay, Rose, I'm out of time. I know you and Phil have been working hard on this, but I need something now. I at least need names, addresses and area of expertise. If you know what they're gonna say, great. But at least give me the essentials."

Rose sat up a little straighter, stared right at me and slightly smiled. She had been waiting to tell me this since late morning. "We have ourselves a teratologist, Terry, a real teratologist. Phil spoke with him this morning. We had sent him a packet of material weeks ago, but he just finished reviewing it yesterday."

"You're kidding! And he's agreed to testify?"

"Yep. He'll be flying in from Detroit next week."

"Great! What's his name?"

"Perrin, Eugene Perrin."

At this point, there could not have been better news. "Well, what's he gonna say? Have you talked to him?"

"No, Phil has, but I don't know what was said other than he felt he could help us and was willing to fly out for the trial. I've got his number if you want to call him."

"Sure, who else you got?"

Rose proceeded to give me the remaining names. She had little detail about their testimony, but at least I had something to give Fredricks in the morning. For the next hour we discussed what she had learned about each witness and when they would be available. They would need to be sequenced such to avoid any dead time. Trial judges, even Tom Fredricks, hated to have a dark courtroom. We needed to fill each day with testimony until we rested, then it would be Belanger's problem.

We also discussed Rose's role throughout the trial. It would be her responsibility to line up each witness every day and arrange my meeting with them prior to their testimony. The meeting would take place, if possible, after trial concluded each day, either in the late afternoon or early evening. Absent that, it would have to take place at the courthouse early morning, probably in the coffee shop. If the need for any legal research popped up, it would be her task to get me the cases, even if it meant going back to the office while the trial proceeded. Other than that, she would simply take notes each day, make observations of jury reactions and be my sounding board. Everything else would be my responsibility. She was quite content with this assignment. Rose had no desire to examine any witnesses, make argument in open court, or in any way be a co-trial attorney. Occasionally she might assist me in arguing a matter in chambers, but that was it. I shared the same view. Rose had little experience at the time in a courtroom, and one big blunder could send us to the bottom.

I returned to my office and immediately got Dr. Perrin on the line. I first went over his credentials. He was eminently qualified as a teratologist. He had also reviewed Mark and Ingrid's medical records, the package insert, the animal studies I finally obtained from Richardson-Merrell and reports the company had received about birth defects that occurred following Clomid pregnancies.

We also talked about the high spontaneous abortion rate during the pre-marketing studies. Whereas various studies on spontaneous abortion rates in the general population ranged from ten to fifteen percent of confirmed pregnancies, following use of Clomid the rate was at *twenty percent*. One in every five pregnancies during Merrell's clinical investigations resulted in a spontaneous abortion. This was important. A spontaneous abortion was the body's natural rejection on an embryo or fetus. First trimester abortions are of particular importance because they are highly associated with abnormalities of the product of conception, usually caused by abnormal chromosomes. Perrin felt evidence was there that Clomid might be a human teratogen.

There was just one problem. He would only state on a witness stand that there was a reasonable medical *possibility* that Mark's congenital anomalies were caused by Clomid. Perrin was a scientist and scientists require strong, sometimes overwhelming, proof to be convinced of a given conclusion. I respected this, but pressed him. I explained that in California our burden of proof was to establish that the drug was the *probable,* not a possible, cause. But this meant we only had to prove that it was more likely than not the cause – 51% likelihood, if you will. He was sympathetic to the problem, but *reasonable medical possibility* was the best he could give me. He wanted to know if he should still come out and I assured him that his testimony would be of value and I would look forward to seeing him the following week.

I recalled recently reading a published appellate decision[21] on this very issue. Although a plaintiff was required to prove that a given injury was probably caused by the defendant's conduct, a jury's decision could still be based upon an expert opinion of reasonable medical *possibility*. In arriving at a decision of *probable* cause, a jury can take that expert's opinion into consideration along with evidence of all the other circumstances as well. Ingrid had not been exposed to any other drugs, radiation, trauma, or any other known teratogen, during the critical period of organogenesis. Nor had she suffered from any maternal illnesses during pregnancy, and these birth defects were not due to heredity. All other known causes of birth defects could be eliminated. These were all additional considerations. Dr. Perrin's medical opinion and the appellate decision might barely get me by a nonsuit, but it was all I had at the moment.

Jury Selection Begins

Tuesday, March 12, 1974. The back of the courtroom was packed with a panel of prospective jurors; men and women, young and old and in between. There were about 40 in the group. At the moment, not one of them had any idea what the case was about. Some of Belanger's trial team were squeezed into a corner of the room, looking a little uncomfortable, uncertain how they should behave with prospective jurors almost in their laps. I was sitting on the left end of the counsel table, closest to the jury box, with Rose and Ingrid seated to my right. Belanger and Swanson were at the other end of the table. At the moment, there was no representative of the company present. We were waiting for Judge Fredricks to take the bench.

Earlier all of the rulings on the motions had gone pretty much as expected. A few losses and a few victories for each side; but nothing earthshaking that would have any impact on the ultimate verdict. A few crumbs for the plaintiffs and a few for the defendant. Two rulings included an order that prevented me from mentioning that Richardson-Merrell had attempted to market thalidomide and had manufactured and sold Triparanol. "Relevant but too prejudicial," Fredricks had said. Expected rulings; but a disappointment. One of my crumbs included a ruling excluding any reference to the auto accident.

The motions, however, had dragged on and jury selection pushed into the afternoon. Now was when the real trial work started; selecting a jury, then opening statements and presenting evidence. I rotated my chair around and looked back at the many faces, wondering who in the group would be the best or the worst for the plaintiffs' case. Where did they come from, what were their backgrounds, their jobs, their histories?

Did any have a hidden agenda, a vendetta, anger about the tort system and high verdicts? Did any of them or close friends or relatives have any birth defects? Had they ever worked for, or held stock in, a pharmaceutical company or large corporation, or worked in upper management? Were they, or any loved ones, dependent upon drugs for their survival? What views did they have about animal testing, including the value of them in predicting the human experience? Had they ever had problems conceiving, taken fertility drugs? Had they ever adopted after the frustration of infertility? These were just a few of the questions that I would shortly be posing. The answers would ultimately dictate the shape of the jury, but would they be candid answers? What would be the body language? In the end, it seemed so often that a decision to challenge or accept a juror was based more on instinct, more on how the question was answered rather than the content of the answer – and at other times like the roll of the dice.

Just then, the Honorable Tom Fredricks entered the courtroom, wearing a black robe for the first time. The bailiff shouted out the instruction for everyone to rise and about 50 people simultaneously rose to their feet. Fredricks sat himself down, then had everyone else be seated. He looked at the audience in front of him for a quiet moment, nodded his head a couple times, as if he was quite pleased this was all happening. He then said, "Counsel, you want to introduce yourselves and your clients? Mr. Belanger, why don't we start with you?"

All four counsel rose, along with Ingrid, and faced the back of the courtroom.

"Yes, thank you, your honor," said Belanger, as he smiled to the panel. He was a seasoned trial lawyer, probably in his late fifties at the time. His brownish hair was peppered with gray. He wore glasses, but seemed to use them more as a tool of his trade, removing them at times while making a point, and looking over the top of them on other occasions. He had an excellent command of the English language, used it with ease and was polished to a bright shine. He had taken many scalps over the years, and one could understand why. He was very good at what he did. Yet in spite of this well-crafted package, there was a certain stiffness and formality to the man. "I am Fred B. Belanger," he announced, "and this is my associate, Charles R. Swanson. We are both members of the firm of Schell & Delamer and represent the pharmaceutical company, Richardson-Merrell."

Fred B and Charles R? That couldn't have been more formal if it had been a wedding announcement. A strategy struck me like a lightening bolt. Whatever the other side was, I would be just the opposite. "I'm Terence…or Terry Mix," I countered, "and this is my co-counsel, Rose Chapman." I motioned to Ingrid. "…and this is our client, Ingrid Breimhorst. We also represent her husband, Heinz, and their three-year old son, Mark."

"Thank you," said Fredricks, as we all returned to our seats. After Elma swore in the panel, Fredricks read them a statement of the case; a brief summary of the nature of the lawsuit, the claims against the defendant, Merrell's defenses to the lawsuit and a general description of the birth defects. He inquired whether any of the prospective jurors knew anything about the case or were acquainted with any of the parties or their attorneys. No one raised a hand. He next read each name from both witness lists and inquired whether anyone knew any of the witnesses. Still no hands. Next he estimated that the trial could last as long as 30 trial days, a month and a half, although he expected it to be shorter. Fredricks wanted to know if it would impose a hardship on anyone to serve that long on the jury. That got their attention. About one-third of the audience raised their hands. The judge then went to work on each one individually, to assess the exact nature of the hardship and how legitimate the reasons were for not serving. By the time he concluded, about ten prospects had been excused. We were now ready to draw the first 12 names.

While this was going on, I subtly inspected Team Merrell. To the side of the room they had about a dozen storage boxes, no doubt filled with company records and exhibits, which had been numbered and neatly stacked. I would attempt to bring in no more than one box each day, along with what I could carry in my briefcase. Any additional boxes would be left in my car. They also had an equal number of 48 x 60 inch charts, graphs and photographic blowups of documents, leaning against the wall. I would use the wide sheets of paper supplied by the court and hand-write information and numbers for exhibits. The only expensive exhibit we would offer would be Mark's day-in-the-life-of film, which had been prepared by professionals at my request. Everything else would look home made. In addition to Belanger and Swanson at the counsel table, there was another firm attorney, plus Fred Lamb and a gofer – to haul boxes and exhibits and perform other chores – behind the railing. On our side there were only the two of us. The other contrasts would be exhibited by me as the trial progressed.

Judge Fredricks turned to Elma and instructed her to, "Fill the box." Elma shook a small box containing the remaining names of the panel, then reached in and drew a name at random, read it out loud, and repeated the process 12 times. Twelve jurors, one by one, passed through the gate and took their chairs in the jury box. After some preliminary questioning of the twelve by Fredricks, he turned the *voir dire* examination over to the attorneys. "Mr. Mix," he said, inviting me to inquire. I casually stood, stepped in front of the jury and smiled, my notes in my hand. Rose would be taking down important responses.

I was now in my element. I have always felt comfortable in front of juries. I love them and the system in which they were participating. Even when they turned me down, I held no ill feelings. Many hold biases and prejudices which they cannot overcome in attempting to reach an impartial decision, and it was my job to discover this and let them off the hook. This would be done in the form of a challenge. With some exceptions, the vast majority of jurors take their oaths and obligations quite seriously and sincerely attempt to do the right thing. I would speak to them as if we were neighbors chatting over the fence. I would use the technical and medical words and terms that they would be hearing during the course of the trial, but then break them down into lay language. I would attempt to educate without speaking down to them. I now was about to hopefully find out who would be the best or the worst for the plaintiffs' case.

I began my *voir dire* examination with an apology. I would be asking some of them very personal questions, but it was unfortunately necessary in order to select a fair and impartial set of jurors. If anyone had any problem answering such questions in open court, I urged them to call it to my attention and we would retire to the judge's chambers. This, of course, had already been cleared with Fredricks. I then launched into my questioning, yet taking all precaution to avoid it sounding like an interrogation. A whole series of questions were first posed to the entire panel, asking for a show of hands if anyone had a positive response to make. Rose duly noted each juror that had raised a hand and the issue it involved. After reviewing Rose's notes, I then went down each row, asking questions of every juror, insuring that no one would feel neglected. Many times the questions were probing, but always in an apologetic tone. Surprisingly, no one found a need to retreat to chambers.

Occasionally I resorted to levity. This had a few benefits. First, it loosened everyone up and got them to relax. Answering questions in court could be quite intimidating. They also, hopefully, would see me as personable and friendly, rather than as a stuffy and detached lawyer. And not infrequently I used it to highlight important covenants I made with the jurors. I was now about to end my questioning.

"Can each and every one of you assure me, that if you are accepted as a juror, you will not under any circumstances speak to anyone about this case until you begin deliberations, and then only with other jurors; would you be able to do that?

"Okay, I see everyone one nodding, but here comes the hard part...it includes your spouse!" I could see several smiles and even a few nods of the head. "Now if your spouse is like my wife, this is not going to be very easy." Even more smiles now. "I mean, I could lock myself in the bathroom and she would be pounding on the door demanding to know what I was hiding from her, why I won't tell her about the case." Now some are actually laughing. "Well, if I was a juror, I still wouldn't be able to tell her, because this promise is that important. It is inviolate. Your decision will have to be based only upon evidence that you hear or see right in this courtroom, not from someone who might even unwittingly influence your vote. Now can you all make me that promise?" At this point everyone is giving me a pronounced nod of the head. Point made. And if possible, always leave on a high point.

I looked up at Fredricks, who was also smiling. "Pass for cause, your honor." Although we each had 6 peremptory challenges, which could be exercised without a need for justification or reason, each party had unlimited challenges "for cause," which would only occur if the judge was convinced that the juror was prejudiced or otherwise could not render a fair and impartial verdict. Civil judges are notorious for resisting challenges for cause. I had just informed the judge that I had no basis for such a challenge. With our fifteen minute break, I had taken up almost all of the afternoon. Fredricks announced that we would break for the day. Next up tomorrow, Fred B. Belanger.

Wednesday, March 13, 1974. Belanger treated the jury with his own set of questions, trying to avoid any repetition of mine, yet following up on some of the answers I had left hanging. Two or three jurors had hinted at possibly being sympathetic to a child with birth defects. I had quickly dropped the line of inquiry, not wanting to give the defense any ammunition for cause. Further questioning by Belanger failed to be productive, although I still expected them to get the boot. Neither of us had yet to use a peremptory. He continued with other expected questions. Could they treat a corporation with the same fairness as a living person? Plaintiffs have the burden of proof to establish that Clomid actually caused Mark Breimhorst's birth defects. Could they send him away without one dollar if they failed to meet that burden? We all have sympathy for Mark Breimhorst, but would you let that influence your ability to weigh the evidence fairly? Would you be able to stand in front of his mother and father at the end of this trial and say, "I'm sorry, but you just didn't prove your case"? He proceeded to phrase it several different ways, but the message was always the same. Sympathy had no business in a courtroom and it was plaintiffs' burden of proof to establish Clomid as a teratogen, not Merrell's to prove it was not.

Belanger abruptly finished after only about forty minutes. "Pass for cause," he announced. I was a little surprised at the brevity. I had expected more extensive questioning. I suspected that this was some kind of strategy, but was at a loss to figure out what it was.

"Very well," said Fredricks. "Peremptory is with the plaintiffs."

I quickly reviewed my notes, as well as those that Rose had handed over to me. She had placed question marks next to two of the jurors, one of which I had significant concern about myself. I tapped my pen on the name of the one and she nodded her agreement with me. "Plaintiffs would thank and excuse juror number six, your honor." I stared at him apologetically as he rose and departed.

Elma pulled another name out of the box and filled chair number six. I generally went through the same series of questions with the new juror number six, and then passed for cause. Belanger did likewise. Fredricks looked at the other end of the counsel table.

"Peremptory is with the defendant," he said. The tennis match back and forth was about to continue – or so I thought.

A Stunning Surpise

Belanger rose slowly, with a hint of a smile. For a brief moment he scanned the twelve jurors. "We accept the jury as presently constituted, your honor."

This decision almost knocked me to the floor. He was prepared to accept the jury without exercising one peremptory – not one. What was he up to? What did he know that I was totally missing? There were several prospective jurors that I was quite pleased with, but then I had been doing this for only 7 years and Belanger had been standing in front of juries for at least three times as long. Then it hit me. That wasn't a smile, it was a smirk. That arrogant son of a bitch...

"Your turn, Mr. Mix," I heard from the bench. Fredricks was staring down at me as if to say, "Okay, fella, *now* what are you gonna do?"

"Just a moment, your honor." I hurriedly ran through my notes. There were a couple more prospects I had some concern about, but I didn't feel strongly about them. I could challenge one or both of them, but who would be their replacements? One might be a claims adjuster for Allstate or an executive with a pharmaceutical company. All I had to do was accept the present panel and Belanger would be stuck with them for a whole month. It was too tempting.

Rose mouthed to me, "What's he up to?"

"He's sending a message," I whispered. "Fred B is telling everyone he'll take any twelve." I looked up at Fredricks. "Plaintiff will accept the jury as well," I said with equal confidence.

And just like that I called Fred B. I locked him in. He was so convinced that we could never prove our case, that he let it be known he would take any 12 jurors that were pulled from the audience. A calculated gamble? Perhaps. But what did he know. He knew he was dealing with a relatively inexperienced young attorney, who appeared unprepared for the task. He knew we had barely scratched the surface of the Clomid IND and NDA records and had conducted very little meaningful discovery. He knew there were a number of employees holding critical knowledge about the drug that were never deposed and would never set foot inside this courtroom. He knew the pre-marketing clinical studies had given Clomid a clean bill of health and that the drug had the FDA's stamp of approval. He knew from the company about every published study involving

51

Clomid to date, and according to Merrell none had shown an increase in the incidence of birth defects. And he knew that any legitimate expert I would bring in to testify would have very little on which to hang his expert opinion. I am sure that Fred B was convinced, at least at this time, that there was very little chance that this case would ever reach a jury. In his view, it had "nonsuit" written all over it.

After Elma swore in the jury, Fredricks let us go for the morning break. We were to return in fifteen minutes to select the alternate jurors. I suggested to Rose that she go on the break without me. I would spend the rest of the time reviewing my notes. Jury selection was going quicker than expected, and I needed time to refine my opening statement, which no doubt would take place shortly.

Within 20 minutes we had two alternates. Neither of us exercised one challenge. If Belanger was going to accept anyone, then I would too. Want to play chicken? Okay, let's play chicken. Since I was more or less unprepared anyway, this recklessness actually felt good. But I needed to maintain control. I couldn't be seduced into a careless trial.

Opening Statements

Fredricks then invited me to give my opening statement. Time to give another performance. Showtime. Going to trial has been likened to creating a play or a movie, with the trial lawyer the composite of the producer, director, writer and actor. I rose from the counsel table.

"May it please the court…counsel," I said, looking over at Belanger and Swanson, then directed my attention to those to be deciding our fate, "…ladies and gentleman of the jury." It had become my standard introduction, although it seemed antiquated and I had no idea where I got it.

I then opened with my usual explanation of the purpose and benefit of an opening statement, explaining that due to the unavailability of witnesses and occasional breaks to discuss important matters with the judge, they would be getting the evidence in pieces and not always in the sequence that we would like. The opening statements would allow them to see an overview of the entire case, much like the picture of a puzzle on the outside of the box, before the pieces are assembled throughout the course of the trial. I also explained how the trial would procedurally progress. Although trying to be informative, this customary beginning to opening statement was designed to allow me to become more relaxed in front of the jury, to get my sea legs, before launching into the evidence I would be presenting.

I explained to the jury that the evidence would establish that the defendant, Richardson-Merrell, negligently designed and monitored its pre-marketing clinical investigations with Clomid; that prior to designing those studies, the company was well aware that a number of drugs were capable of reaching the developing embryo and causing congenital malformations; that in 1962, the Endocrinology Department at Merrell had conducted teratology studies with rats and rabbits that had clearly established the drug's ability to cause malformations in the offspring of those animals; that even though the drug was intended only to be ingested prior to conception, half-life studies with the drug, both with animals and humans, had shown that the drug still carried over after conception and remained in the maternal circulation for weeks later, to a period when the limbs and other organs began to develop; that in spite of this knowledge, Merrell never made an effort to design the study to ascertain whether the drug presented a risk for causing birth defects; that it never used a control group as part of its study, a standard practice with epidemiology studies, and did no more than record the outcome of the pregnancies; that even when it learned, during the study, that spontaneous abortions were occurring at up to twice the rate in the general population, Merrell still avoided setting up a properly designed epidemiology study; and even when it learned that birth defects were occurring at twice the frequency when the drug was administered during pregnancy, it still withheld conducting a properly designed study.

I told them that the evidence would also establish that as the reports came to Richardson-Merrell from the clinical investigators, it was quite evident that many of them contained incomplete information about the dates of Clomid use and dates of conception, and when they occurred in relation to one another, information critical to learning whether the drug might be related to any adverse event; and that in spite of this knowledge, Merrell failed to follow-up and obtain accurate data from the study.

I added that Merrell also failed to provide an accurate warning of the risks of birth defects associated with use of the drug, and even made the representation that there was absolutely no evidence that Clomid had a deleterious effect on the human fetus; and that said representation was made with full knowledge that its clinical investigation was not designed to make that assessment.

I then moved into the issue of causation. I first stated that the evidence would show that as a consequence of all of this conduct, Mark Breimhorst was born with horrendous birth defects that have devastated not only his life, but the lives of his parents. This statement drew the necessary link between the negligence of the defendant and the plaintiff's birth defects, a critical element to avoid a nonsuit. I detailed the reasons for implicating Clomid; that all other known causes of birth defects were eliminated; that Mark's birth anomalies were not hereditary in origin; that Ingrid had not been exposed to any other teratogenic drugs, x-rays or other radiation, physical trauma or maternal illness during the critical first three months of pregnancy; and that at the time Mark's hands would have otherwise started to develop, this drug – that had produced congenital malformations in animals – was still circulating in Ingrid's body. I also recited a list of birth defects that had been reported by concerned physicians since Clomid was initially marketed, avoiding any discussion on the excessive number of anencephaly cases. That would only be exploited when I hit Merrell's experts with cross-examination.

I concluded with a detailed description of Mark's anomalies, and how they impacted his infant life, as well as the lives of his parents. Throughout the entire opening statement I defined each medical and scientific term in lay language, thus starting the educational process. After thanking the jury for their attention, I sat down and anxiously awaited an overview of the defendant's case from Fred B. By this time it was mid-afternoon and Fredricks suggested that it was a good time for our break.

When Belanger rose and began his opening, I eagerly began taking my own set of notes. Rose was writing as well, but I couldn't take a chance of her missing anything. This was my first opportunity to really assess where the defense would be challenging our case, and even the most innocuous statement might reveal a strategy I would have to prepare for. I was also looking for comments of "what the evidence will show," to determine whether I could later shove it down Belanger's throat when such promised evidence did a no-show. No lawyer wants to be embarrassed by failing to prove what he or she promised in the opening statement.

I also mentally noted that Belanger chose not to make a motion for nonsuit following my opening statement. I had adequately covered all of the legal issues, and Fred B no doubt knew that it would have been a useless act at this time. He would wisely wait until after we rested our case; after we had put on all of our evidence.

Belanger began by giving an overview and history of the drug, starting with Clomid's synthesis and following its subsequent development at Merrell, naming certain key people that he would be calling to testify. Since he was running short on time, he shrewdly touched on the use of animal studies with Clomid and explained that what a drug might cause in one animal was not necessarily transferable to another. For example, although Clomid had a *fertility* effect in humans, stimulating ovulation, it had an *infertility* effect on rats. He was beginning to distance the rat teratology studies from the human experience with Clomid. He also wanted the jury to chew on that comment overnight after we broke for the day.

Thursday, March 14, 1974. Fred B immediately launched back into the history of Clomid. He explained how it had been exhaustively studied in animals and humans; that their records numbered over 80,000 pages on the drug; and that it had been under study for 11 years when the FDA gave its approval on February 1, 1967. He cited a number of different studies involving the incidence of birth defects from the general population, all of which had higher birth defect rates than were reported in the Clomid clinical investigations. He pointed out that birth defects similar to Mark's had been reported in the scientific literature years before anyone ever thought about Clomid or fertility drugs.

As to warnings, he explained that the package insert expressly contraindicates Clomid's use after conception; that all of the statistics from the clinical studies are set out in detail and a description of every type of birth defect reported, both before and after marketing; and that the animal teratology studies were also referred to, even though the dosage that caused malformations in the rat and the rabbit were many times the human dose. "The dosage given to humans was miniscule by comparison," he emphasized.

Then with a little fanfare – you could almost hear the drums roll – he brought to everyone's attention that the Clomid records had been reviewed by no less authority than James G. Wilson, a world renowned authority on birth defects – a teratologist. In fact, he reviewed them on two separate occasions, once in 1965 and again in 1968. On both occasions he determined that there was no evidence that Clomid was a cause of birth defects in humans. Dr. Wilson would also be called to testify right here in this courtroom. Belanger then concluded by noting an inescapable fact; that the critical period of organogenesis was at least a month after last taking Clomid, which could not have in any way contributed to Mark's unfortunate birth defects.

Now it was time to start calling my witnesses.

Let the Testimony Begin

First up would be *Nicholas Richards, M.D.* He was a hostile witness, but the jury would never know it because during the motions *in limine* I had excluded any reference to not just the settlement, but also that he had ever been a party to the lawsuit. This was a calculated gamble, because Richards had no desire to do anything that would help our case. It would be better if the jury viewed him as our enemy. My examination of him would have to be tight and closely follow the testimony he gave during his pretrial deposition. I would bring out the essential facts that only he could provide, then stop my questioning and hope he didn't give away the store on cross-examination.

I carefully traced with him each examination he performed on Ingrid, using his medical chart, and brought out the important facts concerning the timing of treatment, the dosage, and the date of conception. I also used Richards to establish that no potential teratogenic events occurred during the first 3 months of pregnancy. Richards had previously been admonished not to refer to the auto accident, which had occurred 3½ months after conception. I then established that he had reviewed the package insert before prescribing Clomid, which was identified as an exhibit and introduced into evidence. I had him testify that after reviewing the insert, he was left with the understanding and opinion that Clomid was not a risk for causing birth defects in humans; that because of this conclusion, he never informed Ingrid that there was any potential for such a risk. Nor did he even inform her of the teratology studies with animals. I had him read out loud the statement that "no causative evidence of a deleterious effect of Clomid therapy on the human fetus has been seen," and acknowledge that he had read it before prescribing the drug to Ingrid. I had him explain his understanding of what it meant to him in his capacity as a prescribing doctor. Finally, I had him follow the pregnancy through to term and describe the congenital anomalies observed at time of delivery. It was now time to turn the witness over to Belanger and hold my breath. Fortunately, it was also time to break for the day. I could still breathe for another 17 hours.

Friday, March 15, 1974. Overnight we lost juror number five to a family emergency. She was replaced by one of the alternates, but now we only had one left and we perhaps had still a month to go. If we lost two more, we would be down to 11 and an automatic mistrial unless both sides stipulated to go with less than the required twelve. Given my circumstances at the time, I thought that I might welcome this possibility with open arms.

Now it was really time to cross my fingers and hope for the best. Belanger stood up and began his cross-examination. His first series of questions were somewhat innocuous, other than bringing out that fetalgrams were performed on June 5, 1970 and June 18, 1970, the day before delivery, which revealed that Mark was in a persistent transverse lie. This ultimately led to a C-section. Belanger attempted to draw from Richards that this may have accounted for the clubfoot, or maybe even the facial palsy. But Richards would not buy into it, no doubt concerned that it would reflect upon how he had handled the pregnancy. He did, however, get Richards to concede that ovulation – and conception – could have been as late as September 25, 1969, and that no one could say for sure when Mark was conceived. This would push treatment further away from when the hands would begin to form.

He then hit the highlight of his cross-examination. He posed a hypothetical question to the witness factoring in all of the relevant information from his medical chart and the histories of Ingrid and Heinz Breimhorst. This is the customary way attorneys solicit expert opinions from their witnesses.

"Tell us, doctor, can you state with reasonable medical certainty, given all of these circumstances, whether or not Clomid was the cause of these birth defects?"

"No, Clomid had nothing to do with these birth defects."

"And is it generally accepted in the medical community that Clomid does not cause birth defects in humans?"

"Yes, I would agree with that."

"Do you still prescribe Clomid?"

"Yes, I do."

"Would you continue to prescribe it to your patients if you believed there was any possibility that it could cause birth defects?"

"Absolutely not."

I knew this was coming. I was also sure that, before posing these questions, Belanger had spoken to Richards' attorney. A seasoned veteran such as Belanger would never violate the cardinal rule: never ask a question of a witness to which you do not know what the response will be. Worrell would have gladly shared his client's views with Belanger before the testimony. My time for damage control would be on redirect examination.

He continued to use the treating doctor as one of his experts. Richards was familiar with the period of organogenesis. It is generally accepted that teratogens must be introduced during this period in order to produce birth defects. The development of the limbs occurs approximately 4 to 6 weeks after conception. Mark's hands normally would have otherwise developed long after his mother last used Clomid. Finally Belanger concluded and sat down. It was now my turn again. I would attempt to use Richards as another victim of Merrell's failures.

"Doctor Richards, your experience with Clomid is somewhat limited, correct?"

"Yes, I would agree with that."

"You are not a fertility specialist?"

"No."

"Nor are you a teratologist?"

"No, I am not."

"Your opinions about Clomid are based primarily upon what you have read about the drug?"

"Well…, I have some experience, but I guess I would agree with that."

"And before you ever prescribed Clomid, you carefully read the entire package insert, correct?"

"Yes, I did."

"In fact, to a great extent you have relied upon the information provided to you in the package insert?"

"Yes."

"And as we have already brought out, that same package insert told you that there is no evidence that Clomid has a deleterious effect on the human fetus?"

"Yes."

"And you believed that to be true and relied upon it, correct?"

"Yes, that is true."

Many of these questions had been asked of Richards during his deposition, when Worrell's strategy had been to portray his client as an innocent physician relying upon what he had been told by the drug company. I then went into the issue of half-life and had him read out loud the statement in the package insert.

"Doctor, you would agree, would you not, that if Clomid was still hanging around 6 weeks after Mrs. Breimhorst last took one of the pills, then it would still be there well into the period of organogenesis?"

"Well…, yes, if it was really there."

"That's what it suggests, doesn't it?"

"Yes, I guess it does," he reluctantly conceded.

It was time to sit down. I had gotten as much mileage as I was going to get, and I would be ending on a high note. The weekend had finally arrived, and I couldn't have been happier. Somehow I had survived the first week. On Monday I had Heinz and Ingrid waiting in the wings.

Monday, March 18, 1974. As expected, *Hienz Breimhorst* went about as smoothly as I could possibly have hoped. Rose and I had spent about 3 hours with Ingrid and Heinz on Sunday, preparing for their testimony. It paid off well. He was attentive to all of my questions, gave full and complete answers without going off on a tangent or volunteering unsolicited information. He was also personable and came across as sincere with every answer he gave. My original hunch was right on; the jury could not help but like him and identify with what he and Ingrid were going through. By the morning break, I had brought all of his relevant medical history, including the absence of birth defects on his side of the family, and then finished with his day-to-day life with Mark and his lost dream sharing his life with a son lacking the multiple handicaps. Belanger very prudently cross-examined almost apologetically, and finished without scoring a point.

Now it was time for one of my star witnesses, *Ingrid Breimhorst*.

Ingrid stood, walked to the stand and stiffly sat down. I sensed that she was nervous. After she was sworn in and officially gave her name I changed my game plan. I customarily sat and inquired of my own witnesses from the counsel table. This allowed the jury to focus on the witness, without distractions from the examiner, and gave me easy access to my notes and exhibit book. But Ingrid was uncomfortable and needed a security blanket. I rose and approached her about half way to the stand.

"Morning," I smiled, as if we had just seen one another for the first time.

She nervously smiled back. "Good morning." Ingrid's hair was as blonde as hay, short and curled, her features naturally attractive.

"Kind of nervous, are you?"

She nodded. "Yes, I am."

"That's all right, so am I."

I got a questioning stare back.

"Okay, well then maybe just a little bit."

This seemed to break the ice, as I got a big grin from Ingrid.

"Could you give us your date of birth?"

"April 21, 1935."

"You understand, of course, that this is the only place I can get away with asking a lady her age?" Another big smile. "Now, then, why don't you tell us where you came from, and how you managed to make your way into the United States?"

Ingrid proceeded to relate the history of growing up in Sweden, her move to the United States in 1959, meeting Heinz and getting married. I then inquired about her use of birth control pills, their decision to have children, their inability to conceive and, finally, her first appointment with Dr. Richards. With each question and answer she seemed to be more and more relaxed, and I gradually worked my way back to my seat. By the noon recess, I had covered all of her relevant family and medical history and was prepared to explore the life of Mark Breimhorst. There was just one last point I wanted to cover.

"Now tell me, if you had been informed that Clomid posed even the slightest risk of causing birth defects, would you have taken the drug?"

Belanger jumped up. "Objection, your honor. Calls for speculation."

Fredricks looked at me for a response.

"Your honor, it would not require speculation if one were to ask me whether I would allow my two-year old daughter to play on the San Diego Freeway at three in the afternoon."

"Overruled," Fredricks quickly replied.

I again fixed on Ingrid for her reply.

"Absolutely not!" she firmly stated.

"Even if it meant going without your own children?"

"We would have adopted. I…we never would have taken such a risk," she added with conviction. "Never." It was time to stop for lunch.

The three of us had a quick lunch in the coffee shop, and spent some additional time reviewing Ingrid's testimony for the afternoon session. The remaining questions would focus on Mark's disabilities and how they impacted his day-to-day life. We would also lay the foundation necessary to introduce the film. I reminded her that when we stopped, Belanger would start his cross-examination, and would probably be a little more aggressive than he was with Heinz. Ingrid was more important on the critical issue of causation, and he would have to go after her – although with kid gloves. I told her to concede the obvious and to be truthful at all times, but on the important facts to avoid equivocating.

"If you make a mistake," I assured, "don't worry about it because I will straighten everything out on redirect. That's why I'm here. More importantly, don't loose your composure or temper, even if you feel attacked. I would rather the jury see you as Belanger's victim than a fighter. So if it happens – which is unlikely – just sit and take it, okay?"

"Okay," she smiled.

An hour and a half later she had concluded her testimony and was off the stand, undamaged and thankful to be sitting back at the counsel table. Belanger had drawn out a few concessions, but nothing that would impact the ultimate verdict. Her father's brother had a minor birth defect, a cleft lip, but there were no other birth anomalies on either side of her family, and the cleft lip was not in any way similar to any of Mark's defects. And yes, she occasionally would get migraine headaches, but had not taken anything for them during the first three months of pregnancy. Fred B attempted to shake Ingrid on the timing of intercourse in relation to using Clomid, but Ingrid would not back away from her prior testimony. She had recorded those dates on her calendar and those entries were made long before she knew anything about Mark's birth defects. Conception was only 4 to 5 days after last taking Clomid, and Ingrid made it clear that those dates were caste in concrete.

My first three witnesses had gone well and I was feeling quite comfortable with our case. But now I would start calling our expert witnesses; now would be the real test. Little did I know that disaster was right around the corner.

A Disastrous Day

First up was *Frank Briganti, Pharm. D.*, a Doctor of Pharmacy. I had first spoken to Dr. Briganti over the weekend, and something in my gut told me that this was not the right witness for the job. He appeared younger than his true age. He was a handsome man, with dark hair and features, but lacked the lines and grey that only comes with years and maturity. I wanted a college professor, but got what appeared to be a college freshman. I also sensed that his was not the right specialty to sell causation in a birth defect case; that I was doing nothing more than trying to force that notorious square peg through an unalterably round hole. Yet I was desperate to get an expert – any expert – to render an opinion that Clomid was the probable cause of Mark's birth defects, an opinion Briganti was prepared to give.

What tipped the scales in favor of calling him as a witness was the fact that Briganti had some experience with a number of animal studies involving assessment of side effects from pharmaceutical products. None of them, of course, had anything to do with teratology studies. But in preparation for testifying, Briganti had also read a number of papers on animal and human teratology and was quite convinced that he was qualified to give the opinion I was after.

With some trepidation, I called Briganti to the stand and began my examination. We first covered in detail his education, training and experience leading up to his Doctor of Pharmacy, spending a good part of the time on his animal studies. We then reviewed his post-degree training and experience, including seminars and symposiums touching on studies related to human reactions to drugs. By the time I finished, I felt we had laid sufficient foundation of expertise to overcome the inevitable objection from Belanger when I asked the big question. But first I needed to establish Briganti's comprehensive review of Merrell's animal teratology studies, a key piece of evidence upon which his opinion was based.

"Now, Dr. Briganti, did you have occasion to review a number of animal studies conducted by Richardson-Merrell during the 1960s?"

"Yes I did."

"May I approach the witness, your honor?"

"Yes you may," responded Fredricks.

I approached Briganti and handed him a full set of copies of the studies that had been previously marked as an exhibit. "Are these the studies that you reviewed?"

After a cursory examination he stated, "Yes they are. These appear to be identical to the set of animal studies given to me about a month ago."

"Can you please describe the nature of these studies?"

"Yes, these are *tetrology* studies, studies designed to determine whether Clomid could cause birth defects to the offspring of rats and rabbits exposed to that drug during pregnancy."

As soon as I heard the word "tetrology," my heart sank to the floor, which was exactly where I wanted to crawl. If I had been standing, rather than sitting at the counsel table, I am sure my knees would have buckled beneath me. My college freshman expert on *teratology* had just described a set of animal *tetrology* studies. For a moment I froze, not knowing what direction to go or how to mend the fence. Do I correct my witness on the stand or ignore the *faux pas*? Had he simply made a nervous error in pronunciation or was this his understanding of how to pronounce the word? If I corrected him on the stand or took a break, this would only magnify the problem. But if I asked another question requiring use of the word again, a second mispronunciation would establish his absolute lack of expertise on the subject and hand Belanger a truckload of ammunition for his cross-examination. I opted to ease away from the subject of teratology and wait for a break to talk privately with my witness. Instead I would cover some areas for which I knew he had some level of expertise. For a few uncomfortable moments I stared at my own set of animal studies trying to collect my thoughts.

"Tell me Doctor, do you have any criticisms about these studies?" This was an area we had previously discussed.

"Yes, I do."

"Would you please give us the benefit of your opinion, in that regard?"

I had expected Belanger to jump all over this with a number of objections, but he sat silently waiting for the next gift from the stand.

"I believe that Richardson-Merrell should have used monkeys in their studies. The results from the rat and rabbit studies are strongly suggestive of what the drug is capable of doing in humans, but simians are the closest species to man and the best evidence in animal studies to tell us what the drug is capable of doing to humans."

"Over the years since you began studying about adverse reactions to drugs, have you learned about the practice of pharmaceutical companies concerning their use of animal studies?"

"Yes I have. This has been a big part of my studies. I am frequently reading papers about animal studies in the industry."

"And are monkeys used for animal studies in the pharmaceutical industry?"

"Yes they are."

"Is this a standard of practice in the industry?"

"Yes it is."

This was as far as I wanted to go. I had a whole line of questions tying this opinion into the teratology studies, but I was terrified that the word "tetrology" would rear its ugly head again. There had been a set of guidelines, recommending use of primates in teratology studies, promulgated in 1966 by the FDA. I had discussed this with Briganti and it had been my intent to bring it out at this time. But not now. I had made my decision. As far as I was concerned, that door had been permanently closed. I would have to get at this testimony through another witness.

I concluded my direct examination right at the time that we broke for the day, finishing with a topic on which my witness had significant expertise and knowledge; the half-life of drugs. He explained that all drugs are studied for their half-life effect. Not only how long it takes them to be eliminated from the body, but also how long their therapeutic effect lasts after last exposure to the drug. This is critically important on the subject of overmedication, since added doses can build on top of earlier ones. He testified that based upon his review of the package insert, Clomid had a half-life of 5 days, and that every 5 days thereafter another half of a half was eliminated. He pointed out that as long as 6 weeks after last using the drug, some measurable level of Clomid and/or its metabolites would still have remained in Ingrid Breimhorst's body, well beyond a month after she conceived. With that we concluded, and I could not have been happier to get Dr. Briganti off the stand. But tomorrow was another day and I could sense Belanger salivating at the thought of his cross-examination in the morning.

As everyone was wrapping up for the day, Rose mentioned that she had a matter to deal with and would see me back at my office at 5:00 PM, as previously scheduled. She quickly disappeared, Ingrid rushed off to relieve the babysitter, and I cornered Briganti in the hallway for some additional prep time. I immediately brought up the subject of the mispronunciation. Briganti assured me that it was nothing more than a nervous oversight, but he didn't sound too convincing; certainly not enough to prompt me to reconsider my decision. After a final shot at damage control, anticipating with my witness where Belanger might attack, we concluded our discussion and agreed to meet in the coffee shop at 8:00 in the morning.

At exactly 5:25 PM, Rose entered my office and eased into one of my client chairs. At the moment I was stuffing a number of papers into my briefcase. I had promised Janet that I would be home by quarter of six. For the past two months I had been so consumed by the case that I had ignored family time. My twenty-three-month-old daughter, Jennifer, had seen little of her father and I assured my wife that I would spend some time with her this evening before she went down.

"Where you been?" I asked, glancing at my watch. "We were supposed to meet 25 minutes ago and I've got to get home ASAP."

"Sorry. I had to talk to someone. It took longer than expected."

It finally dawned on me that something was not quite right. Normally calm and in control, she appeared somewhat anxious. I examined her for a moment then asked, "Alright, Rose, what's going on?"

"Nothing, really."

"Don't give me 'nothing.' Who were you talking to?"

Rose looked away. "Well, if you must know, Belanger. I had a discussion with Fred after trial today."

"You what! You talked to Belanger without me? Why?"

She sighed, still looking away, and then stared at me apologetically. "Today was a disaster, Terry. I wanted to find out if the $75,000 was still available."

My jaw dropped open and I stared incredulously at her for a moment. "You talked to Fred Belanger today about possible settlement at $75,000?"

"Yes," she nodded. "I'm afraid I did."

"You, of course, cleared this with Ingrid?"

"No, I didn't."

Now I was beginning to boil. "Damn it, Rose! What the hell were you thinking?"

"I...I guess I wasn't. I just panicked."

"Damn it! I'm busting my ass on this case night and day, and you panic..."

"We got killed today..."

"Yeah, we got killed today, and maybe we will again tomorrow or the next day, but this is a thirty-day trial, and if you had some goddamn experience you would know that every trial has its ups and downs. Good days and bad days, they're all part it. But what I want to know is whose side you're working on? Either work with me or stay at home, but don't go behind my back!"

My last remark hit home and it was painful. Her eyes began to gloss over with tears and she again looked away. And suddenly I felt guilty. My own frustration with the day had prompted me to take it out on Rose. She was inexperienced and her panic should have been expected. I should have discussed the matter with her before my chat with Briganti. Talking to Belanger without my knowledge, however, was an issue for which criticism was justified. Still, my approach could have been more tactful.

"Look, I'm sorry, Rose," I said in a calmer tone. "I was probably too harsh, but we need to be working together here, and that means no communication with the other side without the agreement and knowledge of both of us….Okay?"

She forced a smile, nodded and got up from her chair. "It won't happen again, Terry, I promise."

"Good. Look, meet me at the coffee shop at eight tomorrow. I'm meeting Briganti there and we can talk some more."

"Fine," she said. "I'll see you at eight." Rose started for the door.

"Oh, and Rose." She stopped and turned.

"What was Belanger's response?"

She shook her head. "No luck. He called corporate office and came back with fifty thousand."

"Doesn't surprise me. Don't worry about it," I assured. "We'll have some good days ahead. I guarantee it."

Tuesday, March 19, 1974. Today was not one of those good days ahead, at least in the morning. Belanger could not wait to get to Briganti, and my only hope was that the jury would see the cross-examination as abusive. The skilled defense attorney stood in front of the jury box, eyeing his victim for a few uncomfortable moments.

"Good morning, Mr. Briganti." Belanger apparently was not going to afford Briganti his professional title. I would deal with it on redirect.

"Morning," responded the nervous witness.

"I was quite interested in these animal studies you looked at, these…*tetrology* studies," he added, looking at his notes.

"Teratology studies," Briganti corrected.

"Teratology?" Belanger looked at his notes again, adjusting his glasses. "I could have sworn you said, 'tetrology.' I mean…that's what I wrote down, anyway," he said, indicating his notes. "But I guess we can check with the court reporter, if necessary." Belanger had already arranged with the reporter to pre-mark the testimony.

"No, that won't be necessary. I did say 'tetrology.' But I misspoke. I intended to say, 'teratology.'"

"Then I take it, this is not a word you are accustomed to using?"

"I was nervous. I am not accustomed to testifying in court."

"I understand that, but my question was whether this word, 'teratology,' is a little foreign to you?"

"I have used it before."

"Really! You mean in preparation for your trial testimony?"

"Well, yes, but I have used it before as well; long before I thought of testifying in this trial. I have reviewed teratology studies."

"You mean studies given to you by Mr. Mix?"

"No, well before I ever met Mr. Mix."

"So Mr. Mix never gave you any teratology studies to read?"

"Well, his associate, Mrs. Chapman, did."

"And you didn't read them?"

"Yes, I read them…"

"Oh, I see, then this is where you got your education on teratology studies?"

"No, I have studied teratology before. It's part of my education as a practicing pharmacist."

Belanger was just warming up and enjoying every minute of the experience. He was like a cat playing with a trapped mouse. I wanted to throw some form of a lifeline to my witness, but was completely helpless and regretting that I had not gone with my initial gut feeling about whether to call Briganti to testify.

"Well then, let me see. Are you a teratologist?"

"No, I'm not."

"A specialist in obstetrics and gynecology?"

"No."

"A neonatologist?"

"No."

"A pediatrician?"

"No."

"A pathologist?"

"No."

"In fact, you're not even a physician, are you?"

"No, I'm a Doctor of Pharmacy."

"You fill prescriptions?"

"My responsibilities go beyond filling prescriptions."

"Is that right. Well, then have you ever participated in any form of a teratology study, animals or humans, anything that dealt with teratology?"

Briganti hesitated, no doubt trying to recall something that might be remotely related to the subject. "No, I haven't," he finally responded.

"Have you written any papers, review articles, anything, on the subject of teratology?"

"No, I haven't."

Nothing improved over the remainder of the morning, as Fred B meticulously dissected and tore apart each topic I had covered with the witness. Other than thalidomide, Briganti could not name another drug which had been used in teratology studies with primates. "Not one drug out of the thousands on the market?" Belanger had asked, almost rhetorically. Additionally, a number of the articles he had read on teratology were written by no less than Dr. James G. Wilson, Merrell's own teratology expert. Did Briganti know that Dr. Wilson had reviewed the Clomid records on two occasions and concluded that it did not cause birth defects? No, he hadn't. Belanger had even dealt with the half-life issue, though not as effectively. What the studies had measured was the C_{14} marker, not the actual drug or its metabolites. It thus could not be stated with absolute certainty that the drug was still around after 6 weeks. Briganti, with little fight left by this time, countered that this was how drugs were measured, and generally considered in the pharmaceutical industry as presumptive evidence of measuring the actual drug. Finally, Belanger concluded his cross-examination and sat down.

Not wanting Briganti on the stand any longer than necessary, my redirect was brief and of little value. After being excused, our eyes briefly met as Briganti passed the counsel table. I wanted to apologize to him at that moment, but of course could say nothing. The decision for calling Briganti to testify was mine and mine alone, and however ineffective or damaging his testimony, the fault was likewise mine and not that of the Doctor of Pharmacy. Due to my relative inexperience, I had made a poor decision. But I was learning. As the trial progressed, my skills and professional judgment would hopefully improve.

The remainder of the day went better than expected, although at the time I was uncertain whether it just seemed so because of the disastrous morning. My next witness was *Ronald Curfman*, who had shot the film of Mark, and testified about the authenticity of the scenes of Mark Breimhorst experiencing an average day in his life. To sit and watch the film was quite refreshing, and although it had not been part of any plan or strategy, was an effective follow-up to Briganti's testimony. The jury could not help but be reminded about the personal tragedy of the case.

In the afternoon I called my specialist in obstetrics and gynecology, a *James Davis, M.D.* Dr. Davis testified about spontaneous abortions. The generally accepted rate in the general population, depending upon the study, ranged between 10% and 15% of confirmed pregnancies. The Clomid pre-market studies reported an incidence of 20%, or a rate of up to 100% higher than that seen generally. Additionally, a high percentage of the products of spontaneous abortions are abnormal, especially those occurring in the first trimester. He had seen some studies reporting as high as 97% congenital anomalies in first trimester spontaneous abortions. Although he was not a fertility specialist, based upon his personal experience over the years, infertility patients had no higher incidence of spontaneous abortions than seen in the general population.

Davis also concluded from his review of the medical records and Ingrid's testimony that the date of conception was September 20, 1969, and that he saw no evidence of exposure to any environmental agent during pregnancy that would have caused the birth defects. I avoided asking Dr. Davis the all-important question: Was Clomid the probable cause of Mark's birth defects? He had relied upon the representations in the package insert and would occasionally prescribe Clomid himself. Belanger drew little blood on cross-examination, just before ending for the day.

Wednesday, March 20, 1974. This was a day primarily used to further build my case on damages. In the morning I called *Irla Zimmerman, Ph.D.*, a clinical psychologist. She had given Mark a full array of tests, designed specifically for young children. Her conclusions were that Mark had an average IQ and mentally was progressing normally for a child 3 years and 9 months of age. However, he scored below average for memory and attention span. Her prognosis was that because of these difficulties and his handicaps, Mark would gradually experience more and more learning problems as he got older. He would also be exposed to prejudicial treatment from others and frustration over his disabilities.

Sam Bumpas, a specialist in vocational rehabilitation, was called in the afternoon. He was of the opinion the because of his handicaps, Mark would essentially be unemployable. In fact, he probably would not qualify for most programs designed for training the disabled. Mark's facial palsy and absence of hands would essentially eliminate any job dealing with the public. There would also be employer prejudice because most people with such handicaps present a safety risk, lack mobility and are prone to absenteeism.

Belanger made a half-hearted stab at cross-examination of each witness, but wisely asked few challenging questions, not wanting to lose credibility over a plaintiff that had obvious major disabilities.

Thursday, March 21, 1974. Another good day, as I continued putting our case together, piece by piece. My next witness was *Barbara Crandall, M.D.*, a geneticist. She would be important in establishing that Mark's congenital anomalies were not hereditary; not some familial abnormality passed down to him from a blood relative through genetics. Dr. Crandall testified about studies that had been performed on samples of Mark's blood, all of which established that he had normal chromosomes. That based upon her examination of Mark, the family history provided by the parents and the nature of the birth defects, she was of the opinion that his anomalies were not hereditary. She added that the cleft lip of Ingrid's uncle was not in any way tied to Mark's birth defects. A cleft lip would hereditarily be expressed down the line as another cleft lip, and she saw no facial abnormalities on Mark that were in any way related. Additionally, Moebius syndrome, as Mark's anomalies are sometimes described, is generally not considered to be hereditary. Belanger drew out a few concessions, but otherwise did little to shake Dr. Crandall's testimony.

Margaret Jones, M.D., a specialist in pediatric medicine and one of Mark's treating doctors, was my next witness. She generally went through each of Mark's examinations over the years and described in detail each of his congenital malformations. I also used Dr. Jones to introduce all of Mark's medical expenses and establish the reasonableness of the charges. She then estimated his future medical costs. I concluded the day with *Robert Schultz, Ph.D.*, a forensic economist, who calculated the present value[22] of the future medical expenses and Mark's future loss of earning capacity. Fred B did little to challenge either witness.

Friday, March 22, 1974. Myron Koch, M.D., an orthopedic surgeon, was next in line and again used to establish my case on damages. He gave a specific assessment of Mark's orthopedic problems, his prognosis, the nature of the future treatment needed for the club foot (metatarsus varus), and estimated the future costs for replacement of Mark's prostheses every two to three years. Cross-examination again had little impact on the opinions offered by the orthopedist.

My Star Witness

By late morning it was time to call my man of the hour, week and month, *Eugene Perrin, M.D.* I had spent time with Dr. Perrin the night before. He not only looked like the professor I had been after a few days earlier, he in fact *was* a professor – complete with a closely trimmed grey beard, a ready smile and warm personality. It was also immediately evident that he came prepared to deal with the subject of Clomid and its potential teratologic risk. Although he would not give me more than *reasonable medical possibility*, the conclusions he held on the subject were well-thought-out and supported by strong and persuasive reasons. His opinion might not be sufficient to sell my case on causation, but I had little doubt that the jury would be quite impressed with Gene Perrin as a man and a professional.

At the outset, I spent a substantial amount of time on Perrin's qualifications in the field of teratology. His background was in pediatric pathology, and as part of this specialty he had been studying the causes of birth defects since 1955. He had published numerous papers in the field of teratology and had even taught on the subject. His experience with animal studies was also extensive. He had participated in many experiments assessing the reactions of various species of animals to drugs, including a number of teratology studies. His degrees included a Ph.D. in zoology. He had also acted as a consultant to pharmaceutical companies in the past.

Dr. Perrin first attacked the animal teratology studies. Merrell should have used at least 3 species of animals, including primates; there should have been microscopic studies of the abnormal tissue from the congenital anomalies; the studies should have been ongoing, extending well beyond initial marketing, implementing newer teratology techniques; animals with ovulatory dysfunction should have been used; and given the long half-life of the drug, Clomid also should have been administered during the period prior to the beginning of organogenesis.

He next challenged the pre-market clinical studies. Basal body temperature (BBT) charts for all patients should have been maintained, as well as complete charting of maternal illnesses and exposure to radiation or trauma of any kind. Drugs during pregnancy should have been excluded as part of the study, but if absolutely needed should have likewise been accurately charted. All abortuses should have been examined microscopically and assessed for chromosomal abnormalities. Autopsies for all stillbirths and neonatal deaths should have been routinely performed. His principal criticism, however, was the failure to include a control group in the study. Along with the patients exposed to Clomid, a second unexposed group with similar histories should have been part of the clinical investigations. Then, and only then, could a meaningful comparison be made on the incidence of birth defects, and a conclusion drawn on whether or not there was a true increased rate of malformations with Clomid use.

During the remainder of the day I reviewed with Perrin the different stages of development of the human conceptus, from the zygote (fertilized ovum or egg), to implantation on the uterine wall (day 6 post-conception), to the formation of the neural groove (days 18 through 22), to the formation of the arm and leg buds (days 26 and 27), to the formation of the hand plates (days 32 and 33) and foot plates (day 37), and to the formation of the finger rays (days 40 and 41) and toe rays (day 45). Perrin explained that by completion of the eighth week (56 days), all organs have taken shape and are in place, and the embryo officially becomes a fetus. He then zeroed in on a key, if not critical, point related to when Mark could have been exposed to a teratogenic insult. The period of highest susceptibility to teratogenesis likely occurs as early as days 11 and 12 in humans, and *a teratogenic injury can occur to a specific organ even before it begins to form.*

Thus, embryonic damage well before day 32 could have caused Mark's hands not to form. This gave the jury something to think about over the weekend, and it was time to break for the day. The big question on the agenda for Monday morning: Would Fredricks allow the jury to consider Perrin's opinion of reasonable medical possibility? Without it, I would lack the critical link between Ingrid's use of Clomid and Mark's birth defects, and my case would collapse.

Monday, March 25, 1974. Over the weekend I had handwritten my hypothetical question, to be posed to Perrin – it covered 3 ½ pages. As soon as the jury had gathered in the box and everyone else had gotten seated, Judge Fredricks took the bench and directed me to call Perrin back to the witness stand. Gene promptly returned to his seat and waited for my first question. I asked him "to assume the following," and then proceeded to read verbatim my entire hypothetical set of facts. Every fact that could possibly be relevant to the question of causation was included; the histories of both parents, as reflected in the medical charts and deposition transcripts, Heinz' low sperm count, an uncle's cleft lip, the dates of use of both prescriptions of Clomid, the dates of Ingrid's last 9 menstrual periods prior to conception, the date of conception, the lack of exposure to any pharmaceutical products, radiation, maternal illnesses, extremes of temperature, or physical trauma during the entire embryonic period, the medical chart on the pregnancy and delivery, a detailed description of Mark's congenital anomalies, and finally his medical history from the date of his birth on June 19, 1970, to his most recent medical exam. I then ended my recital, drew a breath, and asked,

"Now Dr. Perrin, based upon your education, training and experience, and all of the materials you have reviewed, do you have any opinion, that you can you state with reasonable medical possibility, of the cause of the aforementioned birth defects?"

Belanger immediately jumped to his feet and I held my breath. "your honor," he began, "I do have a number of objections to this question. Should we approach the bench?"

"You might be a little premature, Mr. Belanger," Fredricks responded. "Why don't we first hear his answer."

"Yes, I do," said Perrin.

"And what is that opinion?" was my follow-up question.

"Okay, now I can hear your objections. But first let's excuse the jury for 15 minutes, and then we can take this up in chambers."

The jury retired to the jury room and the four lawyers joined the judge in his chambers with the court reporter. After we had all gotten settled, Fredricks invited Fred B to voice all of his objections.

"Well, your honor," he began, "first, the question is an incomplete hypothetical and assumes facts not in evidence. Second, it lacks foundation. And third, and most importantly, it is absolutely irrelevant and should be excluded under Evidence Code 352. It is totally misleading and confusing to the jury. The test, as your honor well knows, is reasonable medical certainty. I mean, anything is possible."

Fredricks looked at Belanger for a quiet moment, then at me, and again at Fred B and announced, "I'm going to overrule your objections on incomplete hypothetical, assuming facts not in evidence and lack of foundation. I believe Mr. Mix has met the minimum requirements needed to pose the question." He now was back at me. "However, I would like to hear from you, Mr. Mix, about his last objection. Mr. Belanger may have a point. I'm willing to consider what you have to say, but don't we need more than 'possibility'?"

I suddenly had the same sick feeling when I heard Briganti utter "tetrology." "First let me correct Mr. Belanger. The test is not 'reasonable medical *certainty*,' it is 'reasonable medical *probability*.' The plaintiff is not required to prove any fact with certainty. And I would refer your honor to BAJI,[23] if there is any question about the measure of our burden of proof."

"I don't disagree with that, Mr. Mix, but how do you prove your case with 'possibility'?"

"The phrase used, your honor, was 'reasonable medical possibility,' not simply 'possibility.' I would agree that the plaintiff must prove that Clomid was the probable cause of Mark Breimhorst's birth defects. However, that is the burden that we must meet based upon all of the evidence introduced in the trial, not just from expert testimony. A party is entitled to have the jury consider an expert opinion expressed in terms of reasonable medical possibility when considering whether the defendant's conduct was the probable cause of plaintiff's injury…and I have a case that says I'm right."

"Very well," said Fredricks. "Give me your citation and I'll read the case. Mr. Belanger, I'll read any cases you have as well. Give me a few minutes in chambers and you'll have my ruling."

I gave Fredricks the Wardrop case citation. Belanger, always prepared, promptly threw out a couple cases for the judge to read as well. We all then returned to the courtroom…and waited. A half hour later, Elma's phone buzzed from chambers. She listened for a moment, and then asked the bailiff to bring in the jury. I nodded to Gene Perrin and he took his seat on the witness stand. As the jury marched in and seated itself, I stared up at the empty bench with an anxiety unmatched at any other time during the trial. It struck me that the trial might effectively end this very day. We still had two more witnesses to go, but I had yet to talk to either of them and didn't know how much help they would be. Finally, Fredricks entered and took the bench. The tension in the air could have been sliced with a knife. Fredricks first stared directly at me and I held my breath. He then made his announcement to the entire courtroom.

"Objection overruled."

I had been given a reprieve and could breathe again. Fredricks asked the court reporter to read the question to the witness and we were again off and running.

Per my prior direction, Perrin looked directly at the jury. "In my opinion, there is a reasonable medical possibility that all of Mark Breimhorst's congenital malformations are due to his mother's use of Clomid."

"Doctor, could you give us the basis for that opinion?"

"Yes, I can." Perrin then proceeded with his assigned task of educating. He was now the professor and the jurors his students. And he had the full attention of every juror, to the last person including the remaining alternate.

He first determined whether there was any other explanation to account for the birth defects. From his review of all the medical records and deposition transcripts of Mr. and Mrs. Breimhorst, and the nature of the syndrome of defects, he was firmly convinced that heredity was not a factor and that it was more likely that the cause was some environmental factor, either a single teratogen or a combination of them. By "environmental" he meant that it was some event occurring external to the developing embryo. Something happened to damage the embryo prior to November 13, 1969. It could have been some form of maternal illness, such as a virus, or a maternal vitamin deficiency or other nutritional deprivation, or it could have been exposure to radiation, extremes of temperature, hypoxia (reduced oxygen), or a pharmaceutical product or other chemical, all of which have been shown to have a teratogenic effect in animal studies and, to some extent in humans. From his review of all the records, there was no evidence to suggest that any of these other potential causes were responsible, although he cautioned that Mrs. Breimhorst could have been exposed to such a teratogen, including one that we might not yet know about, that was not documented or recalled. In any event, aside from the issue of Clomid, there was nothing else that could be pointed to as the likely cause of the congenital malformations.

He then turned his attention to Clomid. In Dr. Perrin's opinion, there was a reasonable medical possibility that clomiphene citrate was a human teratogen. He based this opinion principally on three factors.

First was the spontaneous abortion rate during the clinical investigations. An abortion rate of 20% was in the range of up to 100% higher than seen in the general population for confirmed pregnancies. Most spontaneous abortions involve abnormalities of the developing embryo or fetus, including a large percentage with abnormal chromosomes. Thus, a significant percentage of the total number of spontaneous abortions from the clinical investigations may have resulted because of a teratogenic effect from Clomid. Yes, there have been papers that suggest that infertility patients might have a higher rate of abortions, but whether that was the case with the clomiphene studies could only be determined by looking at the specific reason for infertility for each patient in the study. A woman with a prior history of one or more spontaneous abortions would be expected to have a higher abortion rate. However, a woman that was having a problem ovulating because she had previously used birth control pills, as with Mrs. Breimhorst, would not be expected to have a higher rate than a normally fertile woman. But apparently this was never studied by Merrell. Also remember that many of the studies on the abortion rate in the general population include infertility patients in the group studied; they are part of the cross-section of the general population.

The second factor related to the animal teratology studies. The studies from Merrell clearly established that the drug was teratogenic in the rat and the rabbit when administered during the period of organogenesis. The rats exhibited a number of different anomalies, although the descriptions lacked desired specificity. The reports referred to elongated snouts, hydrocephalus, "head malformations" and "abnormal" hind limbs. In the rabbit studies there was a "turning under" of the hind paws. Other than the turning under of the paws, none of the malformations were similar to those of Mark Breimhorst. However, this did not bother him since it is frequently seen that the anomalies in animal studies are different than those seen with the same teratogen in humans. Further, the timing of exposure during organogenesis can dictate what organs will be targeted by the teratogen, and none of Merrell's teratology studies involved exposure prior to the period of organogenesis. No, he could not directly extrapolate animal teratology studies to humans; a drug that is teratogenic in rats and rabbits is not necessarily teratogenic in humans. There are many animal teratogens that apparently do not cause birth defects in humans. However, he has not seen the reverse. Based upon his research and review of the literature, every known human teratogen can also produce malformations in animals.

Finally, he considered the question of timing of exposure. Due to the long half-life of clomiphene citrate, the drug would have been in the maternal and embryonic circulation well into organogenesis. In other words, Clomid would have had the *opportunity* to inhibit growth of the hands and produce the other abnormalities. When he considered all of these factors, he was left with the opinion that there was a reasonable medical possibility that Mark Breimhorst's birth defects were caused by Clomid.

It was now time to turn Gene Perrin over to Belanger and hope for the best.

"Let me see if I understand," started Fred B. "You said 'reasonable medical *possibility*'?"

"That is correct."

"Not 'probability' or 'certainty'?"

"No."

"Then would you not agree that it is *probable* that Clomid was *not* the cause of these birth defects?"

"No, I would not agree with that either. There is too much uncertainty about the data to state it as probable one way or the other."

Belanger had not expected this answer. The witness had seemingly turned "possible" into 50/50. "Well...let's move to another subject. You testified about relying upon the animal teratology studies. Isn't it true that those animals received four times the human dose and higher?"

"Yes, that's true, but it's been shown that humans are a lot more sensitive to human teratogens than animals."

Two important questions and Belanger could not have been pleased with either answer. It appeared that Perrin was well-equipped to handle himself on the witness stand. Belanger posed some additional questions related to the animal studies, with little success, then moved over to the clinical investigations.

"Doctor, you would agree, would you not, that one of the criteria for assessing whether or not a drug is a human teratogen is whether a pattern of birth defects is seen?"

"It certainly was with thalidomide and several other drugs, but it is not universal. There are some drugs that can cause a variety of malformations."

"But it is one of the criteria generally used by teratologists?"

"Yes, it is."

"And isn't it true that there was no pattern of birth defects in the clinical investigations?"

"I don't know that I could agree with that."

"Now, doctor, you didn't see an increased frequency of any one of the reported malformations, did you?"

"Again, I don't agree with you. There were five reported cases of Down syndrome in the clinical studies out of 1,886 delivered pregnancies. This equates to one out of every 377 births, compared to an average of about one in a thousand births in the general population. This seems extraordinarily high. But the incidence of Down syndrome increases with advancing maternal age, and I don't know the average age of the Clomid population."

I was now starting to enjoy myself and leaned back in my chair for the first time. Perrin had not shared this observation with me before. This had also caught Fred B by surprise, but he was quick to recover.

"Well, Down syndrome is not a malformation,[24] is it?"

"Many have congenital heart defects, but I would agree with you. They are not malformed. They are, however, birth defects."

"And drugs have not been implicated with causing Down syndrome, have they?"

"Not specifically, to my knowledge, but some drugs are teratogenic and mutagenic as well. Down syndrome is due to an abnormal chromosome, usually trisomy 21. It is possible that a drug could produce three of the number 21 chromosomes prior to fertilization of the egg or ovum."

This is the way it went for the remainder of the morning. Belanger would throw a question at Perrin and the doctor would hit the lawyer with something else unexpected. Jab, parry and counterpunch. By the lunch break Belanger had finished with the witness and was no doubt experiencing the same feeling I had when Briganti stepped off the witness stand.

As Rose and I and the doctor were exiting the courtroom, saying our goodbyes, Perrin handed me a piece of paper. On it were a couple of citations. With a wink of an eye, he said, "You may want to read these before Jim Wilson gets on the stand. Give him my regards, will you," he smiled. With that, Gene was on his way down the hall and off to Detroit. I looked again at the citation. He had written, "Teratology – Principles and Techniques. Edited by James G. Wilson and Josef Warkany. University of Chicago Press (1965). Embryological Considerations in Teratology by James G. Wilson (pp.251-260)." He further added, "See also his 1973 textbook." I had been handed one last gift from my star witness.

Lunch was spent with Rose and my next witness, *Clinton Thienes, M.D.*, a pharmacologist. He had been busy and unavailable over the weekend, and Monday morning was out because of my scheduled meeting with Perrin. Rose had told me earlier in the day that Phil had spent some time talking to Thienes over the phone and felt that he would be quite valuable to our case. I had assumed that he would be used on the subject of half-life and the standards of care for pharmaceutical companies. He could also help reconcile FDA approval of an arguably unsafe drug. I was in for a pleasant surprise. Thienes had some background in teratology – and even knew how to pronounce it. He was also going to give me reasonable medical *probability* on causation!

Most of the afternoon was spent eliciting testimony from Thienes on his extensive education, training and experience in the related fields of pharmacology and toxicology, emphasizing anything remotely related to teratology. He had published between 80 and 100 articles in scientific and medical journals related to the effects of drugs on the human body. Although he was not a teratologist, teratology was a branch of toxicology and a part of his studies. No, he had not conducted animal teratology studies, or participated in epidemiology studies designed to assess the teratological risk of drugs, but he had done a significant amount of reading on the subject as part of his education and training. I then had him identify in detail all of the materials he had reviewed for the case. We then broke for the day and everyone began evacuating the courtroom. As Rose and I were loading up our brief cases, I leaned over to her and whispered, "In case you didn't notice. This was one of those good days ahead."

Rose responded with an enthusiastic smile. "You were right, Terry. You were absolutely right."

Tuesday, March 26, 1974. As with Perrin, I first read my extensive hypothetical and then posed the question, but this time couched in terms of reasonable medical *probability*. Thienes' response, of course, was "yes," and we again received Belanger's barrage of objections. Fredricks promptly overruled and the pharmacologist proceeded to render his opinion and supporting reasons, pretty much following those outlined by Perrin. He also criticized the animal and clinical studies, and spent some time on the half-life of the drug. In total, Ingrid had consumed 250 mg. of clomiphene citrate, of which, based upon his calculations, approximately 100 mg. still remained in her circulation at the time of conception, and at least 25 mg. during the sensitive period of early organogenesis. At this point we introduced into evidence a handwritten graph, prepared by the witness, detailing the dropping concentration of the drug in relation to the days of gestation. The drug concentration line extended beyond day 32, when the embryonic hands would have otherwise begun to develop.

On cross-examination, Belanger was effectively able to extract a number of concessions from Thienes. Yes, he lacked "hands on" experience in teratology. It was all in the form of literary research; reading various scientific publications. Yes, he would agree that you cannot directly extrapolate the animal teratology studies to humans. Different species of animals, in particular rodents, frequently react differently to drugs than do humans. Yes, he was aware that Clomid had an antifertility effect on rats and was incapable of making them ovulate. He agreed that at some point the dissipating drug would lack any potency. No, he did not know what concentration of the drug would be required to produce the birth defects. Fred B continued to challenge the witness through the remainder of the morning. Yet, notwithstanding Thienes' weakened conclusions, for some reason I was not bothered. It was as if Thienes' reasonable medical probability was somehow fused with the stellar testimony given by Perrin the day before. Thienes would likely get me by a nonsuit and Perrin would, hopefully, have sold our case to the jury.

The noon recess was spent with our next and final witness, *William Agnew, Ph.D.*, another teratologist. Since he was not a medical doctor, I decided to stay away from soliciting an opinion on whether Mark's congenital anomalies were caused by Clomid. My experience with Briganti had made me gun shy, even though Agnew had true expertise in this area of study. I was also on the home stretch and was eager to conclude our case. He would be principally used to explain why Merrell's animal teratology studies failed to meet industry standards.

Dr. Agnew received his Ph.D. in physiology, the biological study of the functions of living organisms and their parts. A substantial amount of his education and experience related to conducting animal studies, including a number in the field of teratology. In the past, he had worked as a laboratory technician for a pharmaceutical company. He had also written protocols for teratology studies with animals and had published many articles related to his teratological research.

Agnew was quite critical of Merrell's animal studies. Without question, nonhuman primates should have been used. Not only were they recommended by the

FDA, the World Health Organization (WHO) in 1966 likewise published its standards including recommended use of monkeys. There is a strong correlation between the teratological effects of drugs on monkeys and what can happen to humans. This had been found with radiation, steroids and thalidomide. In fact, the phocomelia (limb reduction) defects seen in humans from thalidomide have also been reproduced in monkeys. Further, because of the carryover effect of Clomid, the animal studies should have also been designed to administer the drug to the rats and rabbits prior to the period of organogenesis.

To test any potential teratological effect, the drug should be administered in increasing doses to different animals during the same period of gestation. The classical pattern of teratogenicity is when one sees an increasing number of animals with congenital malformations following increasingly higher doses of the studied drug. This was never done with Clomid during pre-organogenesis. I concluded my direct examination right at the evening break.

Wednesday, March 27, 1974. Belanger's principal attack on Agnew was to cross-examine him on a Clomid study published by Valerio and Courtney in 1968. Monkeys had been used in the study and the drug administered to some of the monkeys during pregnancy. Not one of the pregnant monkeys had delivered a malformed fetus. Agnew was familiar with the study and had a number of criticisms. First and foremost, it was never intended to be a teratology study. The authors did not follow the WHO guidelines, failed to elevate the dosage and the study involved only a small number of animals. None of the monkeys had any form of ovulatory dysfunction and none of the Clomid was given, as with the Merrell studies, prior to organogenesis. Belanger concluded his cross-examination on something sweet. He got Agnew to acknowledge that even sugar had produced congenital malformations in animals. The teratologist was also familiar with this study. Massive doses of sugar had been used and it was questionable whether it was the sugar that produced the malformations or the maternal reaction to it. Finally, Fred B was finished and the witness excused.

Over the remainder of the morning, I read selected portions of the two depositions of Hoekenga and Holtkamp, introduced a number of documents previously marked for evidence, and then concluded with a few "cleanup" questions with Ingrid. Shortly before noon, I announced that plaintiffs rested and waited for the inevitable motion for nonsuit. Not to disappoint, Belanger rose to his feet and advised the court that he had a couple of motions to make. Fredricks excused the jury until 2:00 PM and asked the four of us to return a half hour earlier, at which time he would hear the motions.

Two hours later we were back in the courtroom. Belanger initially moved to exclude all of the testimony given by Briganti, Perrin, Thienes and Agnew, arguing that it was all based upon speculation. As expected, this motion was quickly denied. Richardson-Merrell's motion for nonsuit took substantially more time. Belanger and his staff were well prepared for the motion and methodically hammered the weakness in plaintiffs' case on causation. In many ways, Merrell had been counting on this motion since the beginning of the trial. As Belanger argued, Fredicks sat and listened and I sat and took notes. My hope was that Fredicks would listen to the defense and then deny the motion without needing to hear a word from Terry Mix. But no such luck. When the defense attorney sat down, the judge turned to me and asked for a reply. My argument was brief and to the point. This was a jury trial and the jury had sufficient evidence from which to render a verdict. Under the Wardrup decision, Dr. Perrin's opinion alone was sufficient to support a plaintiff's verdict. But we also had the benefit of the conclusion from Dr. Thienes. In summary, the evidence was there and the jury had the right to decide the case. I then sat down.

Fredricks considered my words for a brief moment, and I found myself again holding my breath. To my relief his next words were, "I'm going to overrule the motion. I believe plaintiffs have introduced sufficient evidence to submit their case to the jury. So we'll take a ten minute break and then hear from defendant's first witness."

In a moment the judge was gone from the bench and I felt a sudden rush of elation. Somehow we had survived. We now knew that a jury would decide the case. The burden of preparing our witnesses each day, praying for their survival on the witness stand, and worrying about filling the courtroom with testimony every day, had finally been lifted from our shoulders and shifted to the defendant. Now all I had to do was sharpen my skills at cross-examination and go on the attack.

* * * * *

CHAPTER 3

Clomid on Trial:

The Defendant's Case

Fred Belanger seemed organized and structured to a fault, at least to my way of thinking. His first witness for the afternoon was *Frank Palopoli*, the research chemist at Merrell who had discovered clomiphene citrate. This would not have been a problem if the witness had been interesting or entertaining in his presentation. But this was not the case. For a good part of the afternoon, Palopoli delivered a lecture to all present from Chemistry 101. Everything was included in his testimony, from a recitation of the clomiphene family of drugs to actually writing out the formula for Clomid on an exhibit. For good measure he even drew it, with all of the various connected hexagons and their chemical names. By the time Belanger had concluded his questioning, it was my assumption that everyone on the jury panel had either been put to sleep or bored to tears – certainly I was.

So I decided to play it up.

"Did you have any questions, Mr. Mix?" I initially ignored Fredricks' inquiry, while doodling on my note pad. I wanted to draw some attention from the jurors – at least from those who were still awake.

"Mr. Mix?"

I looked up with some surprise. "Yes, your honor."

"Did you have any questions? Mr. Belanger has finished his examination."

"Oh! You mean about that formula thing?" I asked, pointing at the exhibit.

"Only if you feel so inclined," smiled Fredricks.

"Nah. I wouldn't know what to ask. I did horrible in chemistry."

With that I concluded my cross-examination of Mr. Palopoli, all to the amusement of the jury. There was not one item of his testimony that was in any way damaging, and questioning would have served no purpose other than to burden the jury with more boredom. I instead tried to entertain. The next witness, however, would earn a lot more of my attention.

James W. Newberne was another employee from Richardson-Merrell. He had headed its Toxicology and Pathology Department from 1962 through 1970. He was an educated and trained veterinarian with a specialty in veterinary pathology. Newberne recited his educational and training background, his employment history to his current position at Merrell, and a description of the nature of his work. He had conducted hundreds of animal studies over his career, including teratology studies, and had used mice, rats, rabbits, cats, dogs, cows and non-human primates in his work. He was a member of the Teratology Society and had attended numerous seminars on the subject throughout the world. By the evening break, Belanger had concluded qualifying him as an expert in the field of animal teratology.

Thursday, March 28, 1974. Fred B now began to get into the meat of his witness' testimony. Newberne was acquainted with the FDA Guidelines on teratology and had first seen them in January or February 1966. The FDA had indeed suggested use of monkeys in teratology studies in these guidelines. He agreed that primates would be preferable to rodents. Monkeys have spontaneous abortions similar to humans, whereas mice, rats and rabbits resorb their embryos when they are exposed to lethal doses of a drug. Their other bodily functions also more closely approximate those of man. Non-human primates, however, had not been available in sufficient numbers throughout the 1960s and early 1970s. If primates had been available to conduct meaningful teratology studies, Merrell would have used them. He also reminded that the FDA Guidelines were no more than suggestions, not mandates. Besides, the Valerio and Courtney study had established that Clomid was not teratogenic in monkeys.

Belanger then turned to the in-house teratology studies conducted by the Endocrinology Department. Each study was detailed, including a description of the animals and numbers used, the routs of administration (oral or subcutaneous), the level of doses administered, the day or days of exposure during gestation, and finally a description of the anomalies. Newberne was quick to point out that all of the teratological doses were several times the human dose, and in fact were up to hundreds of times higher than the amount used by Ingrid Breimhorst. And none of the animals had limb reduction birth defects.

He had later re-evaluated the earlier studies conducted in 1962 by the Endocrinology Department. It was Newberne's opinion that the studies did not

86

demonstrate a teratogenic effect on either the pregnant rats or rabbits. Likewise, when his department performed teratology studies on rabbits during 1966 (T-66-31), administering the drug orally, they concluded that it had not caused any malformations. His final opinion was that Merrell's teratology studies, at best, only presented "a clue" of what might happen in man. Only human epidemiology studies could answer that question. Direct examination had covered the entire morning and into the early afternoon.

I was eager to commence my cross-examination. It is what I enjoyed most about trial work. Whereas I would sit during direct examination of my own witnesses, I would usually stand during cross. Other than when I was drawing out foundational information or essential facts held by a hostile witness, I was pretty much a "free swinger." Today would not be any different. But I had not taken Newberne's deposition and did not know how he would respond to certain questions. My examination would have to be brief and concise, allowing the witness little room to give explanations to his answers.

"Dr. Newberne, I just wanted to clarify a point. Merrell never conducted Clomid teratology studies with primates prior to marketing the drug in May 1967?

"No, they just weren't available."

"I understand. But not one study, correct?"

"Correct."

"Nor prior to September 1969 when Ingrid Breimhorst used Clomid to conceive Mark?"

"No."

"Nor even up to the present date, March 28, 1974?"

"No, we haven't."

"So I guess they're still not available, huh?"

"Well…no, they're not."

"But Valerio and Courtney were able to find monkeys for their studies, even before 1968?"

"They did not use a large number of monkeys."

"So their study was deficient; it lacked an adequate number of monkeys?"

"I didn't say that."

"So then they *did* find an adequate number of monkeys where Merrell failed?"

"I didn't say that either."

I had the witness boxed, which I was able to do because his testimony was faulty on two points. I now needed to drive them home. "Doctor, isn't it true that when one is conducting an animal study during which higher and higher levels of the drug are administered, one would need more animals than when one is only administering one dosage level?"

"Yes, I would agree to that."

"And Valerio and Courtney used only one dosage level, correct?"

"That is true."

"Because this was not a teratology study, was it?"

"Well, some of the drug was administered during pregnancy, so an assessment of possible teratogenicity could be made."

"Doctor, was this study not entitled, 'Treatment of Infertility in Macaca Mulatta[25] with Clomiphene'[26]?" I asked, reading from a copy.

"Yes, it was."

"So this was an *infertility* study?"

"Yes, it was designed as an infertility study, but one could assess the teratological risk as well."

"Really! Did not the FDA Guidelines – that you read back in 1966 – prescribe that you should administer increasing dosages to determine whether there was a dose relationship to an increased number of malformations?"

"Yes, they did."

"And during your many studies around the world, did you also come across certain teratology standards set out by the World Health Organization in November 1966?"

"Yes, I did."

"And didn't those standards also advocate the same practice?"

"Yes, they did."

"In fact, didn't the Endocrinology Department follow this practice back in 1962?"

"Yes, it did."

"And even *you* followed this practice in 1966 with rabbits?"

"Yes."

Newberne's answers had become almost robotic, as he began to appreciate where I was going. "But the Valerio and Courtney infertility study did *not* follow this practice.?"

"No, it didn't."

"Because it was not designed as a teratology study?"

"No, it wasn't."

I had neutralized the importance of Valerio, but had one more point to make on the subject of monkeys. This would also hit close to home, as it involved one of the company's consultants and a key witness in the trial. "You are, of course, familiar with the work of James G. Wilson?"

"Of course. He is one of the top teratologists in the world."

"Then you were aware, were you not, that in 1966, Dr. Wilson conducted teratology studies using thalidomide on monkeys?"

I knew what his answer had to be, even if he hadn't read the paper. It was an important and timely work in his field, so he couldn't deny he had read it. Still, he hesitated because he didn't know how he wanted to respond to the question. I held up a copy of the study and asked, "Have you read a paper by Wilson and Gavan published in 1967, entitled 'Congenital Malformations in Nonhuman Primates: Spontaneous and Experimentally Induced'[27]?"

"Yes, I'm familiar with that paper," he finally responded. Merrell had even supplied the thalidomide for the study, a fact I was not allowed to reveal.

"So prior to May 1967, Dr. Wilson was able to find a sufficient number of monkeys to conduct a teratology study with thalidomide?"

"I don't know how long he had to wait, where he was able to find them or what arrangements he had with the primate center. He may have been given priority because of the importance of his study."

"But he was able to obtain the primates?"

"Yes, he was."

"For a teratology study?"

"Yes."

"In fact, he only used a total of *six* monkeys for his study, isn't that true?"

I handed him a copy of the paper, which he quickly scanned, no doubt hoping I was wrong. "Yes, that's true," he reluctantly answered.

"And with those monkeys, he was able to reproduce the same malformations seen with humans, namely phocomelia?"

"Yes."

"With monkeys, they were able to extrapolate to humans?"

"Using thalidomide, yes."

"Has Richardson-Merrell used monkeys for tests on any of their other drugs?" It was a calculated gamble since I didn't know. But Newberne was uncertain about my state of knowledge and had already seen two published papers thrown at him. He couldn't take a chance and lie. Belanger decided to come to the rescue.

"Objection, your honor," said Belanger. "Totally irrelevant."

"We're talking about the availability of monkeys, your honor. They brought it up on direct examination."

"Overruled."

I turned to the witness again. "And what's your answer, Dr. Newberne?"

"Yes, we have."

I thought I'd press my luck. "How about other types of studies with Clomid? Use any monkeys for those?"

"Yes we did."

"How about *you*, Doctor? Have *you* used monkeys for any studies during the 1960s or 1970s?"

Newberne hesitated again then said, "Yes I have."

"Thank you."

On that note I concluded my cross-examination. Belanger did his best at rehabilitation on redirect, but had little success. Phil had obtained copies of the two papers because of an earlier discussion with Perrin. Even when he wasn't on the witness stand, our man from Detroit was saving our case.

The third witness for the defense was *John E. Johnson, Jr., M.D.*, a former Merrell employee who had participated in the clinical studies with Clomid. He was board certified in internal medicine and had a specialty in endocrinology, which made him suited to assist in overseeing the Clomid clinical investigations as a medical monitor. He had joined Merrell in September of 1963 and retired from the company in 1972. During the clinical studies, Johnson also had several meetings with FDA personnel concerning the drug, including the Commissioner of the FDA, James Goddard, M.D.

Over 360 clinical investigators had been involved in the study, and records from every one of their 2,635 patients had been submitted to the FDA for its review and approval. These records comprised a total of 45 volumes and thousands of pages of documents. Ultimately, in February 1967, the FDA approved Clomid for marketing. Prior to that time, the FDA also approved the wording on all labeling, including physician brochures and the package inserts. Marketing officially commenced on May 15, 1967, and the approval of the drug and its labeling had never been withdrawn up to the present.

As to the results of the clinical investigations, Johnson readily acknowledged that the spontaneous abortion rate with Clomid was at approximately 20 percent. However, given the condition of the patients that were part of their studies, this percentage was to be expected. When they looked at published rates for other infertility patients, they found a range between 20% and 25%.

The birth defect rate, assured Johnson, was also within the range expected in the general population. Including both major and minor defects in their group, the Clomid population had a birth defect incidence of only about two percent of total pregnancies, and he has seen studies from the general population as high as 7%. At this point we broke for the day. Belanger no doubt felt that this was a nice statistic for the jury to sleep on over night.

Friday, March 29, 1974. Belanger and Johnson picked up where they had left off the day before. Although animal studies are important, their usefulness diminishes with more and more clinical experience, and to date the clinical studies have demonstrated that Clomid is safe. The witness then explained how the C_{14} half-life studies are performed. C_{14} is a minimally radioactive substance that attaches to the

Clomid molecules and is measured periodically in the blood, urine and stools to determine the rate at which the drug is being eliminated from the body. The outcome of these studies is fully reported in the package insert.

He could not see any relationship between the use of Clomid and the 58 birth defects reported during their studies. There had been no pattern of malformations seen; no increased frequency of a single type or syndrome of congenital anomalies. Fifty-eight birth defects from 54 pregnancies out of a total of 2,369, where the outcome was known, equated to only a 2.3% birth defect rate.[28] This is within the range seen in the general population. He thus didn't "think" Clomid was teratogenic in humans. The use of the word, "think," reflected equivocation, which I would attempt to exploit on cross-examination.

Fred B then concluded with a hypothetical question, preliminary to asking whether Clomid was the cause of Mark Breimhorst's congenital malformations. Of course, he emphasized the phrase, "reasonable medical *probability*." Johnson hadn't heard or seen anything to suggest that there was any relationship with the mother's use of Clomid.

It was now my turn with the witness.

Between 1963 and 1972, while employed with Merrell, Johnson had shared the responsibility of evaluating the safety of Clomid. If it turned out that Clomid was teratogenic in humans, it would reflect not only on Merrell, but on him as well. He would also bear some of the guilt for not doing the job right. At the outset, I wanted to establish Johnson's bias.

Johnson agreed that to arrive at accurate statistics on birth defects from the clinical studies, they needed consistency and uniformity in reporting from their investigators. Merrell had used a total of 364 clinical investigators world wide. He agreed that many, with the approval of Merrell, had set up their own protocols, which could possibly lead to inconsistent reporting. However, that was only in the beginning of the studies and had been corrected later with a standard pregnancy outcome report form. Yes, he agreed that this meant some of the earlier investigators would have to dig back through their original records to obtain needed information, but he did not think that this would have been a problem.

He acknowledged that the protocols did not require all investigators to maintain BBT charts on each pregnancy, nor to document all exposure to trauma, x-rays, illnesses and drugs during each pregnancy, nor to evaluate all abortions, nor to perform chromosome studies on each malformed child, nor to conduct follow-up examinations on each live born child. Yes, it would have been useful to have had a control group, but this would have been difficult. The very nature of their problem is infertility, and thus getting a pregnant control group would have been a problem. When pushed, he agreed that many patients in their study had conceived several months after last using Clomid; he didn't say it was impossible, just that it would have been more difficult.

I next reviewed with Johnson all of the deficiencies in the 11 pregnancy report forms I had covered with Hoekenga in his March 1, 1974 deposition. Just as Belanger had replaced Holtkamp with Newberne, he had also substituted Hoekenga with Johnson. A strategy no doubt motivated by a desire to put on witnesses whom I had not deposed prior to trial. He thus hoped to impair the effectiveness of my cross-examination.   The reports were of children born with birth defects which lacked such vital information as the dates of conception and the dates of last treatment in relation to when the patient conceived. One case report did not even contain the year of treatment and conception. Was he "thinking" about these deficiencies when he "thought" that Clomid might not be teratogenic in humans? When Belanger objected that this question was argumentative, I withdrew it, having made my point.

Moving to another subject, I asked Johnson to recall his testimony when he quoted spontaneous abortion rates for infertility patients ranging between 20% and 25%. I had a published report marked as an exhibit and handed it to him.

"Doctor, do you recognize this paper?"

"Yes, I do. It is one of my published papers."

"It is entitled, 'Outcome of Pregnancies Following Clomiphene Citrate Therapy,' correct?"

"Yes, it is."

"This is an interim report that you gave on the pre-market studies at the Proceedings of the Fifth World Congress on Fertility and Sterility, held in Stockholm, Sweden, in June 1966?"

"Yes, it is."

"You reported on 672 pregnancies from the study?"

"Yes."

"And these were all infertility patients?"

"Yes, they were."

"In this report, you separated these pregnant infertility patients into four groups, Correct?"

"Yes."

"Group one, the biggest group, were patients who conceived during a treatment cycle; group two were patients who conceived between one to six months after last using Clomid; group three were patients who received a course of Clomid after conception; and group four involved patients for whom the timing of treatment in relation to conception was uncertain?"

"That is correct."

"So then, group one – patients who conceived within a few days of last using Clomid – had 99 spontaneous abortions out of 402 pregnancies, or a rate of 24.6%, correct?"

"I assume that's correct."

"Well, doctor, take a look at your paper if there is any doubt."

Johnson stared at his publication for a moment, and then said, "Yes, that's correct."

"One out of every four had a spontaneous abortion?"

"Yes."

"But group two – the infertility patients that conceived one or more months after last using the drug – they only spontaneously aborted 27 times out of 175 pregnancies, or a rate of only 15.4%?"

"Yes, apparently so."

"Well, doctor, these are your numbers."

"Yes they are."

"And this group of infertility patients, at 15.4%, had a similar spontaneous abortion rate as seen in the general population?"

"In this one small group of patients, yes."

"Yes. But when conception occurred within a few days of treatment, rather than months away, the percentage rose to almost 25%?"

"Yes, it would appear so."

I concluded my cross-examination by attacking his decision to compare the percentage of Clomid birth defects with a study that reported a general population rate of seven percent. Yes, there were studies out there reporting rates as low as 1%, and others between 1% and 2%, but the one he used was a more thorough and comprehensive study.

"My exact point," I said.

We finished with some redirect and re-cross and then broke for the weekend. It had been a long week. Every night I had been up until midnight, preparing for the next day of trial. I was physically tired and emotionally drained, but was feeling good about the case. I had overcome the motion for nonsuit and, it seemed, efficiently challenged Merrell's first three witnesses. Yes, it had also been a *good* week. On Saturday I would take a total break from the trial and spend some quality time with Janet and my daughter. Sunday, on the other hand, would be devoted to outlining my cross-examination for the next group of defense witnesses.

Monday, April 1, 1974. The defendant's fourth witness was still another employee from Merrell, and currently its Vice President of Research. *Murray Weiner, M.D.* was board certified in internal medicine and had a specialty in biochemistry. After establishing his education and qualifications in the field, Belanger spent some time with the witness on the various studies related to Clomid half-life, which essentially minimized the amount of the drug remaining at the start of organogenesis. He also minimized the importance of the animal studies and minimized the significance of the spontaneous abortion rate in the clinical investigations. This apparently was Fred B's minimizing witness. The only thing he maximized was the importance of this New York study which had a general population birth defect rate of 7.1%. My brief cross-examination attacked his bias as an employee, and generally followed my line of questioning of the earlier witnesses on the same issues. The jury no doubt by now was starting to get a sense of where both sides were lining up on the principal points of the case. I wondered if Belanger was going to engage in the same song and dance with each witness.

William Kroener, M.D., was an obstetrician/gynecologist and Merrell's first independent expert witness. He was currently a clinical professor at the USC School of Medicine. He was also quite familiar with Clomid and had used it on approximately 100 patients, about 50 of whom had become pregnant. He did not "recall" that any of the babies had been born with abnormalities and, based upon his reading of the literature, did not consider Clomid a human teratogen. When asked the same hypothetical question about Mark Breimhorst's congenital malformations, he again gave the same response as Merrell's previous witnesses. Apparently Belanger's strategy was to have as many different specialties as possible testify to the same conclusions. By now my cross-examination could have been phoned in, as for the third time I hammered away with the same questions – then sat down and waited for the next expert to take the stand.

Following the mid-afternoon break, Belanger called his third witness of the day, and sixth overall, *William L. Kuhn, Ph.D.* Kuhn was a pharmacologist and had been with Merrell since 1950. He currently headed its Pharmacology Department. For the remainder of the afternoon he was used to introduce a film about "The Beginning of Life," which, admittedly, I found to be quite interesting.[29] It visually followed the development of life in the human uterus from conception to birth. According to the film, the sperm must meet and enter the ovum within 10 hours after ovulation for conception to take place. Thereafter, the fertilized egg (zygote) embarks on a 6 day journey before attaching to the uterine wall as an actively dividing blastocyst. By day 18 the neural plate begins to form and then evolves, first to a fold and then to a groove – over the next 3 to 4 days – as the beginning of the spinal column.

As I sat observing the film, a thought came to me that grew into some interesting questions. The earliest form of the earliest organ to begin taking shape was the neural groove, which ultimately forms into the neural tube, then cranial vault and spinal column. Was it just a coincidence that there had been a disproportionate series of post-marketing reports of neural tube defects (i.e., anencephaly, spina bifida, etc.)? Was it significant that Clomid, although taken preconception, would be at its highest concentration while the neural tube was being formed, when compared to the level of the drug at the time of later developing organs? If Clomid was a human teratogen, would it not hit the neural tube first and the hardest? The film continued on until we broke for the day, but I found it difficult to focus on the remaining images of the other organs as they formed and grew. Even before the final flicker of the film, I had started to formulate questions for my cross-examination when presented with the right witness.

Tuesday, April 2, 1974. Kuhn picked up in the morning with an overview of the different phases of animal studies – acute, subacute and chronic – and finished off his testimony with a history lesson on Clomid, from the initial discovery of its fertility capabilities to its approval for marketing. When Belanger finished his last question on direct, I was perplexed. What was the purpose for putting Kuhn on the stand? Was he just a filler until the next important witness became available? Did Fred B simply want the jury to see a Merrell employee with a warmer personality? In any event, I perceived no apparent damage from his testimony and had only a few innocuous questions on cross.

An Unexpected Gift

After their teratologists, I concluded that the next witness would be the most important for the defense. His testimony would be critical in establishing the quality of Merrell's clinical studies. *Edward T. Tyler, M.D.*, was a fertility specialist and one of the principal clinical investigators with Clomid. For more than an hour, Belanger had Tyler lay out his qualifications in his specialized field – and they were impressive. He was one of the originators of the Pacific Coast Fertility Society and ran the organization for between eight and nine years. He was also an advisor to the FDA, a consultant to the World Health Organization and a professor at the UCLA School of Medicine. Tyler had published numerous papers in scientific and medical journals and had received a number of honors. He operated his own fertility clinic (The Tyler Clinic) in Westwood, near the UCLA campus.

Tyler was either the first or second physician in the country to use clomiphene citrate as a fertility drug on his patients. To date he had treated over 3,000 such patients. During the clinical investigations alone, he estimated that he had treated approximately 1,000 patients of which about 200 became pregnant. Doses ranged from 50 mg. to 500 mg. per day; some patients had received treatment for up to one and a half years; many had received Clomid for 10 consecutive days during a cycle; and, occasionally, some of his patients received clomiphene inadvertently during pregnancy. Yet through all of this history, including the prolonged and higher doses, he only had one pregnancy result in a congenital malformation.

On the issue of spontaneous abortions, he did not consider a rate of 20% to be either high or unexpected. In fact, he considered it low for infertility patients, and had seen a number of infertility studies with a much higher incidence. On the basis of his extensive experience with the drug, and reading virtually all of the world's literature on Clomid and other fertility drugs, it was his considered opinion that Clomid was not teratogenic in humans. He also felt that the animal teratology studies were of little value because the human experience far out-weighed those studies and demonstrated that there was not an increased risk of birth defects following use of Clomid.

Then came the inevitable hypothetical question. As expected, Tyler concluded that there was no relationship between Ingrid's use of Clomid and her son's unfortunate congenital malformations. Indeed, even if Clomid *was* a teratogen, there would not have been enough of the drug in the mother's system to cause damage at the time the affected organs were developing. With that final answer, Belanger announced that he had no further questions and sat down.

Now it was my turn and I had a number of issues to target. Tyler had recited the same script as every other witness, but I got a sense that he was his own man and would likely express his true opinions, notwithstanding how they might impact the case. Not that he would knowingly do anything to help cast an adverse shadow on his favorite fertility drug, but he seemed so taken with his own importance in the field that he could never see his own actions or conclusions subjected to any legitimate criticism. I scanned my notes one last time then stood up behind my chair.

"Doctor Tyler, you were a clinical investigator for Richardson-Merrell from 1960 until 1967, as far as the drug Clomid is concerned?"

"As far as Clomid is concerned."

"Now, when you were first contacted relative to the fertility study on Clomid, was there any particular type of protocol that was set up for you to use the drug?"

"That is a long time back and in those days I think primarily the clinical investigator himself sort of designed how he wanted to use it."

"So you, yourself, designed your own protocol?"

"Yes."

"And a protocol is kind of a guideline?"

"Exactly."

"Now, at any time did Richardson-Merrell, after you initially set up your own protocol, did they ever send you any guidelines or protocol to follow that you can recall?"

"Yes, there was at one time, and I can't remember the exact year, but they were concerned that in their efforts to market the drug they had to demonstrate that in fact it was a drug that would produce ovulation, so they designed a study."

"Other than that, were there any other protocols sent by Richardson-Merrell to you?"

"No, not to my recollection."

I considered this testimony to be a significant concession. Here was one of the principal clinical investigators acknowledging that the individual physicians in the study were designing their own protocols, rather than uniformly following study designs set by the company. Everyone was apparently off doing his or her own thing. The only exception was when Merrell felt that they had to demonstrate, *for market purposes,* that the drug could actually make women ovulate. I decided to press the issue further.

"When you first received the drug, Clomid, to conduct your clinical investigations, was any mention made to you to investigate whether or not the drug might be teratogenic in human beings?"

"No."

"And in 1962 – there has been testimony that certain animal studies were conducted with the rat and the rabbit using the drug Clomid, and I namely refer to the teratology studies – were you ever given the opportunity to review those particular animal studies?"

"You mean studies from the company?"

"Yes."

"I don't recall that I saw them. I was familiar with the literature but not private company reports. As I say, I don't recall that they sent me those directly."

"But at some point along the line you learned about the animal studies, right?"

"I am sure I must have."

"Okay. My question is approximately what date did you first learn of the animal studies?"

"I don't think I can answer that. I don't remember."

"Assuming that the animal studies were conducted in 1962, can you use that as criteria in estimating when you first heard of them?"

"Well, if there were animal studies that were performed by the company and were not published, I probably didn't see them until they were published.'

"And when you first heard of that, after you first learned of those particular animal studies, did Richardson-Merrell ever specifically request that you evaluate whether or not the drug was teratogenic in human beings?"

"No, because I was using it continuously anyway, and we had our data."

There it was. The studies were first published in 1967.[30] Not once in seven years was Tyler asked to assess whether or not Clomid could cause birth defects. This was Richardson-Merrell's scientific study. This was the "evidence" upon which it represented that "no causative evidence of a deleterious effect of Clomid therapy on the human fetus (had) been seen." Hopefully, it was now evident to the jury *why* such evidence had not been seen.

"Now did you deliver all of the 200 babies yourself?"

"I didn't deliver any of them."

Tyler explained that as a fertility specialist, patients were referred to him by outside OB/GYNs to assist their patients to achieve pregnancy, after which they were sent back to the referring doctors for delivery. His office would only follow them for the first trimester. A few of the patients were delivered by other doctors in his clinic, but the vast majority left his clinic after the first three months of pregnancy.

"Then, if I understand correctly, you were involved in the administration of the drug, not in delivery of the children?"

"Exactly."

"Now, did you maintain records on who delivered all of the approximate 200 pregnancies?"

"No, that would be impossible."

"For the same reason, were you aware of the outcome of all of those pregnancies?"

"Well, I think we have to recognize, and at least I recognize it in my practice, that when patients get pregnant after having come to me, almost invariably they tell me the outcome. So we get letters and birth announcements from our patients, and when we know the obstetrician we ask about it. We send them a note requesting that they tell us when the child was delivered and tell us about the delivery."

This response caught me by surprise. I was stunned at what I had just heard. Other than when they knew the obstetrician, Tyler's clinic was actually making a professional determination of whether each infant was born with a congenital anomaly based solely upon receipt of unsolicited "letters and birth announcements" sent by their patients.

"Then you had no specific routine whereby the OB/GYN who delivered the child, or the GP who delivered the child, would, as a matter of custom, report the outcome to you?"

"Not as a matter of custom. It would not be necessary because, I am sure we are aware, the doctors like to let us know what happened. Some doctors were nice enough to just send us the delivery room report."

"Do you have a list of the doctors, the pediatricians or other doctors that performed the follow-up examinations of these youths?"

"I don't keep a list, but I have a general idea of which doctors would have been included."

"Did you review any of those records of the follow-up examinations?"

"Not from other doctors in a formal way."

"Did you ask, as a matter of course, that any physicians report to you all follow-up examinations of children born following Clomid?"

"No, I didn't."

Nor did Tyler request that chromosome studies be performed on deliveries, nor perform any investigation on abortive material, nor request recording of all medications received during pregnancy. Nor, significantly, would he have learned of spontaneous abortions beyond the first trimester.

"The ones that went back to their own obstetricians, some of them may have aborted and I may not have known about it, but in our facility we definitely knew about it."

"Then do I understand your testimony, that there could have been abortions that occurred that were not reported to you?"

"There could be."

I next directed my questioning to the area of teratology. Tyler had concluded that Clomid was not a human teratogen and was not responsible for Mark's birth defects. I would again test his openness and candor, which was proving to be a disaster for the defense.

"Have you reviewed recent literature in the field of teratology?"

"As a specific purpose I would say no. I am not particularly interested in teratology as such, but I have seen, of course, articles on teratology."

"When you express an opinion as to whether or not a drug can produce birth defects, you are touching upon the field of medicine known as teratology, correct?"

"Oh, I am sure we are touching on it, but I don't propose that I am an expert in teratology."

"Okay. So you don't feel that you are an expert in teratology?"

"No."

With that final and unequivocal response I concluded my cross-examination. Okay, Fred B, fix it! Was I fooling myself, or had the witness destroyed the importance of the clinical studies and disqualified himself on the subject of birth defects? The jury would later let me know. But for now, I was feeling quite good about Belanger bringing Tyler to the party. Fred took a half-hearted stab at rehabilitation on redirect, but had little luck. Tyler was not about to have his previously expressed opinions and conclusions tested by anyone, not even by counsel for Merrell. Had Belanger spent any time with the witness or had any idea how he would answer my questions? With Fred B's level of experience and skill, I am sure he had. But what sometimes happens is the lawyer prepares his witness along the lines of his desired direct examination, and ignores getting him ready to respond to difficult questions on cross. This can happen when one is so convinced of the merits of his case that he cannot even glimpse it from the other side. Had this been the case? I would never know. But Belanger had 363 other clinical investigators to pick from and no doubt had others out there more inclined to join ranks in defense of the drug. Yet he still went with Edward Tyler, M.D.

Next up was *Milo Brooks, M.D.*, a pediatrician from Westwood who had examined Mark twice for the defendant. Under California law, the defendant in a personal injury case can have a plaintiff examined by a physician chosen by its counsel. After being qualified in his field of expertise, Dr. Brooks related the details of his two examinations. He then recited the history of Moebius syndrome, which began with a report of the syndrome by Dr. Moebius in 1888, and again in 1892. The syndrome, however, had been around for "several hundred years." Brooks had seen 5 or 6 cases of it at UCLA over the years. When asked about the known causes of Moebius syndrome, his response was that he hadn't "the foggiest," nor did anyone else. At this point we broke for the day.

As Rose and I exited the courthouse, I turned to her and asked, "What do you think, Rose, another one of those good days?"

"Oh, yeah," she smiled. "A great day. Terry, we just might win this thing."

"Too early to say, and you never know the way a jury is seeing the evidence. Tomorrow could be a critical day. They're bringing in two teratologists that could kill us. Yeah, tomorrow will be a very big day. We'll just have to wait and see."

Wednesday, April 3, 1974. Dr. Brooks spent the first hour in the morning describing the variations of Moebius syndrome, listing the different forms of treatment available – and their relatively inexpensive cost – and explaining that there was really no reason why Mark should not ultimately be able to find employment. After all, he knew of an armless radio announcer. He finished off direct by proclaiming that he had seen no evidence in his readings that Clomid would be capable of causing this syndrome that had been around forever.

My cross was brief. I first had Brooks detail each item of cost into the future, including replacement of Mark's prostheses once every two years until age 18, and then every five years thereafter. I thus established a floor in terms of his future medical expenses. I finished off my examination of the witness by testing what he actually knew about Clomid. What had he read about the drug? As it turned out, only the package insert.

My Biggest Challenge

Next up was *Robert Brent, M.D., Ph.D.*, Merrell's first teratologist. Now things would get really interesting. Now would be my biggest challenge of the trial. The road to victory lane had to go through the next two witnesses, and no doubt my skills at cross-examination would be tested to the limit. I was nervous, yet eager to see if I would measure up.

Brent's medical education was in pediatrics with special training in embryology, which he currently taught. He was president of the Teratology Society and had written over 150 publications on teratology for medical and scientific journals and textbooks. Working from Brent's curriculum vitae,[31] Belanger spent almost 30 minutes detailing each phase and accomplishment of his witness' career in this highly specialized field.

After qualifying Brent as an expert witness on teratology, Belanger inquired how one went about ascertaining whether a chemical agent was a human teratogen. Other than first assessing its chemical makeup and comparing it to known human teratogens, one would first go to animal teratology studies. The process included administering increasing doses during the critical period of organogenesis, when the animal is most susceptible to external agents. With rats, the most susceptible period was from days 9 through 12 of gestation; with mice it was days 7 through 11. If the number of malformations in each litter increases with higher and higher doses, demonstrating a dose relationship, one would conclude that the drug is teratogenic in that species of animal. One would also determine at what dose – measured by milligrams of the drug per kilogram of body weight – it was lethal to the embryo, resulting in its resorbtion, and at what dose the embryos were born normal. The difference between would be the teratogenic range of the drug.

Numerous animal studies have demonstrated that exposure to a teratogenic agent prior to the beginning of organogenesis either produces death (and resorbtion) of the embryo or has no teratogenic effect at all. He assured that a drug cannot have a teratogenic effect when exposure takes place prior to the period of organogenesis. This, of course, was an obvious swipe at the fact that the exposure to Clomid was coming from the earliest period of the pregnancy, even pre-conception.

Brent then followed a human conceptus, from fertilizing the ovum through the period of organogenesis, verbally relating what the jury had seen two days earlier in the film. With humans, organogenesis begins on day 18 post-conception. Consistent with the animal studies, in his opinion exposure to a drug prior to day 18 would not cause congenital malformations. In fact, the most sensitive period in the human embryo was between days 18 and 35, long after Ingrid Breimhorst ingested Clomid. Further, Mark's condition, Moebius syndrome, appears to occur spontaneously without any known cause, and certainly has never been attributed to the use of drugs.

Belanger then posed the hypothetical question, and as expected Brent found absolutely no relationship between the mother's use of Clomid and Mark's birth defects. Based upon his extensive review of all relevant literature and the clinical investigations, he was convinced that Clomid was not a human teratogen. He then parroted the same rationale as every defense expert before him: there was no pattern of a type or syndrome of congenital malformations and the incidence of anomalies from the clinical studies was within the range found in the general population. He also found it inconceivable that a drug taken prior to conception could cause these birth defects.

It was now my turn. On the subject of timing of ingestion, I pounded away on the half-life of the drug. Even if drugs were incapable of causing malformations prior to day 18, Clomid was still around at least as long as 42 days (6 weeks), well past the sensitive period between days 18 and 35. I had more ammunition on this issue, but decided that it would be more effective against James Wilson.

I then turned my attention to the pattern issue. There were 5 cases of Down syndrome out of 1886 deliveries during the clinical studies, an incidence of 1 out of every 377 delivered infants, substantially higher than seen in the general population. No, this did not surprise him. The frequency of Down syndrome increases with advancing age and the Clomid patients in the clinical studies tended to be older.[32] These were also infertility patients and notoriously had defective ova, often leading to abnormalities in their pregnancies. Besides, Down syndrome is not a congenital malformation. It is an anomaly caused by an abnormal chromosome. I decided that it was now time to exploit the Drug Experience Reports of anencephaly.

"Doctor, thalidomide causes a limb reduction abnormality known as 'phocomelia,' correct?"

"Yes, that's correct."

"In fact, thalidomide represents the classical case of a human teratogen with that pattern of defects you referred to?"

"Yes."

"And it was because of the rarity of this abnormality that Doctors Lenz and McBride were able to discover the association between the use of thalidomide during pregnancy and these horrible birth defects?"

"Yes, that's true."

"This occurred when they noticed a significant number of case reports of this very rare abnormality and found thalidomide as the common denominator?"

"Yes, I would agree with that."

"So thalidomide was discovered to be a human teratogen from the use of individual case reports, rather than an epidemiology study?"

"Yes."

"So case reports can be used to discover whether a drug is a human teratogen?"

"It is rare, but it can happen."

I now had him set up for the next series of questions. I first wanted to establish some degree of importance to the use of case reports. I knew that this was accomplished with thalidomide only because of the almost unique nature of congenital malformations that it caused. But I also understood from my own experts that a surge of case reports with a pattern of anomalies should at the very least be viewed as a "red flag" of what the drug might be causing.

"While conducting your extensive review of the records for this case, can I assume that you also reviewed the Clomid post-marketing case reports, also known as Drug Experience Reports or DERs?"

"Yes, I did."

"Then you would have reviewed Merrell's case report number 15252?" I asked, handing him a set of the records.

He scanned the records for a moment. "Yes, I reviewed this case report."

"This case involved delivery of fraternal twins, did it not?"

"Yes."

"Fraternal twins are from two separate eggs or ova?"

"Yes."

"And Clomid can cause multiple ovulation and fraternal twinning?"

"It has been so reported."

"Well, you don't dispute that, do you?"

"No, I don't."

"And one of the twins was born with anencephaly, correct?"

"Yes."

"One of the fraternal twins was born *without a brain*?"

I could almost sense some of the jurors wince at that visual image.

"Yes, anencephaly literally means 'absence of a brain.' "

"And that abnormality is described as a 'suspected adverse reaction with the drug'?"

"That's what is stated on the DER."

"In other words, this reports anencephaly as a suspected adverse reaction with Clomid?"

"It's a form submitted to the FDA by the company. The FDA requires a submission on this form whenever the company receives a report of a possible association, no matter how unlikely it might be."

"But that is what is stated on this official federal form?"

"Yes, even though its association is highly unlikely."

"Right. And you also reviewed case report number 17685?" I handed the witness all of the remaining DERs I would want him to review.

"Yes, I did."

"This is another case of anencephaly reported as a suspected adverse reaction to Clomid?"

"Yes, it is," he responded after viewing the records.

"Another child born without a brain?"

"Yes."

"And you also reviewed case number 19948?"

"Yes, I did."

"Another child born without a brain?"

"Yes."

"And you also reviewed case number 20901?"

Without looking now. "Yes."

"Another child born without a brain?"

"Yes."

"And you also reviewed case number 21915?"

"Yes."

"Another child born without a brain?"

"Yes."

"And you also reviewed case number 21983?"

"Yes."

"Another child born without a brain?"

"Yes."

"And you also reviewed case number 21984?"

"Yes."

"Another child born without a brain?"

"Yes."

"And you also reviewed case number 22796?"

"Yes."

"Another child born without a brain?"

"Yes."

"Doctor, by now did you perhaps start seeing a pattern developing?"

"Not really. One of the earlier reports was published in Lancet, I believe in 1973, which prompted a lot of physicians to focus on this specific anomaly. I thus don't place any great importance on these 8 case reports."

"Eight out of only 34 case reports received to date post-marketing – *twenty-three point five percent of all reported cases* – and you place absolutely no importance on it?"

"Not really."

At this point I cared little about his opinion. To deny that this was a pattern would likely cost him valuable credibility points. And in a trial, credibility is everything. In my view, Brent would have been more believable had he acknowledged the existence of a pattern, and then attempted to pass it off with some reasonable explanation. But this line of questioning had apparently caught him by surprise. Perhaps my decision to ignore this issue during Hoekenga's deposition may have paid off. Only the verdict would give me the answer.

I next went through the deficiencies in the clinical study – highlighted by Tyler's acknowledgments – and finished off my cross-examination with Richardson-Merrell's teratology studies. I compared the rabbits "turning under" of their hind paws with Mark Breimhorst's club foot. I also pointed to the "altered limbs' of the rats, and asked Brent to describe how they were altered. How did he know that they weren't limb reduction defects? He, of course, could not describe them any more than Holtkamp could. He "understood" that they were only soft-tissue anomalies, not skeletal, but could not point to any records to substantiate that claim. Every attempt was made to exploit the ambiguities in the malformation descriptions. I then asked if he agreed that Clomid seemed to be attacking the limbs in both animals. He would not attach any importance to such an observation. With that I sat down, convinced I had held my own with this critically important witness.

Now my biggest challenge of the trial. As Belanger called *James G. Wilson* to the stand, I could feel my stomach muscles tighten. Justified or not, I concluded that the outcome of the case would now hinge on this one man's testimony. His importance in the field of teratology could not be denied. He had also evaluated Clomid's teratogenic risk on two occasions, once before and once after it was first marketed. He no doubt would stand behind his conclusions. For these reasons, I had spent more time preparing to cross-examine Wilson than any other person to take the stand on behalf of the defendant. Yet I was thankful that we were now close to the end of the day. I would still have one more night before being put to the test and would take full advantage of that opportunity.

Belanger spent the time remaining soliciting Wilson's education and training in a number of scientific fields that interrelated with teratology, including pediatrics, anatomy, pathologic embryology, endocrinology, reproduction, and primate biology. He had obtained his Ph.D. from Yale University and was currently Professor of Research Pediatrics and Anatomy at Children's Hospital in Cincinnati, Ohio. Tomorrow Belanger would begin by outlining Wilson's list of accomplishments.

Thursday, April 4, 1974. Wilson founded the Teratology Society in 1959 or 1960. As chairman of a meeting of teratologists in Geneva, Switzerland, in November 1966, he participated in formulating guidelines for animal teratology studies for the World Health Organization. He was also the author of that report. Earlier, in January 1966, he had been a consultant to the FDA and assisted in preparing a similar set of guidelines to be followed by the pharmaceutical industry. Wilson then recited his extensive bibliography, including co-editing a textbook with Josef Warkany and authoring another one by himself.

He had conducted numerous studies with non-human primates. They are anatomically and physiologically similar to humans, and are susceptible to a number of human diseases and react similarly to many drugs – though not all. The availability of monkeys for studies is somewhat limited and comes from primate centers. Each center maintains past histories on their monkeys, which provides baseline standards that are important in conducting studies. With many researchers seeking to conduct a large variety of studies with simians, and a limited supply available commercially, it is often difficult to obtain a sufficient supply for animal teratology studies. Limited studies, however, have been conducted with clomiphene citrate on monkeys. These were reported in the literature in one study by Valerio and Courtney and a second by Morris and others. In neither study did clomiphene cause any abnormalities.

Wilson described his own studies with thalidomide and non-human primates. He was able to reproduce the same syndrome of limb reduction abnormalities seen in humans at the same dose levels. The drug even produced some of the lesser known congenital abnormalities attributed to thalidomide, such as to the ears and jaw and a number of internal organs. An increase in the dose to the monkeys increased the incidence and severity of the defects. But this experience with thalidomide was the exception, not the rule. It is impossible to directly extrapolate from animals to man, even with non-human primates, and the ultimate test can only be with humans. One cannot see the total picture until epidemiology studies have been conducted on a large population of humans.

He was requested to evaluate the potential teratogenic risk of Clomid on two occasions, once in 1965 and again in 1968. On neither occasion did he see any evidence that Clomid presented a risk of causing birth defects. Wilson then recited what had now become redundant to the jury: the incidence of congenital anomalies was comparable to that seen in the general population and there was no pattern of malformations, no increase of a syndrome or other anomalies, in the clinical investigations. Wilson also attacked the individual cases of birth defects from the study. Several had a hereditary background, a significant number had been exposed to other drugs and radiation during pregnancy, and some were not even malformations. Then came the inevitable hypothetical question and its inevitable answer. He also found that it was "very, very remote" that any drug could ever cause congenital malformations if taken prior to conception.

It was now time for Terry Mix to step up to the plate. I finished off the last note on Wilson's testimony and rose from my chair, still scanning my outline as I stood. No sooner had I looked up at the witness than I heard Fredricks' voice from the bench announcing that it was 10 minutes of twelve and a good time to take our noon recess. Another reprieve. I would gladly use the opportunity to update my line of questioning from the morning testimony. For the first time during the trial I passed on lunch.

At promptly 1:30 PM Fredricks took the bench and invited me to question the witness. For a second time I stood with my outline in hand. I was sure that each and every juror was quite anxious to hear what I had to ask this key witness – and how he would respond to those questions. My own assessment was that Wilson took pride in his stature within the scientific community and would not compromise that standing by selling out to Richardson-Merrell. Every opinion he expressed would be something he truly believed and could be backed up scientifically. I thus would largely be relying upon statements he had previously made in his numerous writings. Additionally, if I expected him to back away from any of his conclusions, I needed to provide him with an escape route.

"Doctor, when you conducted your reviews in 1965 and 1968, you relied upon *summaries* of the animal and clinical studies, correct?

"Yes, that's true."

"In other words, you did not review the original records, the original raw data?"

"That's true."

"And those summaries were prepared and submitted to you by Richardson-Merrell?"

"Yes."

"And if those summaries were inaccurate, then your opinions might be wrong, isn't that true?"

"Well, that would depend upon what was inaccurate and to what extent."

"Exactly. So if an important fact was significantly in error, then you might have a different opinion?"

"Yes, depending upon what it was."

"So if rather than, say, 58 birth defects, there were 100 or 150 of them, you might have a different opinion on whether Clomid was a human teratogen?"

"Yes, it is possible. But I would have to know a number of other facts as well."

"Of course. But you are relying upon the accuracy of the information that was provided to you by Richardson-Merrell, correct?"

"Yes, of course."

"And when it comes to the number and type of congenital malformations that resulted from the Clomid clinical investigations, you not only are assuming that they were accurately counted and described, you are also relying that the study was properly designed to thoroughly examine each delivered infant and document the findings of that examination; is that not true?"

"Yes, that's true."

"So if you heard that rather than relying upon a thorough exam of each delivered infant, the study depended upon receipt of unsolicited letters and birth announcements from the patients, you might have some problem with the study?"

For a moment I thought I detected Wilson cast a quick glance over at Belanger. I was sure that this acknowledgment by Tyler had not been shared with the witness. "Yes, I might have some concern with such a study."

It was now time to move on to some important admissions made by Wilson from his many writings. "Would you agree that comparing the incidence of birth defects following Clomid with incidence figures from the general population might be somewhat unreliable?"

"It could present some difficulties, but I wouldn't totally disregard their importance."

"Well, one of the difficulties would be that there can be significant differences in malformation rates from country to country, and even from city to city; would you not agree?" I made sure that Wilson could see I was referring to his own text book.[33]

"Yes, I would agree with that."

"So the birth defect rate in Japan could be significantly different than in Italy?"

"Yes, it could."

"And that would also apply to *specific* malformations – such as, let's say, anencephaly – as well as total malformation rates?"

"Yes."

"So it would not be advisable to compare a birth defect rate from a world wide population of patients with a rate from a single city such as, let's say, New York?"

Another quick glance at Belanger. "No, such a design would not be preferable."

"Another problem with comparing incidence figures in the general population is that there is a lack of agreement as to what constitutes a birth defect; correct?" I again stared at a page in his book as I posed the question.[34]

"I would agree with that."

"Then it would not be advisable to compare the rate of birth defects of two groups unless they both used the same definition of birth defects?"

"It would be preferable to use the same definition."

"Another problem is underreporting of birth defects, including inadequate examinations and failure of follow-up exams?" Another glimpse at the book.[35]

"I would agree."

"If one study conducted a thorough examination of every delivered infant at birth, and follow-up examinations for a year, one would expect a higher rate of defects than another study where the investigators relied upon letters and birth announcements from the parents and performed no follow-up exams?"

Wilson appeared almost amused at the question. "Yes."

"In fact, it is because of these problems that epidemiologists use control groups; isn't that true."

"Yes."

Now it was time to address another issue that had been hanging around for awhile. "Doctor, you commented on direct about the lack of a pattern of defects. Do you recall that testimony?"

"Yes, I do."

Holding up his book again I asked, "Well, would you agree with the following statement: 'It is likely that truly unique or highly characteristic syndromes are not always induced by environmental teratogens, either in the laboratory or in man. At least it would seem *unwise* to depend upon sentinel defects as an unfailing criterion in the recognition of induced teratogenesis.'[36]?" I had read directly from his textbook.

"I guess I should."

"Because you wrote it?"

"Yes, I did."

Wilson agreed that the anticancer drug, folic acid antagonist, a known human teratogen, did not produce a pattern of defects.

"So it would be *unwise* to conclude that Clomid was not a teratogen simply because of the lack of a pattern of defects?"

"I would agree with you if this was the only criterion being used. But the lack of a pattern can be useful when considered along with other factors."

"But lack of a pattern alone cannot eliminate a drug as a human teratogen?"

"No."

I would now move to the timing of exposure. I first went through the same series of questions I had posed to earlier witnesses related to the half-life of Clomid. Wilson generally conceded he was unable to assure that neither Clomid nor its metabolites would be present during early organogenesis, including the highly susceptible period. Nor could he tell me the quantity of the drug that would be around at this time.

"Doctor, would you agree that the onset of teratogenic susceptibility could be as early as days 11 or 12 in man?" I was now referencing a paper he had authored.[37]

"Yes, I would. Something else I have written," he smiled. He was now getting the idea. I came armed.

"Then if Clomid was still present on days 11 and 12, because of its half-life, you could not discount it as a possible teratogen simply because it was taken before conception?

"Not solely for that reason, no."

"In fact, it has been demonstrated in laboratory animals that malformations can be induced well before the beginning of organogenesis, correct?" [38]

"Yes, it has."

"This includes such teratogens as hypoxia – reduced oxygen – hypothermia and radiation?"

"Yes, it has been so demonstrated in the laboratory."

I next highlighted the limitations of the Valerio and Courtney study, as I had done previously with Newberne, and addressed the same limitations with the study published by Morris and colleagues.[39] Morris only exposed 3 monkeys to Clomid during pregnancy, two subcutaneously at the same dose and one orally at a single dose late in organogenesis. Neither study met the teratology guidelines Wilson had helped to promulgate. Finally, I finished by referencing the 8 reports of anencephaly post-marketing, although this time identifying them as a group. Wilson conceded that this "might" represent a pattern and would justify further study. He also agreed that Clomid would be near its highest concentration during pregnancy when the neural tube was being formed.

When I sat down, I felt a sense of relief and satisfaction. The witness had not been destroyed in any fashion, but instead neutralized – at least that was my hope, since one never knows how a jury has perceived the evidence. Belanger's redirect did little to help his case, because every concession made from the stand was an honestly-held opinion of James G. Wilson. And he was not about to compromise on those opinions. We finally broke for the day. Next up tomorrow, two more witnesses for the defense and then the defendant would rest. We were nearing the end.

Friday, April 5, 1974. The first witness to be called was *Stephen Cederbaum, M.D.,* a medical geneticist from UCLA. In my view Cederbaum offered little to the defendant's case other than providing an introductory course on genetics and explaining how Moebius syndrome occurred "sporadically" as a new mutation. Apparently Fred B felt compelled to call a geneticist because we had called one as part of the plaintiff's case.

My cross-examination was short.

In the afternoon Belanger called his last witness, *John R. Marshall, M.D.,* an obstetrician/gynecologist. He had extensively studied Clomid; why it works, how it works and its effect on the female reproduction system. It was "thought" to work on the pituitary gland, causing it to produce gonadotropins, including luteinizing hormones (LH) and follicle stimulating hormones (FSH), which in turn stimulate the follicles of the ovaries. This relationship is referred to as the "pituitary-ovarian axis." He then reviewed the statistics from the clinical investigations. After setting out all of the numbers on a chart, and *this time deducting out the abortions*, he came up with a birth defect rate of 3.1%, which he considered to *still* be within the range seen in the general population. It "did not give rise to a suspicion that Clomid was a human teratogen." He also began analyzing each of the anencephaly case reports, passing them off as chance occurrences having no relationship to the coincidental use of clomiphene citrate. As Fred B concluded for the day and week, it was becoming evident to me that this was his "clean up" witness. Any remaining matters leaving Belanger a little unsettled would be addressed with Marshall. Coming down the home stretch, I was grateful for a weekend off to prepare for my final cross-examination and closing argument.

Monday, April 8, 1974. Marshall picked up where he left off on Friday, completing his assessment of the anencephaly DERs. He testified that four of the 8 cases of anencephaly occurred in England, and that this type of neural tube defect occurs 2 ½ times more frequently in the United Kingdom than in the United States. This condition is often genetic in origin, being transmitted through heredity. He then turned his attention to the Clomid spontaneous abortion rate. He cited one study involving infertility patients in which the incidence of abortions was reported at 22.3%. These women were notorious for not maintaining pregnancies. He then made an analysis of the clomiphene half-life. Using a chart he attempted to minimize the level of Clomid present at the time of organogenesis. He concluded with the expected opinion that Clomid had nothing to do with Mark Breimhorst's congenital malformations.

On cross-examination I went right to the anencephaly case reports. I first had him read the language from each of the federal forms describing the defect as a "suspected adverse reaction" to Clomid. Next up was a report on two of the cases in the British publication, *The Lancet*.[40] I again had him read aloud from the text: "We think, however, that the possibility of a causal relationship between ovulation-stimulating treatment and C.N.S. (central nervous system) abnormality should not be dismissed lightly."

I had carefully reviewed each case report and knew how the witness had to answer my next question. "Would you agree that none of the physicians who reported these cases expressed a view that heredity was the cause of the anencephaly?"

"It would appear not."

The remainder of my cross was familiar ground to the jury, but was again repeated to at least induce equivocation in Marshall's conclusions. I was even able to solicit a concession that it was "possible" that Clomid was a human teratogen. Many of the concepts I was espousing were complex, and the more they were repeated the greater the likelihood that most, if not all, of the jurors would understand them. Repetition bred understanding. It was how I educated myself on clomiphene citrate and birth defects, but I had the benefit of two years of opportunity – the jurors only four weeks. Hopefully I would be able to tie everything together in closing argument, which was just around the corner. By noon, I had concluded my cross and Fred his redirect. All of the testimony the jury would ever hear on the case was now history. Subject to introducing into evidence previously marked exhibits, the defendant rested. I announced to the court that the plaintiff would not be calling any rebuttal witnesses.

Judge Fredricks released the jury until 11:00 A.M. the next day, with counsel to return after lunch to discuss the introduction of exhibits and begin the task of deciding which jury instructions would be given. But when we finished with the exhibits, it was mid-afternoon and Fredricks wanted to start fresh on Tuesday with jury instructions. We were asked to return at 9:30 AM the following day.

Tuesday, April 9, 1974. When the jury arrived at eleven, we were already an hour and a half into jury instructions and had just scratched the surface. They were asked to come back at 9:30 AM on Wednesday and they would hear argument from counsel at that time. We then rolled up our sleeves and went back to work.

At the beginning of every trial, all parties submit to the judge a written request for jury instructions that they desire the court to read to the jurors at the conclusion of the case. In California, many come from a text entitled, "Book of Approved Jury Instructions" (BAJI), which are pre-printed and previously approved statements of the law. All are numbered, and all the attorney needs to do is request the specific number of each desired instruction. Once the judge approves giving these instructions, the clerk pulls them out of a file drawer and provides them to the judge for reading to the jury.

In addition to the BAJI instructions are *special* jury instructions, the text of which has been prepared by trial counsel. Appellate cases supporting the proposed statement of the law are cited on the instruction. Many times all of this involves comparing the special instruction to what is included in BAJI in order to determine whether it is even necessary. Frequently the cited cases are read by the judge and argument submitted by counsel. Added jury instructions are also provided during the trial when new and unexpected issues arise. All of this is on the record in front of a court reporter and can consume a lot of time, depending upon the nature of the case. Because drug product liability cases were infrequently tried, and even fewer appealed, there were very few cases on the subject at the appellate level. And other than the standard instructions used in every personal injury trial, BAJI was of little use. Judge Fredricks was also inclined to give free rein to all counsel in hearing their arguments – a trait I admired.

As a consequence a substantial amount of time was consumed on jury instructions. We finally wrapped up at 4:45 PM, and I was out the door to put a final polish on my sermon in the morning.

Closing Arguments

Wednesday, April 10, 1974. I rose from my seat and stood in front of the jury, with structured outline in hand – my security blanket in case I forgot something. It was also used to keep me on track. By this point I had so much information bouncing around in my head, that the difficulty was not whether I had something important to say, but how and when to say it.   It was my first opportunity to talk directly to the jury since my opening statement, about four weeks earlier. All 12 jurors and the remaining alternate stared right at me, pens poised over their notepads, eagerly waiting to hear what I had to say. I took a breath, smiled at them for a moment, and then began.

"Today I'm going to tell you a story. The year is early 1492 and the world is flat. Talk to the guy on the street, and the world is flat. Talk to the shop owner, and the world is flat. Even if you asked the educated, the opinion is that the world is flat. Almost everyone held that point of view. Why? Because nobody tried to prove otherwise. It was just accepted as the gospel truth.

"Well, Richardson-Merrell wants you to believe that the world is flat.   They represent to you, to the medical profession, and to every female patient with a fertility problem, that there is no evidence that Clomid causes birth defects in humans; that there is *no* evidence that Clomid therapy has a deleterious effect on the human fetus. But what has been done to prove or disprove that representation?

"Since Richardson-Merrell first began testing this drug, up to the present day, it has totally neglected to make a thorough – even a meaningful – evaluation of whether or not Clomid causes birth defects in humans. What has it done? When clomiphene citrate was first being developed, it had been known for years that certain drugs could produce birth defects in man. Yet in 1960, *without the benefit of any animal teratology studies*, it sent the drug to clinical investigators, the world over, to be used in humans. Why? Why would they expose hopeful mothers to the risk – even a remote chance – that Clomid might cause a malformation in their babies without doing such studies? Because it was not *required* by the FDA at the time. Hey, it's not required, so why should we do it?

"Then came the revelation of the terrible tragedy of thalidomide. In late 1961 it was learned that thousands of babies had been born without limbs because of the exposure of that drug to pregnant mothers. Finally, the following year – in 1962 – Merrell conducted teratology studies with the rat and the rabbit. And what did they find? Clomid was capable of causing congenital malformations in those animals. Even their own Dr. Newberne acknowledged that this was at least a *clue* as to what might happen in humans. But *still* they continued to use this fertility drug in their human clinical investigations without a design to assess the risk of birth defects.

"Significantly, in 1964 and again in 1966, it was demonstrated that when one administered thalidomide to pregnant monkeys, using the same dose and at the same time of gestation as in humans, it produced the same type of birth defects. In January 1966, the FDA suggested use of monkeys in teratology studies. In November 1966, the World Health Organization strongly recommended use of monkeys in teratology studies. Yet up to the present time, Richardson-Merrell has still not conducted teratology studies with Clomid using monkeys. If truly interested in what this drug might do to the human fetus, why not? What were Richardson-Merrell's excuses?

"Well, they're just simply not available. We can't find enough monkeys to do primate teratology studies with Clomid. But Dr. Wilson found them, didn't he? Valerio and Courtney found them. Merrell found monkeys to do tests with other drugs, even other types of tests on Clomid. Even Dr. Newberne used monkeys in other experiments at Merrell. Yet they couldn't find them for Clomid teratology studies.

"Another excuse. Hey, those studies have already been done, so what's the need? Valerio and Courtney did them. But that was designed as an *infertility* study, with only one dose level, using only a small number of monkeys. The monkeys were not given the full range of doses as recommended by the FDA and the World Health Organization. Nor was exposure to the drug earlier than organogenesis.

"Then, of course, was the final excuse: that the ultimate test is in man anyway, and there is absolutely no evidence from human studies that Clomid produces malformations in man. But let's take a good look at those human studies – the Clomid clinical investigations. Between 1960 and 1967, Clomid was sent to over 360 clinical investigators world wide.[41]   And how were those studies designed?   Certainly not to evaluate whether Clomid could cause birth defects.   No one was required to examine spontaneous abortions following Clomid use; nor to record all medications taken during pregnancy; nor record traumas during pregnancy; nor record x-ray exposure during pregnancy; nor record maternal illnesses during pregnancy; nor to conduct chromosome studies on deformed babies – needed information to eliminate other causes when a child was born deformed.   And most important of all, the investigators were not required to perform follow-up examinations of all Clomid babies.

"Indeed, it is highly likely that a large number of Clomid babies were *never even examined at all as part of the study*.   Recall the testimony of Dr. Edward Tyler, one of Merrell's principal clinical investigators.   Since he was a fertility specialist, patients would be referred to him by outside OB/GYNs who had been unsuccessful in helping their patients conceive.   Once a patient had conceived with Clomid, Dr. Tyler would follow that patient for a few months. Then he would send the pregnant mother back to the original OB/GYN for delivery of the baby.   The problem?   The OB/GYN was not part of the study and was under no obligation to report to Merrell, or even Dr. Tyler, the outcome of the delivery.

"At this point, of course, a pediatrician takes over care of the new baby. Unfortunately, none of the pediatricians who saw the babies from the 1,866 deliveries were included in the pre-market clinical investigations either.   So they had no obligation to report their findings to Richardson-Merrell, or to the fertility specialist, or even to the delivering OB/GYN.   This situation evolved because performing a follow-up examination was never part of the study.   Another glaring deficiency.

"Why is this important?   As you have heard from the witnesses – and there would appear to be no dispute over this statistic – when examinations are performed on a group of infants one year after birth, one will find approximately twice the rate of birth defects as were seen at the time of their deliveries.   Yet, notwithstanding the poor design of this study, Richardson-Merrell wants you to believe that all congenital malformations from the Clomid patients were *observed* and all observed malformations were *reported*. This is absolutely absurd!

"For example, consider Dr. Tyler, himself. He was one of the original clinical investigators and, according to his own testimony, the Tyler clinic was responsible for producing approximately 200 pregnancies. Since the overall birth defect rate of the clinical investigations was 3.1% of delivered pregnancies, this means that Dr, Tyler's clinic alone should have reported approximately 6 infants with congenital malformations. Yet he reported only *one*!

"How, under these circumstances, can Richardson-Merrell come before you and the medical profession and claim only 58 children were born with birth defects? They want you to believe that each OB/GYN and each pediatrician *voluntarily* reported each and every birth defect and *voluntarily* conducted follow-up exams on each and every child. Let me refer you to Dr. Tyler's actual trial testimony, which we had transcribed.

At this point I read verbatim from the transcript. I highlighted the testimony that demonstrated the clear deficiencies in the investigations: that he was never asked by Merrell to investigate whether Clomid had a teratogenic effect on his patients; that he had not learned of the rat and rabbit teratology studies until he saw them published in 1967; that the vast majority of all his patients did not deliver their babies in his clinic; that instead he relied on getting "letters and birth announcements from (his) patients" to assess the outcome of the pregnancies; that he did not even keep a complete list of the numerous OB/GYNs who had referred the patients to him; that when they knew the obstetrician, they would "send them a note requesting that they tell (Tyler's staff) when the child was delivered and tell (them) about the delivery;" that he was never requested to report on follow-up examinations of the infants and had no knowledge what was done in that regard; and that he had never been requested to record all medications received by his patients during pregnancy, nor record exposure to x-rays, maternal illnesses and trauma, nor to do chromosome studies and investigate abortive material.

I then turned my attention to the issue of causation.

"Did Clomid cause Mark Breimhorst's congenital malformations? Have we met our burden of proof? Remember that the plaintiff's burden is not beyond a reasonable doubt, as in a criminal case, or with certainty. Plaintiff need only convince you that, considering all of the evidence introduced on the issue, it is probable – more likely than not – that Clomid was a substantial factor in causing the birth defects.

"Consider the proof that has been presented. You heard Dr. Thienes testify that there is a *reasonable medical probability* that Clomid was the cause of the birth defects. You also heard from Dr. Perrin, a demanding scientist, that there was a reasonable medical possibility that Clomid was the cause – an opinion that you can consider, along with all of the other evidence, in determining whether it was the *probable* cause. What is the other evidence you should consider? As Dr. Perrin stated, these birth defects resulted from some damage occurring to the embryo at some point prior to November 13, 1969. Something happened to the embryo between September 20, 1969 and November 13, 1969.

What happened over that eight-week period that could have accounted for these horrible malformations? It wasn't from heredity. We know that. You heard from our geneticist, Dr. Crandall, that this was not a genetic defect. We also know that there were no drugs ingested, no trauma, no x-rays, no extremes of temperature, no nutritional deficiencies and no maternal illness during this critical period. All other known causes of birth defects could be eliminated as being responsible for Mark's anomalies. Nothing was there to cause these birth defects. Nothing, that is, except for Clomid.

"Was Clomid there? I mean, after all it was never taken during pregnancy, so how could it possibly be responsible? Well, ladies and gentlemen, we have all learned something during this case about drug half-life; how fast a drug is eliminated from the body. And with Clomid, quite frankly, it simply takes its time. We know from studies conducted by Richardson-Merrell that Clomid and/or its metabolites, can be around for up to 6 weeks, and maybe even longer. Ingrid conceived on or about September 20, 1969, only four days after last ingesting Clomid. Clomiphene citrate, and/or its metabolites, were there after conception, they were there at the beginning of organogenesis, they were there during the highly susceptible embryonic period, described by Dr. Wilson during cross-examination, and they were there on day 32 when the hands were to begin forming. Thus, if Clomid was teratogenic in humans, it certainly had the *opportunity* to cause Mark Breimhorst's congenital malformations. We also know that on September 20, 1969, the date that she conceived, Ingrid Breimhorst called Dr. Richards and complained of pain in the area of her ovaries.[42]

"The remaining question, of course, is whether it is *probable* that Clomid is a human teratogen? Unfortunately, because Richardson-Merrell failed to design the clinical studies to assess the risk of birth defects, including use of a control group, we are limited in what we can look at. This is a problem, I might add, created by the defendant.

But what *do* we know? We know that during the pre-market clinical investigations there was a 20% spontaneous abortion rate for confirmed pregnancies, which was at least one-third higher than seen in the general population. We know that the majority of spontaneous abortions are caused by abnormalities of the embryo or fetus. We know that a reasonable inference could be drawn from this that clomiphene citrate was causing such abnormalities, and thus producing the abortions. We know that when Clomid was given only prior to conception, the birth defect rate in the clinical studies was 2.5%. However, when the pregnancies were inadvertently exposed to the drug after conception, the rate rose to 5.1% – there was twice the frequency. Even Merrell's own expert, Dr. Marshall, admitted that there was a possibility that Clomid could be a human teratogen.

"What about the animal teratology studies? What do they tell us? We know that the package insert, published by Merrell, reports that Clomid was teratogenic in the rat and the rabbit when administered during the period of organogenesis. This was further acknowledged in the deposition I took of Dr. Holtkamp, who oversaw the studies. We also know, according to what Dr. Newberne told us, that animal studies give us a clue as to what may occur in man. But maybe, just maybe, there are some *questions* that tell us even more about the value of these animal studies. For example, we know that there were, quote, "limb abnormalities," but why weren't they given an exact description? We know that photographs were taken of the malformed animals, but why haven't they been produced here in this trial? We know that monkeys have been used on other studies, but why haven't they been used by Merrell for teratology studies with Clomid? And most importantly, why did Merrell bring Dr. Newberne to this courtroom and try to convince you that Clomid was *not* teratogenic in those very same animal teratology studies?

"In fact, Richardson-Merrell has consistently demonstrated in this trial that it is not beyond trying to mislead you about the evidence. Consider this. First, Merrell represents that as proof that Clomid is not teratogenic, you should consider that there has been no pattern of birth defects in their clinical studies; that there is not an excess of a certain type of congenital malformation. Yet during the cross-examination of Dr. Wilson, he admitted that folic acid antagonist – a known teratogenic drug – does not produce any basic pattern or syndrome of defects; and he further acknowledged that it would be *unwise* to rely upon this as a sole criterion.

"Second – and this is a big one – the incidence of birth defects following Clomid use is the same as in the general population. Well, we know how much care Merrell took in *counting* those birth defects. So who knows what the real rate is following use of Clomid? But what is the rate in the general population that is to be used for comparison? Depending upon how and where that study was done, the numbers are all over the board. Nobody really knows what that birth defect rate should be. Some surveys report a rate of less than one percent, whereas others report between 1 and 2%. Why not use those studies to compare with? Why, indeed. We can't use those, because our rate is 3.1%. Hey, there's this New York study where they found a rate of 7.1%. Let's use *that* study. Never mind that they conducted thorough follow-up exams of all infants for *two years* after they were born. This is the very reason why epidemiologists use control groups as part of the same study. It's a shell game, ladies and gentlemen, and they have been playing it since Clomid was first marketed in 1967.

"Third. The rat and rabbit teratology studies have little meaning because we had to use several times the human dose before we could produce malformations. Well, you have all heard testimony that, unlike primates, it took many times the human dose of thalidomide to produce malformations in the same animals. So why should this be used to minimize the value of Merrell's teratology studies?

"Fourth – and we have already covered this – there were no monkeys available to use for primate teratology studies with Clomid.

"Fifth. Mark's combination of birth defects, known as 'Moebius syndrome,' were seen over one hundred years ago, so how could Clomid be the cause? Yet, as you've heard, congenital heart defects were also seen 100 years ago, but can be reproduced by teratogenic drugs. Cleft palate was seen over 100 years ago, but can be reproduced by drugs. So what's the point? Only a slight of hand, ladies and gentlemen, that's all it is. Get you looking off in one direction so that you won't see the real story.

"And sixth. In order to produce birth defects, a drug must be introduced during the period of organogenesis. This, of course, ignores the half-life factor, which is exactly what they want you to do. As you have heard, even though taken before conception, Clomid *is* around during the period of organogenesis. You have also heard from their own teratologist, Dr. Wilson, that teratogens, introduced *prior* to organogenesis, have produced malformations in animal studies. He also testified that damage to the embryo, well before limbs start to form, could result in malformed limbs, and that the susceptible period for the human embryo starts as early as day 11 or 12 after conception. Just more slight of hand, ladies and gentlemen. So don't be taken in."

At this point I concluded my closing argument discussing Mark's malformations, the impact they have had on his life, and the lives of his parents, and reminding them what they had seen in the film shown to them weeks earlier. I talked about his medical expenses, past and future, and the impact his disabilities would have on his future earning capacity. I then suggested a number of ways that they could arrive at a fair and just figure for his past and future pain and suffering. Finally, I thanked them for their attention on this important case, not only during my argument, but throughout the lengthy trial. As I sat down, I felt a sense of burden being lifted from my shoulders. I would stand up and talk in this trial only one more time, during my rebuttal argument, and then it would be over. Judge Fredricks would read the jury instructions and the case would be turned over to twelve people to decide the most important case in my career. Next up after the afternoon break – Fred B. Belanger.

At exactly 2:40 PM, Fred B stood, offered the jury his own little smile, and began his pitch. And as Belanger presented his case to the jury, I hurriedly noted each important comment and outlined my response for rebuttal.

His first statement was what I had been waiting a month to hear: he asked that the jury's decision be made without sympathy or passion. This was what the plaintiff was banking on and it should be rejected. My response would be that neither Mark

Breimhorst nor his parents wanted sympathy; they wanted justice. If I had wanted to base our case on sympathy, they would have seen Mark right here in this courtroom. But they never saw him, did they? That's because we have proven our case on its merits.

Belanger next challenged the value of the animal teratology studies. There was a serious question of whether they even produced malformations in either the rat or the rabbit. But they certainly could not be extrapolated to humans. And what was the purpose for insisting on the use of monkeys? If the drug had already proven to be teratogenic on the rat and the rabbit, it would serve no purpose. Besides, Valerio and Courtney did the studies and were unable to produce birth defects.

I would ask, if they were unimportant, why didn't they describe the "limb abnormalities" in the rat studies? Why weren't the photographs of the deformed animals produced? Why didn't they call Dr. Holtkamp, who oversaw the studies, as a witness? *What didn't they want you to see or hear about?* As to the value of primate studies, what did they tell us about thalidomide? Using the drug at the human dose level, at the same time during pregnancy caused the same malformations as experienced by humans. And referencing Valerio and Courtney is another slight of hand. It was a fertility study where only a couple of monkeys were exposed to the drug during pregnancy at a single dose level. James Wilson, there own witness, would not even call it a teratology study.

There was no such thing as a safe drug, Belanger urged. They all have side effects and every prescribing physician in the country will tell you the same thing. On this comment Fred B left himself wide open. All we wanted was a reasonable and adequate warning of the risks of the drug. Telling every prescribing physician and their patients that there was no evidence that Clomid therapy had a deleterious effect on the human fetus did not meet that responsibility.

He dismissed the importance of the case reports after marketing. They lacked the numerator and denominator that existed in the clinical investigations. "Plaintiff wants to make an issue out of a handful of anencephaly cases, which are frequently hereditary, when there are tens of thousands of women out there who have conceived with Clomid over the past seven years."

I would acknowledge that since marketing started, we currently lack the ability to calculate a rate or percentage of anencephaly cases following Clomid. Thus, the eight cases may be just the tip of the iceberg; there may be dozens, even hundreds of unreported cases out there. What was important was that these eight Drug Experience Reports, suspected by the reporting doctors as possibly related to the use of Clomid, might represent that *pattern* that the defense has been talking about throughout this trial. And as we can see, they are refusing to even acknowledge to this day that this might be a *red flag* that needs to be investigated.

Richardson-Merrell brought to testify before the jury two noted and experienced teratologists, Robert Brent and James G. Wilson. Both are respected the world over as eminent experts in their field. Both have analyzed all of the records available, not just from the clinical investigations, but from the world literature as well. And both have concluded unequivocally – not in terms of a *possibility*, as stated by the plaintiffs' sole teratologist – but with certainty, that Clomid is not a human teratogen. Belanger reminded the jury that Clomid was given prior to conception, long before the critical period of organogenesis. Any Clomid that was still present at that time would have been miniscule. The percentage of defects from the clinical studies was the same as in the general population. The few criticisms leveled by plaintiffs about those studies would not have made a meaningful difference in the rate of birth defects and plaintiffs have not presented any evidence that it would. In fact, as Dr. Wilson explained, many of the conditions referred to as "birth defects" are not really congenital abnormalities.

Again I quickly noted my rebuttal. Aside from the obvious embarrassment to Dr. Wilson if Clomid proved to be a human teratogen, my response to the testimony of Wilson and Brent was quite simple. A building, no matter how well otherwise constructed, was only as strong as its foundation. If the foundation was faulty or defective, then the building could still collapse when its integrity was challenged. The results from the pre-market clinical studies provided the primary foundation to Wilson's and Brent's conclusions. But did they examine the actual studies – the original records? No, they reviewed *summaries*. Summaries, I might add, that were prepared by Richardson-Merrell, a company with an obvious bias to receive a clean bill of health. Neither Wilson nor Brent could have known from those summaries all of the deficiencies in the study design, including investigators relying upon birth announcements and letters from the patients to calculate the number of birth defects. Nor would they have known that Merrell calculated the birth defect rate from total pregnancies rather than deliveries to reach a lower percentage.

Humans are more sensitive to teratogens that laboratory animals, and it is absurd to suggest that a given quantity of Clomid circulating in the mother and embryo at 11 or 12 days after conception would be incapable of producing a malformation. Clomid, as we all know now, was the only known environmental element that was present when the cells that could evolve into hands were damaged. Maybe Dr. Wilson chooses not to describe certain infant anomalies from the clinical studies as "birth defects," but Richardson-Merrell has described them as such in its package insert.

At 4:00 PM we broke for the day while Belanger was still in the middle of his closing argument. I would have overnight to refine my comments for rebuttal.

Thursday, April 11, 1974. Today was my fourth anniversary, and it was comforting to know that Janet and I would be able to enjoy the evening with the case finally put to bed and submitted to the jury. Fred B also appeared to be in higher spirits. Perhaps he too appreciated that the trial was drawing to a close. He seemed energized as he stepped up to the podium with his notes, almost out of character for his laid-back and methodical style. But maybe someone had spoken to him. A trial lawyer never wants to telegraph concern if a trial is not going as expected. Was that how he perceived the case at this critical stage? I would never know. Not once had we been approached about discussing settlement.

Belanger's next comments were directed to Tyler's suggestion that he had never been informed of the animal teratology studies prior to marketing of the drug. These studies, and their results, were described in pre-market brochures that were disseminated to all of the investigators. The documents were entitle, "Physician's Drug Monograph," and they were dated January 11, 1965. I would ask, "Where were they? Why did we not see one introduced into evidence?" It is true that an employee of Merrell testified about such an alleged distribution, but Tyler was never shown one and there was no evidence from any investigator of having received one.

Then came the "greatest gift" argument. Clomid was as valuable to society as insulin and penicillin. Without Clomid, thousands of families would never have babies of their own. It was almost a miracle that women, incapable of ovulating and having children of their own blood and lineage, would be able to conceive and deliver their very own babies.

I would respond that insulin and penicillin were life-saving drugs, the lack of which could result in death. It was unfair and unjustified to compare a fertility drug with other pharmaceutical products that were absolutely essential in order to continue living. Clomid is an *elective* drug, which is not essential to one's health. In fact, it is for this very reason that having a comprehensive warning about *all* risks associated with its use is critical. Unlike a drug one might die without, one should be able to make an *informed* choice when considering use of Clomid, or any other fertility drug. I would emphasize that I was not minimizing the joy at having your own child, nor were we contending that every Clomid child would be born with a birth defect. But if using the defendant's product doubled or tripled the risk of a malformed child, the users of Clomid had the right to know this going in.

After Belanger concluded, I stood in front of the jury for the last time and recited my rebuttal, just as I had outlined in my notes. Twenty minutes later, Fredricks was reading the same jury instructions we had all spent a full day crafting. As I listened to the law of California being delivered from the bench, I could not help but feel that with all of the objections, argument, concessions, give and take and agreements between the attorneys and the trial judge, the statements coming from His Honor were balanced and fair to both sides. If I ended up on the losing side of this trial, it would not be for the reason that the jury had been given erroneous or unfair instructions on the law.

Fredricks would read one page, then turn it over and read from the next. They had all been organized into a logical and understandable order. And with each page that he turned, I could feel the tension of the month-long trial slowly peeling away. More and more I was becoming relaxed as it sank in that there was nothing further to be done on my part that could in any way affect the jury's verdict. At 11:40 AM, the case was submitted to the jury for deliberation and decision.

And I had no desire to stick around. My office was only 10 minutes away from the courthouse and the clerk, Elma Ota, had my telephone number. I would be called as soon as the jury had a verdict. I had never enjoyed sitting and standing around the

130

courthouse waiting for a verdict, knowing what was taking place on the other side of the door to the jury room. And today would be no different. Rose, on the other hand, was happy to stay and wait with Ingrid. That was fine with me. It was always nice for the jurors to see, as they filed in and out on their breaks, that the plaintiff and her attorney were interested enough in the outcome that they were still hanging around. Did I truly believe that such strategy would ever impact the final verdict? Not really. But then, why take the chance?

Nervous Time Begins

If the verdict came in this afternoon, it likely would be a defense verdict and I would have no desire to be present. Quick verdicts, especially after a lengthy trial, were almost invariably in favor of the defendant. This was because the plaintiff had to carry the burden of proof, making it more difficult to persuade the panel of jurors to say "yes," and easier for them to say "no." Then, should they find in favor of the plaintiff, they would need to explore the evidence on damages and at least nine of the 12 agree on the same amount to award to that prevailing party. All of this would take time, and after a one month trial, certainly more than an hour or two. No, I would not be there to take the verdict if the jury came in today. Rose could have that dubious privilege. At 4:10 PM the jury broke for the day, not having reached a verdict.

Friday, April 12, 1974. Today was Good Friday, and the jury would be released by Fredricks at noon if they still did not have a decision. As I had on Thursday afternoon, I remained in my office all morning anxiously waiting for a call from the courthouse, probably from Rose. And each time the phone would ring my heart would quicken its beat and I would feel a rush of anxiety. My secretary, more often than not, would be able to deal with the matter from the caller. On other occasions she would buzz me on the intercom, which would raise my level of anxiety another notch. Yet not once did I get the call, and with each added hour I felt that we had an increased chance for a victory. At about 12:15 PM I got a call from Rose to tell me that the jury still had not reached a verdict and had been released for the weekend. For the next two and one half days I would be able to breathe again.

Monday, April 15, 1974. It was income tax day, but that was the last thing on my mind as the jury commenced deliberations again at 9:15 AM. Again, just like Friday, I would jump with every phone call. I didn't have to wait long. At precisely 11:30 AM I got the call from Rose. They had a verdict. I hurriedly got down to my car and drove over to the courthouse.

I greeted Rose and Ingrid at the entrance to Department "D." It seemed that they were not doing much better than I. I asked Rose whether there had been any requests or questions from the jury during deliberations. Sometimes a jury would ask for testimony to be read or a jury instruction explained. This would often provide a clue as to where they were going. There had been none. Rose queried me about the length of time the jury had been out. All combined, it had been less than a day and a half. I told her I was a little uncomfortable about the brevity of the deliberations, but who knows? We hurriedly took our seats at counsel table, joining Belanger and Swanson. The Merrell entourage was also present, seated in the back of the courtroom. With all counsel present and accounted for, Elma called in the jury.

The Verdict

As the jurors filed out of their sanctuary, taking their seats in the jury box, I was frozen, unwilling to look at their faces. Instead I stared at the empty bench. I was almost holding my breath, my breathing somewhat shallow. We were all standing, as had been the tradition when the jurors entered and exited the jury box. My knees felt weak, waiting to be relieved of holding me up.

Taking a verdict had always made me feel a little anxious before, but I had never experienced anything like this. What was going on? I concluded that I had wanted this verdict more than anything else in my professional life. Careers had been made on less important cases. I also thought of little Mark Breimhorst back at home with the babysitter. If Rose and I were able to hand him a large check, it wouldn't magically reproduce his hands, but it no doubt would help make life easier in the difficult years ahead. Perhaps I would have played a major role in brightening his future. Yes, I wanted this verdict so bad I could taste it.

With the jury seated, Fredricks promptly entered and took the bench. He noted for the record everyone that was present and turned to the jury.

"I understand you have a verdict?" he asked, with his ever-present smile.

The foreman, Clifford Kette, rose from his seat and said, "Yes we have, your honor."

"Very well. Hand it to the clerk, please."

Elma went over to the box and accepted the verdict form, then took it over to Judge Fredricks for his review. I am sure that this all occurred with relative quickness, but to me it was all happening in slow motion. My heart was pounding so hard I could almost feel it in my chest. Fredricks scanned the verdict and then stared down directly at me. Was he saying, "Sorry, fella, you just got dumped"? I couldn't tell. It was straight deadpan – and only for a brief moment. But it was as if he wanted to say something to me. Instead he handed the form back to Elma and instructed, "The clerk will read the verdict."

Elma turned to everyone, with the verdict held in front of her like the town crier of old. My heart rate by now had to be up to 120, as she read:

" 'We, the jury in the above entitled action, find for the plaintiff, Mark Breimhorst, by and through his Guardian ad Litem, Ingrid Breimhorst, and against the defendant, Richardson-Merrell, Incorporated, a corporation, and assess damages in the sum of $530,000.00, and we further find for the plaintiffs, Ingrid Breimhorst and Heinz Breimhorst, and against the defendant, Richardson-Merrell, Incorporated, a corporation, and assess their damages in the sum of $40,000.00.' Signed by C.D. Kette, Foreman."

I suddenly felt a rush of emotion – not to mention relief – and immediately wanted to hug my two partners, Rose and Ingrid. But the ritual was not yet over. Fredricks next had the jury polled. Each juror was asked by name if this was his or her verdict, and each responded with a "yes." Although a verdict of only nine of 12 was necessary, the decision had been unanimous. Fredricks complimented and thanked the jurors for their service and informed them that they were released and now could talk about the case, if that was their choice. His Honor then vacated the bench[43] and I finally had the opportunity to do my hugging and congratulating.

In the midst of all this jubilation, someone suddenly approached me and extended his hand. It was Fred B. Belanger. "Congratulations," he said. "You did a very good job for your clients."

This was an act of class I had never experienced before. And it no doubt hurt. Especially after the earlier thalidomide verdict, Fred and his firm would likely lose Merrell as a client. Yet there he stood congratulating and complementing his adversary. It would not be something I would soon, if ever, forget. I was so stunned that all I could do was take his hand and say, "Well, thanks, Fred." He then disappeared into the crowd.

As we started for the door to catch up to the jury, I began to wonder about the amount of the verdict. After hearing that the jury had found for the plaintiff, the numbers had become somewhat obscure. I asked Rose for clarification. It totaled $570,000,[44] she enthusiastically assured. This had been the best day of them all.

* * * * *

CHAPTER 4

The Chromosome Factor

Mark Breimhorst had been born without hands, a partial palsy involving the left side of his face, and metatarsus varus of his right foot. But like the vast majority of infants born with congenital malformations, he had *normal* chromosomes. Thus, when it was discovered that there was twice the expected frequency of Down syndrome during the pre-market studies, it had been seen at the time as something important but of little use in the case. Down syndrome is always caused by an *abnormal* chromosome.

By the fall of 1974, Breimhorst had settled in lieu of an appeal of the plaintiffs' verdict. Although I had been retained on two new cases at the time, they likewise did not involve chromosomal anomalies. Yet the possible association between use of Clomid and Down syndrome still loomed as an important question. Was Clomid capable of damaging or altering chromosomes? If so, it did not seem to be a stretch to assume that it might also be capable of damaging genes (within the chromosomes) or otherwise inhibiting the growth of embryonic organs. As I would later learn, whether a drug is *mutagenic*[45] is a factor that is used in assessing its likelihood of being a human teratogen. For the first time, I began to immerse myself into serious medical research on Clomid and other fertility drugs. I started by hiring the services of a medical researcher.

Down Syndrome

Merrell reported 5 cases of Down syndrome (mongolism) during the clinical investigations. The incidence thus equated to *at least* one in every 377 deliveries (5 out of 1,886). Preliminary research revealed that the incidence in the general population ranged between 1 in every 600 to 1,200 births, depending upon the study and the average age of the population studied. The incidence was, at a minimum, approaching twice the expected frequency. The numbers were also *statistically significant.*

Although I did not know it at the time, Drs. Oakley and Flynt from the Centers for Disease Control (CDC) had done a statistical analysis of the combined cases of Down syndrome occurring during the pre-market investigational series with Clomid (5 cases) and Pergonal (1 case). Pergonal is human menopausal gonadotropin (hMG) and another fertility drug used to induce ovulation. They reported their findings in abstract form in 1972.[46] An "abstract" is a summary of the full-blown study. Since the incidence of

Down syndrome increases with advancing maternal age, Oakley and Flynt calculated the expected rate after adjusting for the average age in the two populations. They determined that there had been 6 cases reported when only 2.6 would have been expected. Based upon their statistical calculations, the probability of these numbers occurring by chance were less then five percent (P = .049). Five percent or less is generally accepted as the threshold for concluding that the results of an epidemiological study are "statistically significant." The higher-than-expected rate was thus not due to age. But two[47] of the six cases involved mothers who had not conceived during a treatment cycle. For this reason, they surmised that "the increased risk may not be a function of the therapy but may be a function of the abnormal physiology for which the women were treated." This would become a frequent argument I would hear over the years: women with infertility problems have a physiological abnormality to begin with, and are more inclined to have abnormal embryos than women without infertility.

However, when Oakley published another paper in 1979,[48] he seemed a little more concerned about a causal association between Down syndrome and the use of fertility drugs.

> "Clomiphene citrate is an ovulation-inducing drug. Chromosomal anomalies (Down's syndrome) are more common among infants born to women *treated with ovulation-inducing agents*. * * * The association with *treated* infertility has been strengthened by two other studies which reported three infants with Down's syndrome among 373 infants born to treated women. Thus in the pre-marketing studies and the two additional cohort[49] studies, 9 of 2702 (3.3 per 1000) infants born to women treated for infertility had Down's syndrome, which is about *three times the incidence in the general population*. The incidence of Down's syndrome in this group is therefore similar to that in 36 year old women. Hard data for risk of Down's syndrome among infertile women by age do not exist. A working hypothesis is that the risk lies in the range between three times the risk at a given age and 3.3 per thousand." [Emphasis added.]

Oakley's later uncertainty about the role of infertility is reflected by his comment on the lack of data about the incidence of Down syndrome among women experiencing that condition. The only accurate way to assign infertility as a risk factor for Down syndrome is to conduct a properly-designed study to make that assessment. Until controlled studies have clearly demonstrated ovulatory dysfunction as a risk factor for Down syndrome, it would seem unwise to *assume* that to be the case. As will be seen later, there are other reasons to exclude ovulatory dysfunction as a cause of chromosomal anamolies.

From this early research, I learned that as many as 95% of the Down syndrome cases are caused by trisomy of chromosome 21. Except for the germ cells (ovum and sperm), there are normally 23 pairs of chromosomes in every cell of the body. Each pair is numbered from 1 to 23, with the smallest being assigned the highest number. Trisomy 21 exists when there are three, rather than two, of the number 21 chromosomes. The abnormality is not considered to be an inherited condition and can develop in the ovum (egg) at or near the time of ovulation, but prior to conception.

Trisomy 21 occurs when one of the pairs of number 21 chromosomes fails to divide (nondisjunction) during meiosis[50] and forms one single cell egg with 22 chromosomes and another with 24 chromosomes (rather than 23). Upon conception with the 24-chromosome cell, there are 47 chromosomes (three 21s) in the resulting conceptus, now called a "zygote." Thus, when Down syndrome is caused by trisomy 21, it can be precipitated by some event or condition in the maternal environment occurring at around the time of ovulation.

As mentioned above, there is also a direct correlation between maternal age at the time of conception and the incidence of Down syndrome. As women become older, the frequency of Down syndrome in their pregnancies increases. Up to age 25, the incidence is approximately 1 in every 2,000 deliveries. However, when conception occurs at 45 years of age, the incidence is at least 1 in every 50 births.[51] The closer women get to menopause, the more frequent the occurrence of Down syndrome. Among the possibilities I initially considered was whether Clomid was capable of reproducing an environment in the ovaries and/or fallopian tubes that approximated the condition of those organs in a woman approaching menopause.

On this question, my research assistant came up with an important discovery. In 1973, a Dr. Judith Ford published a study entitled, "Induction of Chromosomal Errors."[52] She demonstrated through in-vitro (test tube) studies that by elevating the pH[53] in cultures of actively dividing fetal fibroblasts (connective tissue cells from a fetus), she was able to induce numerical chromosomal errors, including *trisomy 21*. She suggested that these errors could occur soon after ovulation, producing an abnormal gamete or after conception, "giving rise to chromosomal mosaicism in the zygote." She noted that *reduced estrogen levels* can lead to an increase in the pH in the oviduct (fallopian tube). This condition, she postulated, could produce chromosomal errors in vivo (within the body). "I now suggest that low maternal estrogen levels very early in pregnancy may be of clinical significance in determining the risk of fetal chromosomal abnormalities." This proposition is consistent with the increased frequency of Down syndrome as older women experience a decline in the production of estrogen.

Recalling the testimony from Edward Tyler during the Breimhorst trial, I was aware that Clomid initially acted as an *antiestrogen* at around the time of ovulation. That Clomid has both *antiestrogenic* and *estrogenic* actions is verified in the drug's current package insert. "Available data suggest that both the estrogenic and antiestrogenic properties of clomiphene may participate in the initiation of ovulation. The two clomiphene isomers have been found to have mixed estrogenic and antiestrogenic effects, which may vary from one species to the other."[54]

It was no surprise when I learned that Clomid could produce a side effect quite familiar to most women entering menopause.

"A common side effect of Clomid therapy is the vasomotor phenomenon designated as hot flashes, *similar to those associated with menopause*. Hot flashes occurred in 271 patients; this symptom was present in 11% of women who had multiple short courses of Clomid (7 days or less), but in only 3% taking only a single short course."[55] [Emphasis added.]

Not only does Clomid cause antiestrogenic action (e.g., inhibition of estrogen production), it is involved in the process of initiating ovulation. It would thus occur at or near the time the ovary releases the ovum (egg) for its journey down the fallopian tube.

Could this be causing chromosomal errors in the ovum at this critical point in time? Could the antiestrogenic effect of Clomid produce an increased pH in the oviduct, in turn causing chromosomal anomalies in the egg? If so, Clomid would also be responsible for producing first trimester spontaneous abortions (SAs).

Spontaneous Abortions

A high percentage of SAs occurring during the first 3 months of pregnancy have abnormal chromosomes and other abnormalities of the embryo and fetus. In fact, abnormal chromosomes are responsible for up to to 60% of early SAs in women not using fertility drugs.[56] About half of the remaining abortuses with normal chromosomes have observable anomalies of the embryo/fetus.[57] First trimester SAs are thus nature's screening mechanism to purge the body of a human conceptus that either could not survive at term or would be born with major abnormalities. Later SAs tend to be more related to the inability of the uterine environment to maintain the pregnancy, rather than anomalies of the fetus.

The question of whether Clomid is mutagenic would seem to be addressed and answered in another critically important early study. Joelle and Andre Boue of France reported in the March 24, 1973 edition of *The Lancet* (pp.679-680) on a chromosomal study they had been conducting on the products of human first trimester spontaneous abortions. [Exhibit 1] When sent to me by my medical researcher, the title of the paper quickly caught my attention. "Increased Frequency of Chromosomal Anomalies in Abortions After Induced Ovulation."

Looking only at these early SAs, the patients were divided into four groups. Group one involved women who had conceived during a treatment cycle with fertility drugs, including clomiphene citrate; group two conceived 1 cycle after last treatment with these drugs; group three conceived 2 or more cycles after the last treatment; and group four included women who had *not* been treated with fertility drugs. The results were striking. Of the abortuses from groups one and two, 83% and 86%, respectively, had abnormal chromosomes, whereas only 61% and 60% of groups 3 and 4, respectively, had abnormal chromosomes. There was a one-third increase in abnormal chromosomes when conception occurred within one cycle of being treated with a fertility drug. The mean age of all four groups was the same and the differences were statistically significant.

The increased errors included trisomies, as seen with Down syndrome, although the numbers for this subgroup of anomalies were not large enough to be significant. Group one included 23 abortuses with trisomies out of 47 SAs (48.9%); group two had 7 out of 14 SAs (50.0%); group three had 9 out of 23 SAs (39.1%); and group four had 441 out of 1374 SAs (32.1%). Importantly, group three was comprised of infertility patients and had the same percentage of total defects as non-fertility patients. This would tend to argue against the underlying infertility condition being responsible for the increase. The authors suggested that the fertility drugs were responsible. "A prospective study of 473 women has shown that (induction of ovulation) may increase the risk of having a conceptus with chromosomal anomalies."

The association between the use of Clomid and damage to chromosomes finds further support in another study published during the enlightening year of 1973. This one was entitled, "The Endometrial Karyotypic Profiles of Women after Clomiphene Citrate Therapy."[58] The authors of the study (Charles, et al.) examined tissue from the endometrium (lining of the uterus) of women exposed to Clomid (clomiphene citrate). The tissue was examined for any chromosomal anomalies both before and after treatment with the drug. They reported "a highly significant increase ($P<0.01$) in abnormal chromosome counts...." The odds of the abnormalities occurring by chance were less than one in a hundred. The authors concluded that the clomiphene therapy was the cause of the chromosomal alterations. "It therefore appeared that clomiphene therapy changed the relative frequency with which structurally altered chromosomes were observed and induced a statistically significant transformation to a heteroploid (abnormal number of chromosomes) profile." They termed the drug a "clastogen" (capable of causing a genetic mutation or chromosomal breakage).

This study takes on added significance when one considers that a high correlation has been found between presence of a chromosomally abnormal endometrium and the occurrence of a chromosomally abnormal abortus. In a paper published in 1970,[59] Arakaki and Waxman reported on a study in which they examined the chromosomes of endometrial tissue and abortuses of pregnancies resulting in spontaneous abortions. Although the numbers are small, they found that when the endometrium was chromosomally abnormal, 100% of the abortuses from the same women also had chromosomal anomalies. At the very least, this might suggest that a drug capable of inducing chromosomal anomalies in the endometrium may also be capable of inducing similar abnormalities in the unfertilized egg at or near the time it is being expelled by the follicle of the ovary.

For about three months now, I had been accumulating medical research. I would send my researcher a topic or medical question and she would hit Medline, a research tool containing a database of medical abstracts. She would then send me a list of citations, along with copies of the abstracts. After an assessment of each abstract, I would order the complete paper on the ones I considered useful. The whole procedure was time-consuming and frequently resulted in a dead end. I would struggle through a paper, invariably reading it two or three times – often referring to my medical dictionary. When I finally grasped a full understanding of the text, the vast majority of the time I would end up tossing it aside with an appropriate expletive reflecting my frustration. Yet every once in awhile I would come across a gem. The Boue and Charles articles were a couple of diamonds.

Neural Tube Defects

When I had gone as far as I could on Down syndrome and SAs, I decided to explore the possible association between Clomid and *neural tube defects* (NTDs). By the end of 1974, Merrell had received a total of 52 Drug Experience Reports (DERs) from the medical profession related to birth defects. Out of that total, 14 (26.9%) of them involved NTDs (including 11 cases of anencephaly). Considering the multiple types and forms of congenital anomalies described in the medical literature, it still seemed that NTDs represented an excessively-high proportion of the total defects reported. Each DER also reflected an opinion of the reporting physician that there might be an association between the use of Clomid and the resulting NTD.

Some of the NTD reports even found their way into the published literature. One such paper was by Drs. Dyson and Kohler, who reported on two separate cases.[60] The first patient (Merrell no.21983) had taken 100 mg. of Clomid per day for 5 days during the conception cycle and later delivered an anencephalic female with cervical (neck) spina bifida. The second patient (Merrell no.21984) had ingested 100 mg. of Clomid per day for 5 days one cycle before conception, but also took two similar courses *after* she had conceived. She delivered an anencephalic male at approximately 37 weeks. After discussing some of the possible causes of these two cases, the authors made the following comments.

"We think, however, that the possibility of a causal relationship between ovulation-stimulation treatment and (central nervous system) abnormality should not be dismissed lightly. If additional evidence is found for this hypothesis, the question arises whether, in case 1, the ovum was damaged before implantation or even before fertilization."

Additional reports in the literature followed. On August 18, 1973, another NTD case history involving Clomid appeared in *The Lancet*,[61] this one reporting on a male anencephalic baby with "very severe spina bifida extending down as far as the lumbar spine." The author postulated that perhaps the anomaly was caused by an abnormal delay between ovulation and conception, since the manufacturer had assured that there was no evidence that Clomid could cause anencephaly. Yet another case report appeared in the same publication two months later,[62] involving a male infant with anencephaly. The mother had conceived during a treatment cycle with Clomid (100 mg/day for 5 days).

I also reviewed the cases from the Clomid pre-market investigations. Because of the numerous deficiencies in the design of the studies, the numbers would have little meaning. But I wanted to be assured that there were at least *some* NTDs included among the reported 58 birth defects. There were three of them: two cases of meningomyelocele (incomplete closure of the vertebral column with resulting exposure of the meninges and spinal cord) and associated hydrocephaly (accumulation of cerebrospinal fluid in the brain);[63] and one case of spina bifida occulta.[64]

By January 1975 my researcher was working on the new assignment.

The most compelling evidence related to a correlation between the incidence of anencephaly and dizygotic (fraternal) twinning. There is little question that Clomid and other fertility drugs cause multiple ova to be expelled at the time of ovulation. When conception occurs with two or more of the eggs, you have fraternal twins – or worse. Out of 1,886 delivered pregnancies during the clinical investigations, 186 (9.86%) of them involved multiple births; one out of every ten. Of that total, 165 were twins; 11 were triplets; 7 were quadruplets; and 3 were quintuplets.[65] Cases of sextuplets have also been reported.[66] If there is anything all fertility specialists can agree on, it's that fertility drugs can cause multiple ova and multiple births.

As early as 1966, Stevenson and others took a close look at the incidence of anencephaly and its relationship to dizygotic twinning. In this major study on birth defects,[67] they found a positive correlation between the two. The importance of this finding was highlighted 8 years later by a Dr. J. Mark Elwood, an epidemiologist out of Ottawa University in Canada. Responding to the suggestion that subfertility was possibly responsible for the above-reported cases of anencephaly, he made the following statement.[68]

> "(D)izygotic twinning rates and anencephaly incidence would be expected to be negatively correlated between populations, whereas in the only international study where both were ascertained by similar methods a positive correlation of 0.578 (P<0.01) between 24 centres was found. This latter finding suggests the alternative hypothesis that dizygotic twinning, which is due to double ovulation, and anencephaly may be associated, and *perhaps clomiphene acts via a mechanism which increases the risk of both.* * * * Obviously more information on the relationships between twinning, fertility, and neural-tube defects is desirable, and *the possibility of a teratogenic effect of clomiphene should not be ignored.*" [Emphasis added.]

If anencephaly occurs more frequently in the presence of dizygotic twinning, it would indeed be suggestive that both are being produced by a common mechanism. Could Clomid and other fertility drugs be that mechanism?

Only a month after the Elwood paper, another article seemed to add strength to the premise. Although it appeared in a psychiatric publication,[69] the reported history of the patient was stunning. The 26 year old woman had conceived with the use of human menopausal gonadotropin (Pergonal) and began to deliver in her sixth month of pregnancy. Her attending physician had suspected that she might be carrying triplets. But as it turned out, he wasn't even half right. On March 17, 1972, she delivered septuplets, *two of which were anencephalic.* Two of the seven were stillborn, and the other five died within 12 hours.

Like clomiphene, Pergonal is used to stimulate ovulation. However, it is a much more potent drug. Whereas Clomid is administered as a tablet, hMG is injected. It also has twice the frequency of multiple births (20%), of which twenty-five percent involve 3 or more concepti.[70] And it shares the common side effects of ovarian hyperstimulation syndrome (OHSS) and elevated estrogen levels.

As I analyzed the literature, I recalled the theory I had developed during the Breimhorst trial. In terms of the drug itself, Clomid would be at its strongest concentration at the earliest stage of any pregnancy it had produced. One of the first organs to form is the neural groove (days 18-22), which folds into the neural tube and later becomes the spinal column and skull. If clomiphene citrate and/or its metabolites are indeed teratogenic, it would likely attack the neural tube the hardest, and inhibit its closure when the drug was at its most potent level. It would thus not be surprising to see these cases appearing first in the literature.

But from my reading I learned that NTDs were considered to be caused by several different factors. The etiology (cause) of NTDs was said to be "multifactorial." Could one of the factors be *abnormal chromosomes?* If so, NTDs might be caused – at least some of them – in the same manner as cases of Down syndrome. Again my researcher provided me with some valuable information.

Although chromosomal *triploidy* (three sets of 23 chromosomes) had been found in embryos with isolated neural tube closure defects,[71] most reported cases associated with abnormal chromosomes involved *trisomies*.[72] At the time, we were unable to discover any incidence figures; the percentage of NTDs that could be attributed to chromosomal defects. But more recent studies have shown that 7-10% of NTDs involve abnormal chromosomes, most of them with trisomy 18.[73]

Maternal age was also a risk factor. Epidemiologic studies had shown that there was an increase in the incidence of NTDs above the maternal age of 35.[74] Although this increase was not as pronounced and dramatic as that seen with Down syndrome, it was large enough to be significant. Since it was accepted that there was a multifactorial etiology for NTDs, including chromosomal anomalies, one would not expect the large increase that one finds with Down syndrome – which is *always* related to abnormal chromosomes. Perhaps Clomid was capable of causing NTDs in two separate and distinct ways: one as a *teratogen* acting directly on the developing embryo; and one as a *mutagen* acting indirectly on the ovum.

To my simplistic way of looking at things at the time, all of the pieces of an otherwise complex puzzle were falling into place. Everything I was putting together made sense; it all seemed to fit. In a certain percentage of women exposed to Clomid, the antiestrogenic effect created an environment in the sex organs similar to women approaching menopause. This condition in turn produced chromosomal anomalies in the ova, prior to conception, leading to an increase in first trimester spontaneous abortions, Down syndrome and, to a lesser degree, neural tube defects.

But what was I going to do with this? Neither of my cases involved Down syndrome nor NTDs, nor did either child have abnormal chromosomes.

Actually, the answer was quite simple. In early 1975, hundreds of thousands of women were using Clomid to conceive. And all of them were facing an unknown risk of having a child born with birth defects. Whether it was a fifty percent increased risk, or twice the risk, or three times the risk, I did not know at the time. But everything was telling me that there was evidence about the drug's potential teratogenicity that was not being disseminated to the ultimate user, or even to her prescribing physician. A 27-year-old woman using Clomid would not appreciate that she was facing the same risk of delivering a Down syndrome child as a 36 year old woman without the drug. A young couple might want to know that they may have to face the emotion of delivering an anencephalic child or the medical expense of a surviving infant with spina bifida. More importantly, many women using Clomid to conceive could actually become pregnant without the drug. It might be more difficult and take longer, but there is little question that many physicians were prescribing Clomid to simply *facilitate* pregnancy; to make it easier to conceive. What if it was possible to save infants from being born with congenital anomalies?

Bottom line: however high or low the increased risk of having a child with a birth defect, every patient had a right to know the true level of that risk. Maybe I might be able to reach a sympathetic ear at the FDA. Maybe I had accumulated enough evidence to reach someone that might insist on some form of a warning. I had absolutely no idea of what I would be facing, but I knew I had to make the effort.

* * * * *

CHAPTER 5

An Invitation to Rockville, Maryland

In January 1975, I began to hammer the FDA with a series of letters requesting that Clomid be pulled from the market. Based upon evidence presented at the Breimhorst trial and later medical research, I was convinced that it was causing birth defects. I was also determined to do something about it. It was my view back then that all I had to do was collect some persuasive evidence, forward it to the FDA, and the federal agency would take it from there.

Looking back now, I was quite naïve.

My effort to generate action out of the FDA, however, is illuminating and worth a brief history lesson. At the time, I had a good idea of who I wanted to talk to. Her name was Frances Kelsey, a pharmacologist that had been with the FDA for over 14 years. I was aware of her name and reputation, and was convinced that she was someone that might take action. Her history[75] with the FDA will explain why.

Frances O. Kelsey, M.D., Ph.D.

Kelsey joined the FDA in August 1960 as a medical officer. One month later, Richardson-Merrell (the same company) submitted an application for approval of its drug, Kevadon, which was assigned to the newly-arrived pharmacologist. The drug was to be used for the treatment of insomnia. Under federal law at the time, the FDA only had 60 days to review the drug application. However, if the medical officer determined that the submission was inadequate, the pharmaceutical company had to resubmit it with additional data and the 60-day clock would start again.

Kelsey was having legitimate concerns about the drug. The clinical studies had been poorly designed, the chronic toxicity studies had not covered a long enough period of time, and the absorption and excretion data were inadequate. Each time Merrell would submit additional data Kelsey would find problems with it and reject the application. Soon she began receiving complaining calls from Merrell, and even visits from its representative. All were designed to put pressure on her. Complaints were lodged with Kelsey's superiors, urging that she was being unreasonable and the drug's approval delayed unnecessarily. But still she resisted.

Merrell pointed out that the drug was already marketed in Europe and there were no problems in spite of its widespread use. In some countries it was even sold over the counter. But in December 1960, Kelsey read an article in a medical journal that reported some cases of peripheral neuritis in patients using the drug. She suspected that if Kevadon might be damaging nerves, it might also pose some danger to a developing fetus. Many women in Europe were also using it for morning sickness. Kelsey became even more resistant to Merrell's continuing pressure, and insisted on still more studies to satisfy her that the drug was safe.

By late 1961 Merrell was beside itself. This had now been dragging on for over a year. What more could Kelsey want? As part of a pre-market clinical study, it had distributed Kevadon to over 1,000 physicians throughout the United States without any demonstrated ill effects. She was being absolutely unreasonable, and a single low-level medical officer should not have the power to stop an important drug in its tracks without proof that there were significant adverse reactions from its use.

But in November 1961, the world would learn that Kevadon did indeed have serious side effects. A German pediatrician, Widukind Lenz,[76] made a startling discovery about a series of children who had been born with a rare, if not unique, congenital malformation. Many had shortened and absent limbs. Some had toes extending from their hips, others with hands protruding from their shoulders. Malformations of internal organs, eyes and ears were also seen. Lenz had found a common denominator. All had been exposed to Kevadon during the first trimester of pregnancy.

The generic name for Kevadon was *thalidomide*.

This single low-level medical officer had prevented a national disaster. Although 17 children had been born in the United States with congenital anomalies due to thalidomide, the number in Europe and other countries was over a staggering 10,000. On August 7, 1962, President John F. Kennedy awarded Kelsey with the Distinguished Federal Civilian Service award, the highest honor that can be given to a United States civilian.[77]

The actions of Kelsey had also been a catalyst to the enactment of new laws related to the safety and efficacy of drugs. Recognizing that the country had just ducked a bullet, Congress took immediate action in 1962, when it (unanimously) passed the

Kefauver-Harris Amendments to the Federal Food, Drug and Cosmetic Act. For the first time ever, pharmaceutical companies now had to demonstrate not only that the drug was safe,[78] but *effective* as well. Measures to insure safety were also improved. Patients used in clinical trials were required to sign informed consent forms, advising them of all possible known risks. Adverse reaction reports were now required to be reported to the FDA and laws on drug advertising mandated that complete information on a drug be set out in the text, including its risks. Additional FDA regulations were created to implement the changes in the law.

Yes, I was well-acquainted with the name of Frances Kelsey. And on January 13, 1975, I sent her the first of several letters to the FDA.

I explained who I was, including my involvement in the Clomid litigation. I then summarized my reasons for believing Clomid to be a human teratogen. Among other things, I cited the high incidence of spontaneous abortions during the pre-market clinical investigations and the published study out of France which found a higher incidence of abnormal chromosomes in abortuses of women treated with fertility drugs. This was followed with a request. "Under all of the above-mentioned circumstances, it is strongly urged that serious consideration be given to removing Clomid (clomiphene citrate) from the market until such time, at the very least, that further studies are conducted to ascertain whether or not this drug is in fact altering chromosomes." I then waited for her reply.

Over a month later (February 25, 1975), Dr. Kelsey finally responded – beginning with an apology for the long delay. She had forwarded my letter to the Division of Metabolism and Endocrine Drug Products, and requested the members of that division to reply to the questions I had raised. She explained that this was the division within the FDA that was responsible for monitoring Clomid. Perhaps now the FDA would take some action.

Again I waited.

By March 21, 1975, I was out of patience and shot off a second letter, this one directed to the Division of Metabolism and Endocrine Drug Products. I now presented a strong argument of why I believed that Clomid was causing Down syndrome, with a full analysis of the data and published studies in support of my contention. My attached 6-

page presentation had the dubious title, "Conclusive Evidence Establishing Clomid (Clomiphene Citrate) as a Cause of Down Syndrome (Mongolism)."

For the first time I also made a commentary on the pre-market clinical studies. "I have a lot to say concerning the gross inadequacy of the clinical investigations done on Clomid, insofar as evaluating its potential teratogenic effect on human beings. As mentioned in my previous letter, I will be pleased to speak with anyone by telephone, in writing or even fly to Washington D.C. to confer with anyone on this matter. I am firmly convinced that the true incidence of birth defects which actually occurred during the clinical investigations is significantly higher than those reported by Richardson-Merrell. This opinion is based upon the method employed in documenting and counting birth defects, rather than any evidence of suppression of records or reports." The letter was sent by certified mail.

And still I waited.

By May 9, 1975, I was at a low – no, medium – boil. It had been almost *four months* since my first letter to Dr. Kelsey. It was time to test my skills at penetrating a federal bureaucracy. The first step was to target a name, rather than a department title. Sending a letter to a division within the FDA provided a built-in excuse for anyone who found it sitting on his desk. "It never got to me," could easily be recited with some degree of credibility. I sought out the identity of the head of the division, and came up with a Dr. Edwin Ortiz.

Next I needed something with some teeth in it. Some form of overt threat. Bureaucrats hate accountability. So I had to set up the potential risk of being embarrassed or, even worse, chastised for ignoring the responsibilities of his job title. After summarizing the frustrating history of my earlier efforts, I concluded with the following promise. "Before submitting this matter to Senator Edward Kennedy's subcommittee on health, it is my sincere hope that some decision be made by the FDA on what course of action to follow concerning Clomid, and that I be contacted relative to the inquiries made in this letter and my prior correspondence. If I have failed to hear from you within two weeks from the date of this letter, I will assume that it is your intention to continue ignoring my inquiries and to continue disregarding the studies and information submitted, and will proceed to seek some action from Congress." The letter was also sent by certified mail.

That got someone's attention.

Within 10 days I was called by a Dr. A.T. Gregoire, the Executive Secretary of the Obstetrics and Gynecology Advisory Committee to the FDA. He informed me that the issue concerning a possible relationship between Clomid and Down syndrome had been set on the advisory committee's agenda for its July 22, 1975 hearing (later changed to July 18, 1975). The material I had previously sent would be distributed to each member of the committee for their consideration.

Oh, and one more thing. I was *invited to make an oral presentation.*

In addition to its employed physicians, scientists, technicians and other staff members, the FDA also functions in conjunction with various advisory committees. For each therapeutic category of drug or device, there is an advisory committee; today approximately fifty of them. Each committee meets 4 to 6 times a year, two days at a time. Every one is composed of a panel of nationally-prominent members of the medical and scientific community, drawn primarily (though not exclusively) from the designated specialty. Its function is to advise and make recommendations, which the FDA customarily follows, although not legally required to do so. I had been asked to persuade this advisory panel that Clomid was causing Down syndrome in the offspring of its users.

Think of a lawyer walking into a neurosurgeon's office and offering advice on how to perform brain surgery. I could already hear the snickers and see the smiles as I pitched my case. Somebody had evidently come up with a great idea. "Want to get rid of this pesty Mix character? Let him plead his position to an advisory committee. He'll be laughed out of the room." It was one thing to submit papers expressing theories and citing medical publications in support of them. It was quite another matter to stand in front of these highly skilled professionals and field their pointed and challenging questions. Was I insane?

Apparently so. Without much thought, I accepted Dr. Gregoire's invitation and committed myself to certain humiliation. My thought was, however, that the more I could give the committee members in writing, the less they would have to inquire about – and the less pain I would suffer. Gregoire agreed that I could send as much written material as

I desired, as long as I provided 20 copies of each presentation. All material had to be received no later than July 3, 1975.

On June 17, 1975, I sent off my fourth letter to the FDA, this one addressed to Dr. Gregoire. Enclosed were twenty copies of a presentation entitled, "Pre-market Testing of Clomid Inadequate and Totally Invalid as a Basis to Determine Teratogenicity." This was my first effort to lay out my case about all of the deficiencies in the pre-market animal and clinical studies. It was also something about which I had some level of knowledge and expertise, and was quite comfortable in presenting. Challenging these studies had been successfully pulled off during the Breimhorst trial, and arguing carelessness and corporate irresponsibility is what trial lawyers do best.

My nine-page paper was broken down into two subcategories: animal studies and clinical studies. Under the subheading, "Clinical Studies," I recited all of the known deficiencies of the clinical investigations I had discovered to date: the impossibility of comparing the worldwide Clomid study with another population using comparable ethnic groups in the same countries; the lack of uniformity in the type and nature of examinations of the babies; the lack of a definition of "birth defect;" the lack of follow-up examinations of the infants; the fact that most of the Clomid pregnancies were delivered by outside clinics and physicians; and, finally, the trial testimony of Dr. Edward Tyler, describing how he relied upon his patients voluntarily informing him about the outcome of their pregnancies.

My fifth and final letter to the FDA was sent on July 2, 1975. Included was further material on the contended association between Clomid and Down syndrome. For the first time, I also argued the likely causal relationship between clomiphene citrate and neural tube defects. By now I was doing my own medical research, and the information and data on NTDs had taken longer than I had expected – but I had still squeezed it in under the wire.

My presentations had also taken the shape of a scientific hypothesis. Not only was I trying to convince the FDA that Clomid was a human teratogen, I was so presumptuous as to suggest *how* it was taking place. To put this in perspective, medical science in 1975 had yet to determine the *mechanism* by which most teratogens exacted their altering influence on human embryos – including thalidomide. They knew from epidemiology studies, and other evidence, that certain environmental agents were teratogenic; they just didn't know how or why. In fact, when teratologist Thomas Shepard set out the "Criteria for Proof of Human Teratogenicity" in his 1992 text,[79] while including as a criterion that "the association should make biologic sense," he added that such proof was "helpful but not essential."

Was I now ready for my encounter with the advisory committee? Probably not, but I had put together the best possible case from what I could find. I was also not a scientist, and was feeling increasingly like a fish out of water as the big day approached. Hopefully, something good would come out of the experience.

* * * * *

CHAPTER 6

Selling the Mix Hypothesis

July 18, 1975 was forecast to be a hot and sultry day in Washington D.C. As my wife and I left our hotel and jumped into the rental car, I could tell that the weatherman was not going to let us down. It was no later than 7:45 AM and the temperature was already pushing into the upper seventies. I also had sweat beading up on my forehead, although I was uncertain if it was from the heat outside – or the heat inside that I would shortly be facing in nearby Rockville, Maryland.

I kicked on the engine and directed the airconditioning vent onto my face, then sat there for a moment staring through the windshield.

"You all right?" my wife asked.

I turned to her and smiled. "A piece of cake," I responded.

"Sure it is. That's why you were tossing and turning in bed all night."

"I couldn't get comfortable," I explained, as I dropped the car in gear and sped off for my appointment. For the rest of my drive to 5600 Fishers Lane I fended off efforts to induce me to talk about my anxieties over the experience. I had always been convinced – and still am – that my wife was a "wannabe" psychologist who had never been given the educational opportunity to achieve that dream. Back at home there was at least a half dozen self-help books stacked on the night stand next to her side of the bed.

At approximately 8:30 AM, we pulled into the parking lot in front of the main building of the FDA complex. I was first up at nine o'clock and wanted to be settled in well before I was called on to speak. We quickly entered the building and were directed by a lady at the information desk to our hearing room.

I had asked Janet to come along on the trip. Neither of us had been to the D.C. area before, and I had suggested that this would be a wonderful opportunity to take in all of the sites. The following year would be the country's bicentennial, which seemed to add a special touch to the timing of our visit. But if the truth be known, I wanted to bring along my own cheering section. There would be at least one friendly face among the sea of strangers.

Inside the room I met Dr. Gregoire. He seated us, then generally explained the format and procedure and quickly departed. As we sat anxiously waiting, more and more attendees entered and seated themselves. Among them was Robert Dickson, who smiled and gave me a brief nod of the head. Dickson was the Los Angeles attorney representing Merrell on all of my new Clomid cases. As expected, Belanger and his firm had been replaced. By 8:50 AM the room was almost packed.

The Obstetrics and Gynecology Advisory Committee was comprised of 11 permanent members, the Executive Secretary (Gregoire) and 4 consultants. Out of those 16, three were absent (two members and one consultant). However, also present were 17 staff members from the FDA (including Dr. Edwin Ortiz). [They must have been selling tickets. "Wanna have some fun this morning? Go on down to Conference Room G and watch a trial lawyer make a fool out of himself."] Along with Dickson, the Merrell contingent was also there in full force. Three expert witnesses were on the agenda and present to testify: Robert Brent, the teratologist who had testified for Merrell in the Breimhorst trial; Luigi Mastroianni, M.D., an obstetrician/gynecologist; and Raymond Vande Wiele, M.D., another obstetrician/gynecologist. Team Merrell also included an in-house lawyer and three doctor/employees from Merrell-National Laboratories. The official agenda for the public hearing was "The Use of Clomid and Down Syndrome."

At precisely 9:00 AM, Dr. Theodore King, chairman of the committee, called the meeting to order. After a brief statement by the medical officer assigned to the drug, I was called to the podium. With my hand clutching my notes, I nervously approached the lectern and faced the panel. All were sitting at a table at the head of the room. Behind me was the audience, including my sole cheer leader. My pounding heart was reminiscent of the Breimhorst verdict. I cleared my throat once and began with a few introductory remarks. One of them was close to an apology.

"Let me first say, before I proceed, that I hope none of you think it's presumptuous of an attorney to come before doctors and scientists and tell or suggest to them a given opinion about medical or scientific problems. I do, however, feel that I have more than a nodding acquaintance with clomiphene citrate. Some of you may know that approximately a year and three months ago I concluded a jury trial in Torrance, California, contending that Clomid was teratogenic in man and that it had, in fact, caused malformations in a child by the name of Mark Breimhorst. The jury in that case reached a unanimous decision in favor of the plaintiff.

"Prior to that time, of course, I had adequate opportunity to investigate records and do medical research. And since that time, especially in the last six months, I have done a substantial amount of medical research on the proposition that Clomid is actually altering chromosomes, a theory I had not totally explored prior to that time."

Mechanism of Action

I was now prepared to discuss the mechanism of action by which Clomid was damaging chromosomes. If I was destined to see smiles of amusement on the committee members, now was when it would happen. I began with a description of the Ford in-vitro study, detailing how she was able to induce trisomy 21 errors by elevating the pH. I then tied the rising pH to the affect Clomid had on normal estrogen levels.

"Thus we start with the basic proposition that an abnormal level of estrogen, whether high[80] or low, can conceivably cause a rise of pH in the reproductive tract of the woman. It is my position that clomiphene citrate does both. It creates an extremely low level of estrogen in manifesting its antiestrogenic effect at the time of treatment, and that thereafter there is a continuous surge in estrogen climbing to a peak at about the time of ovulation, where there is again another abnormal level of estrogen. So you have an abnormally low level and you have an abnormally high level."

A quick check revealed not one smiley face.

"When a woman is actually ingesting the clomiphene there is a reduction of estrogen, probably brought about by the drug having an inhibitory effect on the production of estrogen by the ovaries. This, I believe, is manifested and is supported by the fact that women have been known to have vasomotor flashes, the hot flashes that doctors generally ascribe to menopause and the absence of, and low, estrogen levels. This has also occurred and is dose-related to clomiphene citrate."

Still no smirks or rolling of the eyes.

"I believe there is, at least, a reasonable medical possibility that at this particular time, prior to ovulation, that this low estrogen level could actually cause a rise of pH in the ovaries and actually induce chromosomal anomalies within the germ cells in the ova or ovum right about the time the woman is actually taking the drug."

I now began to appreciate that the men and women I was addressing were professionals first, and would be extending me the courtesy of listening to what I had to say. All were attentive and some were even taking notes – although I might not want to see what they were writing down. I would no doubt be facing some embarrassing questions at the end, but for now I was being treated with respect.

"At this point there is an increase of pituitary gonadotropins and the beginning of a build of estrogen; a surge of estrogen occurs which continues to climb up to the time of ovulation. At its highest peak there are abnormally high levels of estrogen. And very significantly, it has been reported[81] that when exposed to Clomid, existing levels of estradiol[82] can be four to five-fold higher than controls, indicating that there is, at least in some instances, *four to five times the level of estrogen* at its highest point than there would be in normally ovulating women. At this peak…there is literature that indicates an increase of estrogen, high estrogen, causes an increase in pH. Drill's Pharmacology points to the fact that this increase in pH can occur in the oviduct with the increase of estrogen.

"It is my position that when, following Clomid treatment, this surge and high level of estrogen is reached at about the time of ovulation, there's an increase in pH and chromosomal anomalies are induced."

I went on to cite examples of other side effects which were related to the high levels of estrogen, including ovarian enlargement, ovarian cysts, ovarian hyperstimulation syndrome (OHSS), superovulation and dizygotic twinning; they all correlated with elevated levels of estrogen. And every one of these side effects was similarly produced by Pergonal (hMG). That Clomid and Pergonal shared these side effects was a key element in my presentation, because the most persuasive clinical study involved the use of both drugs.

I next launched into the clinical evidence, which admittedly was not all that substantial. But if I was to persuade this group, it would not be on some theory created by a lawyer from California. When it came to proof of teratogenicity, these physicians and scientists would want to see epidemiology studies. They wanted to see numbers. They wanted to see that there was a true increased risk of anomalies in real patients actually using this drug. I opted to go with my weakest case first – neural tube defects.

Neural Tube Defects

"First of all, there is an indication in the literature that neural tube defects can be associated with abnormal chromosomes. The literature indicates that trisomy and triploidy have both been associated with neural tube closure defects. I have referred to the article by Doctor Wright, who has cited many of the authorities that I have set forth in my paper.

"Very significantly, in one of the most widely-cited studies, at least in my reading, namely the Stevenson study in the mid-1960s, there was a finding of a direct correlation between dizygotic twinning and neural tube defects. This is an indication, ladies and gentlemen, that there could be a *common mechanism causing both*.

"One of them, the dizygotic twinning, we know can be caused by clomiphene citrate, human menopausal gonadotropin, et al. The question is: if it is causing dizygotic twinning, is it also causing neural tube defects? There is at least an indication that it is. I would again like to point out that I believe the same vehicle, the same mechanism, is the abnormal increase in estrogen found at the time of ovulation."

It was now time to move on to first trimester spontaneous abortions and hopefully tie them in with NTDs. Here I had a solid epidemiology study conducted by two respected scientists. The rub, of course, was that the study did not exclusively involve clomiphene citrate. But if the members of the panel were convinced that the three drugs used during this phase[83] of the study (Pergonal, Clomid and human chorianic gonadotropin) had a similar impact on the female reproductive system, it might give them cause for concern.

"Another very significant study is that study that was done by Doctors Boue in France between 1965 and 1972, and reported, I believe, in the March 24, 1973 edition of *Lancet*. They examined something in excess of 1,400 abortuses that had occurred in the first trimester, for abnormal chromosomes. These doctors found that as far as the *trisomic* anomalies, there was a 52.8% increase between the groups that were related to treatment with ovulatory-stimulating drugs as opposed to the two groups that were not. They also found a 61.5% increase in *triploidy* between those groups.

"These doctors expressed the opinion that this might be an indication that ovulatory-stimulating drugs could be altering chromosomes. And again, I would like to point out the fact that in the studies that have related neural tube defects to abnormal chromosomes, there is a finding of *trisomy* and *triploidy*, these two major chromosome anomalies that Doctors Boue found during their study.

"Another very significant fact, and one that cannot be ignored, were the teratology studies done with clomiphene citrate; that there were no studies done to determine the effect of the drug on animals during the post-conception up to the organogenesis period. I believe organogenesis begins in the rat at day eight. There were no teratogenic studies done on the rat earlier than day eight. So, of course, I am handicapped. I cannot point to a study that was done to show that this early administration of the drug prior to conception could, in fact, induce anomalies in the animal.

"However, I can point to a study of a drug that has been at least chemically related to Clomid, and that is MER 29, Triparanol, in a study done by a Doctor Roux, I believe in about 1964, 1963, in that area. I have cited it in my text. I might point out that the entire article is in French, but I have gone to the expense of having it transcribed and I do have the transcribed portion with me, which I will make available. Doctor Roux administered the drug, MER 29, a drug chemically related to Clomid, and was able to induce *anencephaly* and *spina bifida*...and a couple others that I can't pronounce.

"Ladies and gentlemen, there is very strong evidence, with this clinical summary on neural tube defects, and with the mechanism of action that I have indicated, that there is a probability, and certainly a reasonable medical probability, that clomiphene citrate and other ovulatory-stimulating drugs are actually causing neural tube defects by altering chromosomes."

At this point, almost as a post script, I referred to the numerous Clomid DERs identifying neural tube defects. There had been a clear excess of these reports, and I emphasized this point. I also reminded every member of the panel that it was from the receipt of individual case reports, not epidemiology studies, from which we learned about the terrible tragedy of thalidomide.

Down Syndrome

At the outset I wanted to draw a comparison between the Clomid pre-market investigations and the previously-identified Stevenson study.[84] Both were international studies conducted during the sixties. Stevenson found an incidence of Down syndrome (DS) at .84 for every 1000 births – one in every 1205 deliveries – whereas during the Clomid investigations there was an incidence of one in every 377 deliveries; a three-fold increase. Further, the mean maternal age of the Clomid DS patients was 31.5 years compared to 34.0 years in Stevenson. The difference could not be attributed to maternal age. I also offered a meaningful observation about the DS patients from the Clomid population.

"Of the two women under 30, women that are least likely to have a child born with Down syndrome, very significantly we had women with the highest dosage. The woman who was 24 took 200 milligrams for five days, which was the last course of treatment and occurred only eight days before conception; in other words, a total of 1,000 milligrams during her last course of treatment prior to conception. The woman who was 29 had 100 milligrams per day for ten days. She also had 1,000 milligrams. Both of these women had very high dosages; in fact, dosages that exceed the recommended amount at the present time. These women who are least likely to have Down syndrome had children born with Down syndrome. We also know from the records that the woman who was 29 conceived during a treatment cycle. So both of the women who were under 30 conceived during a treatment cycle.

"But unfortunately, the records do not disclose the dates of treatment, the dates of conception, or even the date of birth; a reflection, I submit, of the care that was taken during the study. However, from reading the records it can be determined that conception did occur during the treatment cycle.

"I'd further like to point out that trisomy 21, the very cause of Down syndrome, is one of the chromosomal anomalies that was induced by Doctor Ford in-vitro. And also that trisomy was one of the chromosomal anomalies that were actually increased following ovulatory-stimulating drugs in abortuses during Doctor Boue's study."

Pre-market Investigations

"Another comment about the clinical studies. I thought when I started working on the Breimhorst case that these were scientific studies, that they were prospective studies, studies that are geared, that are outlined in advance, where the protocol is set up in advance of the study, and that all expression of opinion, i.e., that there is no evidence that clomiphene citrate has a deleterious effect on the human fetus, all such expressions of opinion were based upon a prospective study.

"I submit that if anyone sits down and takes a careful look at the clinical investigational records, you will find that the first couple of years of records are not prospective studies; that many of these doctors were using this drug believing initially that it was a contraceptive drug, not knowing its fertility effect, and that, to find the information on the earlier pregnancies, the clinical investigators had to resort back to earlier records; that the first couple of years of the clinical studies on Clomid entails a retrospective study, not a prospective study. A very significant fact is that the first case of Down syndrome was not reported until late 1964, even though the drug had been used since, I believe, some time in mid- or late 1960.

"Stevenson's study points out that Down syndrome is not always easily detected at time of birth and that many times, depending upon the race, the ethnic origin of the mother, the child, chromosomal studies are needed to determine this. The fingerprint studies are also needed, and that even the most astute observer can miss a case of Down syndrome. And as Doctor Stevenson pointed out, maybe as much as 25 percent of the cases of Down syndrome may be missed at birth.

"I submit to you that from what we know of the clinical studies conducted on clomiphene citrate, that there very well could have been many more cases of Down syndrome missed, during the earlier period especially. And if this study is supposed to be complete, it is really supposed to be investigating whether or not the drug is causing malformations in man. Why weren't chromosomal studies done on all five, instead of only two of the cases of Down syndrome? We know that the translocation type is generally considered to be inherited, but that this is not the case with trisomy 21.

"Why then aren't we investigating this? Why didn't they do five chromosomal studies? They would at least have then an indication that perhaps something had happened during gametogenesis which may have caused trisomy 21 to occur; some further evidence indicating a common mechanism between multiple ovulation and abnormal chromosomes."

The above statement sought to make three points. First, because the clinical investigators had initially thought they were investigating a *birth control pill*, when the fertility capabilities were later discovered, they had to dig back through earlier records to determine the outcome of each pregnancy; that because the early phase of the study lacked protocols requiring examination of pregnancies, it was highly likely that many congenital anomalies, including Down syndrome, would have been missed.

The second point was that even using the best methods of detection at the time, it is often difficult to diagnose Down syndrome at birth, and as many as 25% of the cases are not detected until later. This statement was made in reference to my earlier contention that the vast majority of the infants from the Clomid study were only examined at birth. And finally, if the investigations were truly designed to assess the risk of potential birth defects, including Down syndrome, why did Merrell only report on chromosome studies for two cases of Down syndrome, rather than on all five. A determination of the *type* of chromosomal defect, suffered by each infant, would have assisted in eliminating heredity as a causal factor in the condition.

Spontaneous Abortions

"Next we come to spontaneous abortions, a very hotly contested issue in the trial of Breimhorst versus Richardson-Merrell. If we have a drug here that is causing congenital malformations by inducing abnormal chromosomes, it would be likely that we might also have a drug which would be causing spontaneous abortions. Doctors Boue indicate that the majority of spontaneous abortions are actually caused by the abnormal chromosomes or the malformations that are created by the abnormal chromosomes. So, one might suspect that if clomiphene citrate is altering chromosomes, there might also be a higher rate of spontaneous abortions in the clinical studies as compared to the general population.

"Ladies and gentlemen, such evidence does exist. The rates of spontaneous abortion, given in the general population, range from ten percent to approximately 15 percent. I would cite Richardson-Merrell's own literature wherein they indicate that in the general population the instance of spontaneous abortion is only ten percent. I would cite the January 1963 clinical investigation brochure, the August 1, 1964 Status Report to Clinical Investigators and their Physician's Drug Monograph submitted to the clinical investigators of 1965. In all of those publications they indicate and acknowledge that the incidence of spontaneous abortion in the general population is ten percent.

"There are some reports wherein it is cited as being higher. I have cited one conducted by Warburton and Frazer, at 14.7 percent. So let's say we're dealing with a range of ten to 15 percent. In the clinical investigations with Clomid we had an instance of 20 percent, twice that of the lower figure, and one third higher than the higher figure."

"Mr. Mix, could you finish up, please, sir?" Dr. King was reminding me that I had been given an allotted time to speak, and that others were also on the agenda.

"One more comment about spontaneous abortions," I added. "Richardson-Merrell has maintained that the incidence of spontaneous abortions in *infertility* patients is in the area of 20 percent. This totally ignores, first of all, a study done by Israel, wherein the incidence was somewhere around ten percent in infertility patients. And it also ignores the fact that the Buxton study that they cite does not involve an international study. It involves one clinic as opposed to 364, was a prospective study as opposed to a partially retrospective study, and that many of the patients in their study had a different type of infertility problem than the Clomid patients we're dealing with, ovulatory dysfunction patients; that the patients in the Buxton study had problems which might also be related to causing abortions other than abnormal chromosomes."

After a few additional comments, I decided to wrap it up before King got on my butt again. My prepared finish was designed to perhaps instill in the panel some sense of responsibility to pick up the baton that I was dropping in their lap.

"Finally, let me say this. A couple of months ago, after spending about three or four full days at the UCLA Medical Library and watching the files on my desk mount, realizing that I should be practicing law and not researching medicine, I asked myself what in the world am I doing?

"It didn't take me long to come up with the answer. I felt that nobody else out there was really interested, and unless I did something about it, nobody would. And so here I am, one week post-surgery,[85] out here at my own expense, asking you ladies and gentlemen to please listen because it's up to you now.

"That's all I'm saying."

"Thank you, Mr. Mix," said Chairman King. "Are there any questions from the panel?"

I held my breath, praying that everyone would pass on the opportunity. But no such luck. Doctor Blye, one of the consultants for the committee, seemed quite eager to get a piece of me.

"I have a few questions for Mr. Mix. Mr. Mix, are you now involved in any litigation or prelitigation activities on behalf of any client who is claiming damage as a result of Clomid administration?"

Had we been in court, I would have objected on the ground of relevancy. I did not come before the committee as an expert, whose bias might be an important consideration. I was simply conveying information I had accumulated along with my personal views about the importance of that information. Although I had hoped that the information would be persuasive, I would have been a fool to expect this body to give any weight to my opinions.

"Yes sir, I am," I courteously replied. "I have presently four cases."

"Thank you," responded Blye. "Would you please provide for us briefly your educational background? I don't wish a complete CV, but just indicate your educational background."

"First of all, I am not a doctor. I am not a scientist."

"I don't want to know what you *aren't*. I want to know what you *are*."

Ouch! This was my first experience with a hint of hostility. Of course, he already knew that I was an attorney. "All right. I'm an attorney. I graduated from the University of Southern California in 1963. I graduated from Hastings College of Law in San Francisco, 1966. I was admitted to the State Bar of California, January 4, 1967. I am presently on the Board of Governors of the Los Angeles Trial Lawyers Association. I am one of the founders of an important arbitration program in the Los Angeles Superior Court system, and act in the pseudojudiciary capacity as one of its arbitrators. I also sit on its appellate tribunal as a member of the grievance committee. I have written articles in legal publications.

"I didn't, of course, come here with a complete resume. Is that sufficient, Doctor?"

"Thank you very much," Blye responded, as he signed off.

Next a Dr. Sarto slightly elevated his hand. "I have one or two questions," he announced. The question, actually, was only a matter requiring clarification. His motive for speaking seemed more designed to educate than to question. He made two points: first, that the rate of chromosomal anomalies in abortuses was determined by the gestational age of the abortuses, with very early stages having the highest rate; and second, women with infertility problems tended to have a higher incidence of infants with malformations. Having made his contribution, Sarto nodded to King that he was finished.

The committee chairman then solicited further questions, first from the panel and then from the audience. After a brief moment of silence, he turned to me and said, "Thank you very much, Mr. Mix."

And just like that, I was let off the hook. Slightly shaken, but not stirred. Before anyone had second thoughts, I was quickly back in my seat accepting an approving nod from my wife.

Next up was Dr. Godfrey Oakley from the Centers for Disease Control (CDC). I was now about to be broadsided – or so I thought. Oakley summarized his findings from the CDC, which pretty much followed his 1972 abstract on the subject. They had been following fertility drugs (Clomid and Pergonal) and chromosome defects since 1969. They had combined the clinical studies from both fertility drugs and found 6 cases of Down syndrome. When they adjusted the data for maternal age, they concluded that there were 6 cases when only 2.6 were expected, over a two-fold increase. This was statistically significant at around the .05 level. They thus could not attribute the difference to maternal age. He noted, however, that 2 of the six cases did not conceive during a treatment cycle,[86] which would tend to argue against the drug, although he admitted not knowing the denominator of the women from both studies that likewise did not conceive during a cycle of treatment. He then pointed to studies demonstrating that infertility patients might have defective ova even without the treatment of fertility drugs. Although he did not conclude that fertility drugs were causing Down syndrome, he certainly left open the door on the possibility.

Dickson then approached the podium and after some preliminary remarks introduced Merrell's speakers. First up was Robert Brent, who only targeted the question of Down syndrome. His argument somewhat parroted Oakley's by referring to the two cases not following conception during a treatment cycle and the high risk of infertility patients due to their underlying condition. Luigi Mastroianni, M.D. was the next to speak on behalf of Merrell. He was critical of the Ford paper because it used fetal fibroblasts rather than cells from human ova. He also challenged that low estrogen levels would increase pH in the oviduct, claiming it had only been demonstrated to occur in the vagina and that the follicles of the ovaries and the fallopian tubes are buffered from such an effect. Merrell's final witness was Raymond Vande Weile, M.D. His arguments principally attacked the claimed half-life of Clomid – what was measured was only the C_{14} and not the active drug itself, which in reality had a biological half-life of just one day; that thus at the critical time for trisomy 21 to develop, Clomid – and its anti-estrogen effect – would be virtually non-existent; and that the level of estrogen had little to do with cell division or abnormal chromosomes in the human ovum. His final point was that the true spontaneous abortion rate in the general population was no different than in the Clomid studies.

By 11:00 AM, the open session of of our segment of the day's agenda had concluded. One or two other items were yet to be covered, after which the advisory panel would go into closed session to deliberate the presentations and come up with its recommendations, if any.

As Janet and I exited the building, the warmth of the sun hitting my face felt therapeutic. All tension was gone – my muscles for the first time in days were relaxed. It had been a novel and challenging experience. But I had not been pleased with my performance. At times I was clumsy – several times stumbling over my words and on a couple of occasions I even misspoke. My knowledge of the material could also have been more thorough. I was satisfied that I had stepped up to the plate. I just wish I had taken some better swings.

Suddenly I realized that the stress of the day was behind me and the two of us would be sharing some fascinating and interesting sites over the next couple of days. I grabbed Janet's hand and asked, "So what do we have planned for the rest of our stay in Washington?"

My wife stopped and looked up into my eyes. Up to this point she had been quiet – unusual behavior for a classic type A. "I was proud of you in there," she said, avoiding my question.

"You were, huh?"

"Yes, I was."

For a moment I was speechless; then gave my cheerleader a big hug and kiss. "Thanks Honey," I weakly uttered. I couldn't have asked for a better accolade.

On August 5, 1975, I sent a letter to Dr. Gregoire requesting a copy of "all Conclusions and Recommendations made by the Obstetrics and Gynecology Advisory Committee." After a month and a half without a reply, I called Gregoire. He apologized for not getting back to me sooner, but said that I would need to make a formal request to the Freedom of Information Office for the conclusions and recommendations and any transcripts I desired from the hearing. On October 8, 1975, I forwarded my request to that office.

Finally, in early November, I received a full set of the requested transcripts. Surprisingly, they came with a cover letter from Gregoire (rather than the Freedom of Information Office). His comment was brief and to the point. "The committee concluded that the evidence presented at the meeting did not allow them to conclude that Clomid is a causative factor in Down syndrome." Nothing was stated about any recommendations.

But sandwiched in the enclosures that included a list of those in attendance, informational material that had been supplied to the committee members, a summary of the oral presentations, and the verbatim transcript, was a letter from Dr. Edwin M. Ortiz, Director of the Division of Metabolism and Endocrine Drug Products, to Richardson-Merrell. It was dated August 15, 1975, and stated in part:

"The Committee recommended that further prospective and retrospective data be collected by your firm regarding the occurrence of congenital anomalies, including Down Syndrome, in children of mothers treated with clomiphene citrate. We are requesting that your firm initiate studies to collect such data. Please submit your proposed protocols for our review and comment prior to the initiation of the studies." [Exhibit 2]

As a consequence of the meeting, Merrell had been requested by the FDA to conduct further clinical studies, designed this time to ascertain the true risk for birth defects. Perhaps I had not convinced the committee members that Clomid was a human teratogen, but apparently a majority of them had cause for concern.

Although implementing a *retrospective*[87] study would not have been a significant expense for a major drug company, conducting a well-designed *prospective*[88] study could only have been done at a substantial cost. Such a recommendation by the committee would not have been casually made. There is little doubt that the panel was having serious reservations about the value of the pre-market clinical studies and wanted to get a true reading on the risk that Clomid might pose to the human embryo.

I may not have been able to sell the Mix Hypothesis, but I had sufficiently dug my spurs into the flank of the FDA to bring about meaningful clinical studies – or so I thought.

* * * * *

CHAPTER 7

Working the System

Dr. Thomas B. O'Dell was stunned as he read the Ortiz letter of August 15, 1975. After all, everything had gone well at the hearing of July 18, 1975. Although he had not been in attendance himself, as recently as three weeks ago Drs. Holtkamp and Kuhn had filled him in. This was followed by an Interdepartment Memo to all personnel involved with the drug. Mix's "mechanism of action" appeared to fall on its face with the advisory panel, and he had very little in clinical evidence to support his argument that Clomid was a human teratogen. The Boue study involved primarily Pergonal and hCG, which made it of questionable relevance. And Oakley pretty much discounted any causal association between the use of Clomid and Down syndrome. Merrell's three experts had also done a stellar job. So what in the hell happened?

As the head of Merrell's Drug Regulatory Department, it was O'Dell's responsibility to liaison with the FDA and to act as a troubleshooter for matters concerning that regulatory agency. His first act was to call Holtkamp, who at the time was the Group Director for Endocrine and Metabolic Clinical Research. Clomid fell directly under his responsibility and was one of his babies. I could just imagine the exchange.

"Dorsey,…Tom."

"Yes, Tom."

"Just got the advisory findings and recommendations from FDA."

"Yeah…." Holtkamp did not like O'Dell's tone.

"Not good. Cleared us with Down syndrome, but still want full blown clinical studies, retrospective…*and prospective*."

"What! What godly reason did they have for doing that?"

"Beats me. As I said, we got cleared on Down syndrome. I'm gonna ask for a meeting. Need some clarification anyway. What kind of designs are they looking for? Maybe I can get a line from Ortiz on what prompted this request."

At the other end of the company intercom, Holtkamp was already thinking strategy. "Good idea, Tom. See what you can set up. In the meantime, let's get our team together. We need a game plan. Check your calendar and get me some clear dates and times. I'll check with everyone else and call you back."

Conducting well-designed studies would be a disaster. There was absolutely nothing to be gained and a lot to lose. The cost for a prospective study would be upwards of two million in 1975 dollars, and although not as costly, a retrospective study could be expensive as well. Merrell personnel would be pulled from other projects to monitor, compile data, analyze, report and generally oversee the studies. The fact that the FDA felt a *need* for clinical investigations might impact sales if it got out – which was highly likely. And the final results would offer little benefit, but could end up catastrophic. A finding of no increased risk for birth defects would essentially give Merrell nothing. It could be used as a marketing tool, but no one believed Clomid to be a human teratogen anyway. Conversely, a finding of a positive association would have a major impact on sales and could even lead to the drug's withdrawal from the market.

On August 25, 1975, O'Dell sent Ortiz a letter requesting a meeting. But the FDA director passed on the idea until such time as Merrell at least had some preliminary study designs to discuss. To provide some guidance to the drug company, two forms were forwarded; a preliminary report and a 16-page follow-up form for pregnancies with an adverse outcome. The suggested detail, especially in the follow-up report, was of concern to the Merrell team. If followed, the study would be quite comprehensive and thorough.

There had to be a way to sidestep the studies.

A preliminary step would be to secure feedback from members of the advisory committee. The minutes of the closed session were likely inaccessible. However, Merrell had a few long-standing relationships with some of the members, who no doubt would be willing to talk. One such member was Dr. Gordon P. Griggs, an OB/GYN from Pasadena, California. *Griggs had been one of Merrell's clinical investigators*[89] in the Clomid pre-market studies. He thus had economic ties to the drug company, and had participated in the very studies that were being criticized as inadequately designed to assess the risk of birth defects – hardly one to be sitting in unbiased judgment. Another former Clomid investigator on the panel was Dr. S. J. Behrman[90] from Ann Arbor, Michigan.

Communication with Advisory Committee Members

In October 1975, Holtkamp met with Griggs at a medical symposium in Palm Springs, California. At the time, they generally discussed the advisory committee's recommendation for further studies. The discussion focused on the difficulty of finding an appropriate control group. Holtkamp complained that patients with ovulatory dysfunction are either incapable of conceiving or can do so only with considerable difficulty. So how do you find infertility patients who can conceive without the use of Clomid or another fertility drug? How can we follow the outcome of their pregnancies if they cannot get pregnant to begin with? Griggs sympathized with Holtkamp about the difficulty of designing such a study, but felt that it could still be done. Because of a shortage of time, they agreed to speak later on the subject.

As a follow-up to the October meeting, Holtkamp placed a call to Griggs in Pasadena on November 14, 1975.[91] Although he was unable to reach the obstetrician at his office, Holtkamp was able to track him down in a hospital delivery room.

"Hello, Gordon?"

"Yes, this is Gordon Griggs."

"Hi. Dorsey Holtkamp here."

"Oh, hi Dorsey."

"Did I catch you at a bad time?"

"No, just finished up. About ready to head on back to the office."

"Good. I wondered if we could pick up where we left off last month. It would be helpful to have some insight into the panel's thinking on this advisory matter."

"Sure Dorsey. How can I help?"

"You wouldn't happen to have any minutes of the closed session, would you?"

Whereas the minutes of the open session were a matter of public record, the deliberations of the committee in closed session were off limits. Knowing that a member's comments could become public information might inhibit him from speaking out and frustrate the process. But in 1975, whether a *drug company* had a right to them fell into a grey area of the law. The FDA had been using advisory committees for only three years at the time. That, of course, would not deter Holtkamp from giving it a try.

"No, I don't, Dorsey. I asked Gregoire for them at the last meeting, but have yet to see them. Ted King may have a copy. He's chairman of the committee, as you know."

Holtkamp would not go to King, who no doubt would first seek to clear it with Ortiz. Merrell's only chance to get a look at the deliberations was through the back door, and that meant Griggs or Behrman.

"I'll just wait until you have a copy. Let me read to you what we got from Ortiz." Holtkamp read the short letter verbatim to Griggs. "So is that how it went?"

"You know, Dorsey, the committee very well may have recommended that. We had the debate, of course, and then King probably dictated a summary and the recommendations. But I believe that's pretty much the way the vote went." Because of his allegiance to Clomid and Merrell, Griggs began to feel a tinge of guilt. "Of course, Behrman and I, in fact most of us, never felt there was any evidence of an association between Clomid and Down syndrome. Your data and Oakley's presentation pretty much supported that."

"But why the recommendation for further studies?" Holtkamp's unhappiness with that recommendation was quite evident, even over the phone.

"I'll tell you, Dorsey, it got started with these two members...I don't know their names, but I believe they are both geneticists. I'll get you their names at the next meeting. December 15, I think it is. Any way, they were both insistent on getting more data...and everyone else just started to go along with the idea. It seemed to be the concensus that ascertainment techniques have improved over the past 10 years and we are now better able to analyze the data than we could back then. So out of an abundance of caution..."

"You see the problem, don't you?" Holtkamp was looking to generate some misgivings about the panel's decision.

"Yeah, I guess I do."

"As I understand, Dr. Shubeck saw you earlier this week." Shubeck was another Merrell employee assigned to the project.

"Yes he did. And I saw the forms. I can see that your study will require a voluminous amount of work."

"Then you can appreciate our frustration here?"

"That I can.... You know, you should be able to go to fertility centers and get some data to clear this all up. There are a number of them scattered throughout the U.S., so you won't have the geographical problem Oakley has in Atlanta." Griggs was referring to Oakley's ongoing follow-up on birth defects at the CDC in Atlanta, which were only being drawn from that area. Studies had shown that birth defect rates varied significantly between different regions of the country, and some of the members of the panel had discussed this problem during the closed session.

"So I take it that the 2,300 pregnancies referred to in our current labeling were not sufficient to satisfy the panel? As you know, they were drawn from a worldwide population."

"I can appreciate that. But as I said, methods and techniques have changed since the 1960s. Everyone seemed to want a fresh look. If you have a different idea on how to deal with this, why don't you contact King or Gregoire? I doubt that it would be fruitful to talk to Ortiz, so you may want to stick with members of the committee."

"So you feel we'd have better luck with the committee?"

"No question. Whatever plan gets submitted to the FDA will be sent to the Advisory Committee for review. I can assure you, it will be the Advisory Committee making the decision on the adequacy of your study design, *not the FDA*."

This was a telling statement. Although the FDA was not legally bound by recommendations from its advisory committees, it invariably followed them. In this instance the Committee's decision would have even more influence over the FDA because it was the panel's recommendation to conduct the studies to begin with. Griggs was assuring Holtkamp that Merrell need not be concerned about the FDA's view on the matter.

"Well, what do you think will sell to the Committee?"

For the prospective study, Griggs recommended one that had already been endorsed by the American Fertility Society. The sponsors of the study were currently seeking a grant from the National Institutes of Health (NIH). Griggs was sure that the Committee would accept this study in lieu of Merrell conducting one on its own. As to the retrospective study, he was certain that securing data from various fertility centers scattered throughout the U.S. would be sufficient, rather than any in-depth control study necessitated by the forms shown to him by Dr. Shubeck. Griggs again agreed that such a study would be quite difficult to complete, and for that reason the panel would not be insistent on employing the forms he had reviewed.

Finally, Griggs urged Holtkamp to get a copy of the actual recommendation from the Advisory Committee, rather than Ortiz' interpretation of the document. It might be very important to have the specific language used should any legal situations arise as a result of it. Both men then said their goodbyes and promised to keep in touch.

As a trial lawyer, I was shocked and appalled when I first read the memo outlining the above conversation. To me, the phone call was analogous to jury tampering. Although it did not violate any laws, Holtkamp was having clandestine dialogue with a member of a panel sitting in judgment of his employer's product. Griggs and Behrman also had a clear conflict of interest[92] as former Clomid clinical investigators. Any criticism of the pre-market studies would have brought their own conduct under scrutiny. For the first time I realized that FDA advisory committees were not objective and impartial panels. Instead they were comprised of prominent physicians and scientists, many of whom had direct ties with the drug industry and were vulnerable to its manipulation.

Letter of December 30, 1975

On December 30, 1975, O'Dell thought he would take another shot at Ortiz. Merrell by now had what it needed from the advisory committee, but still had to deal with the FDA. O'Dell's effort would initially be in the form of a letter directed to Edwin M. Ortiz, M.D., Director of the Division of Metabolic and Endocrine Drug Products. The goal of the letter was to convince Ortiz to agree to a meeting without first submitting an extensive set of study protocols.

"Mr. Frank Korun, of your Division, indicated in conversation any proposed protocols should be submitted prior to a meeting. We continue to believe a preliminary conference is necessary and perhaps we have not adequately explained the reasons for our desire to hold such a discussion.

"In regard to the request for retrospective studies, you are aware that the New Drug Application file for Clomid (NDA 16-131) contains data on over 2,000 cases of Clomid-related pregnancies and the NDA further covers experience for a period of the last 15 years. Apparently the information contained in the NDA which bears on the matter at hand was not made available to the Advisory Committee.

"We believe these data are the strongest retrospective data base regarding the safety of Clomid that is available. For that reason, we do not believe that further retrospective studies are needed and would like to discuss with you the presentation of an appropriate summary of this NDA data for the Advisory Committee in order that they may reconsider their recommendation to the Commissioner in respect to retrospective studies.

"We do not necessarily object to the suggestion that additional data be collected, although we may question whether there is a valid scientific reason for additional new studies."

This was O'Dell's pitch to avoid conducting *any* retrospective study, beyond making a compilation and summary of data already contained in the NDA. He was urging that the pre-market studies be revisited, along with all of the reports of birth defects (DERs) and published Clomid studies received since marketing began in 1967. Merrell wanted to present this summary to the Advisory Committee members in hopes that they might "reconsider their recommendation to the Commissioner (of the FDA) in respect to retrospective studies." Based upon Griggs' discussion with Holtkamp, Merrell was convinced that any summary that its staff could put together would likely satisfy the panel and relieve it of conducting the requested retrospective study. Next item: prospective studies.

"Another study, which would be prospective, is under consideration by the American Fertility Society (AFS). The AFS has endorsed the Battelle Memorial Institute Human Affairs Research Center in Seattle, Washington, to apply for an NIH grant for a controlled prospective study to determine the incidence of and type of birth anomalies in infants born of subfertile women (with and without treatment of Clomid) compared with those in a normal fertile population. The application has been submitted to NICHD,[93] we are informed. We understand a study of this type would cost between $1 and $2 million. We plan to contact the American Fertility Society at appropriate intervals to determine the status of this study."

174

What better way to evade conducting a study, than to pass it on to someone else and have the federal government pay for it. Of course, there would be some uncertainties. The NIH, with its own budgetary limitations, may not approve the grant. At that point the study would either die a quick death or the researchers would seek funding elsewhere – most likely from Merrell. Should the latter circumstance arise, Merrell would have a choice. It could provide the funding, for which it would have total control over the project; or it could decline to provide financing and watch the study evaporate. By the time this process had run its course, the FDA, as it often did, would likely forget about its request, especially if it was no longer being sought by the Advisory Committee.

In the event that the NIH provided the grant, Merrell would likely be asked to supply Clomid for that part of the study. At the very least, this would give the drug company a "first look" at any draft submitted for publication on the results of the study. If the data from the study were unfavorable, criticisms of its design and/or findings would be communicated to the researchers in hopes of influencing the conclusions to be drawn from it. Even better, some of the Clomid pre-market investigators and/or Merrell consultants might be participants in the study.

O'Dell was quite sure that all of their bets had been covered, if only they could avoid preparing all of the protocols for the two requested studies. He just had one more point to make.

"As the public record shows, the allegations made by the attorney who appeared before the Obstetrics and Gynecology Advisory Committee on July 18 were unsupported hypotheses which ranged from the original announced subject of Down syndrome to the broader subject of birth anomalies in general. When the agenda for the July 18 meeting was announced in the Federal Register, the subject was related solely to the questioned relationship of Clomid administration and Down syndrome. Testimony presented on behalf of the company, through recognized experts, was limited to the agenda topic. The Plaintiff's attorney, Mr. Mix, was allowed to speak on matters not covered on the agenda. We believe his presentation, without complete answer, may have influenced the Obstetrics and Gynecology Advisory Committee to make a recommendation beyond the agenda topic without having complete information.

"For the obvious reasons of equity and fairness, we respectfully ask that Merrell be given the opportunity to present data to the Committee which were not made available to them on July 18 because of our planned response only to the announced agenda. The data would include that mentioned in this letter.

"I hope that you now appreciate the basis for our request to meet with you at an early date to discuss this subject more fully and why we do not believe that the meeting should be conditioned on a requirement that the proposed retrospective and prospective protocols be submitted prior to affording us this opportunity.

"May we hear from you in regard to our request for a preliminary meeting?"

O'Dell represented to the FDA director that my presentation at the hearing "may have influenced the Obstetrics and Gynecology Advisory Committee to make a recommendation beyond the agenda without complete information." But Griggs had assured Holtkamp that they had *not* been influenced by my pitch; that the majority felt there was no evidence of an association between the use of Clomid and Down syndrome. He had instead justified the need for further studies because of *advances in ascertainment technology over the past decade*; they wanted to get a fresh look at the data.

So why had O'Dell deceived Ortiz about the panel's basis for requesting further studies? Because in looking at the entire picture, the Advisory Committee's true justification for requesting the studies would have seemed reasonable. By playing the "equity and fairness" card, Merrell had hoped to get another shot at the panel with no more than a summary of old data and literature.

Although it took almost another two months, by February 25, 1976, Merrell had scheduled its meeting with Ortiz and his staff without preparing one set of protocols.

On March 17, 1976, at the appointed hour, Drs. O'Dell and Holtkamp, along with their in-house legal counsel, John Chewning and Frederick Lamb,[94] marched into one of the conference rooms at 5600 Fishers Lane in Rockville.[95] In addition to Ortiz, the FDA was represented by Drs. Ridgely Bennett and B. St. Raymond, Mr. Harold Krzma, a consumer safety officer, and a Missy Davidson from the FDA legal department. This was not by any means a casual meeting to chit chat about submitting a few extra papers.

Everyone was initially introduced and then seated themselves at the conference table; four on one side and five on the other.

As it turned out, Ortiz was an easy sell. He was quite willing to accept Merrell's proposed submission and allow the Advisory Committee to determine whether it still desired the retrospective and/or prospective studies. He just needed to be filled in on some of the details of the summary. Ortiz was also assured that a number of expert consultants had reviewed all of the related material and were convinced that Clomid was not a human teratogen. Further, Oakley had continued to accumulate data at CDC in Atlanta, and had yet to see any indication of an association between use of Clomid and Down syndrome. Merrell presented a full broadside – nothing was left to chance.

Ortiz no doubt saw this approach as the safest way to go. He wouldn't rattle any cages at Merrell and at the same time demonstrated an interest in accomodating the needs of his advisory panel. Like any other bureaucrat, he was always looking for the path of least resistance. Avoid controversy and conflict at any cost and always – always – go by the book. Never deviate from specified procedure and established protocol.

Merrell's written submission would be placed on the agenda for the May 7, 1976 meeting of the Obstetrics and Gynecology Advisory Committee (later changed to May 6, 1976). It was to be filed with the FDA no later than April 1, 1976, and 20 copies supplied for the Advisory Committee by April 15th. The agenda item would be titled, "Clomid – Outcome of Pregnancies." Speakers on behalf of Merrell would be Dr. Robert L. Brent,[96] Chairman of the Department of Pediatrics at Jefferson Medical College and Dr. Raymond Vande Wiele, an obstetrician/gynecologist who had testified (along with Brent) at the July 1975 hearing.

Submission of March 30, 1976

On March 30, 1976, Merrell forwarded to the FDA its 168-page written submission, entitled "Pregnancy Outcome of Humans Following Clomid (clomiphene citrate USP) with Summary of Detail of Reported Information on Birth Anomalies of Offspring." The document included 67 pages of tables, 74 pages of medical citations related to published literature on Clomid, a four-page udate on Oakley's CDC study in Atlanta, and 23 pages of index and text. The cover letter from O'Dell to Ortiz described the report's contents as follows:

"The document now being submitted is a summary of data available on Clomid associated pregnancies from (a) the investigational studies (1960-1970)[97] in a population of known denominator (2,369 delivered and reported pregnancies), (b) worldwide clinical experience during over eight years of United States commercial availability (May 1967 through 1975), and (c) published scientific literature (over 2,100 published papers with a citation to Clomid)."

It concluded that there was no evidence to support a causal relationship between Clomid therapy and congenital anomalies, including Down syndrome.

There can be little doubt that Merrell was quite confident that Ortiz would agree to accept its written submission. After all, it had been dealing with the FDA on a multitude of disputes for decades. This confidence is reflected in the document itself – it was dated *January 16, 1976*,[98] over a month before Ortiz had even agreed to a meeting without protocols.

The submitted report was replete with a number of inaccurate and misleading statistics and statements. It attacked the issue of teratogenicity by looking at its own compiled statistics in three specific areas: (1) pregnancy wastage, including spontaneous abortions; (2) the overall incidence of all congenital anomalies; and (3) the incidence of specific types of birth defects, including Down syndrome.

For obvious reasons, the issue of **Down syndrome** received special treatment in the submission. Merrell's discussion related to this unique birth defect was set out under the heading, *Comment on Down Syndrome*.

"Among the 2082 live born and stillborn infants (single and multiple births) of Clomid associated pregnancies during the investigational studies, 1960-1970, there were 5 reports of offspring with Down syndrome. This calculates to an incidence of 2.40 per 1000. The mean incidence figure for 1968-1973 for the metropolitan Atlanta population was 1.00 per 1000 (Table 9). Of the mothers of these offspring, one (069-014) discontinued Clomid on 9/12/63 and had an estimated date of conception of 2/1/64; one patient (100-176) *discontinued Clomid on 10/21/65* with a record of LMP (last menstrual period) of 12/30/65; one patient (208-033) had no Clomid in the cycle of conception with ovulation induction attributed to prednisone; and one patient (066-233) received Donnatal,

Stelazine, Librium, and prednisone at and near the estimated date of conception of 9/22/65 and later that month. If for reasons presented above, 1 to 3 patients are excluded, then *the incidence for 4 is 1.92 per 1000*, for 3 is 1.44, and for 2 is 0.96.

"At the time of the 7/18/75 meeting of the Ob/Gyn Advisory Committee, Dr. Godfrey Oakley of the Center for Disease Control presented the following information on a cohort of 739 cases, which was updated on 3/11/76 to a cohort of 865 cases as shown by the accompanying figures in parentheses. None of the mothers of the Down syndrome cases (127) had received Clomid.

* * *

"The overall difficulty of trying to determine the incidence of Down syndrome in a general population was recently summarized (Center for Disease control: Congenital Malformations Surveillance Report, July, 1974 – June, 1975, pp. 7-9). The value of 0.93 per 1000 was judged the most likely maternal age corrected incidence.

"At the time of the 7/18/75 FDA Ob/Gyn Advisory Committee meeting on Clomid and Down syndrome, information was given to the FDA for transmittal to the committee on the 5 cases of Down syndrome of the investigational series and on 3 cases of Down syndrome reported by Drug Experience Reports. No additional cases of Down syndrome have been received by Drug Experience Report since that date. 'The committee concluded that the evidence presented at this time does not allow them to conclude that Clomid is a causative factor in Down syndrome.' " [Emphasis added, pp.21-23.]

As is clearly indicated by the above text, Merrell's goal was to challenge the increased incidence by disqualifying as many of the 5 cases of Down syndrome as possible. This was done primarily through the issue of timing of treatment in relation to the date of conception. It argues that 3 of the 5 cases involved women who did not conceive during a treatment cycle. Without those three cases, the incidence would have been 0.96 per 1000, which would compare to the CDC calculated incidence, adjusted for maternal age, at 0.93 per 1000. This would seem quite persuasive, except for a number of problems.

The purported facts related to one patient (100-176) are patently false. Merrell represented to the FDA that this patient "discontinued Clomid on 10/21/65 with a record of LMP of 12/30/65." Contrary to Merrell's claim that Clomid was discontinued on October 21, 1965, the Analysis of Pregnancy form clearly records that the last course of treatment took place from *January 3, 1966 through January 7, 1966* (200 mg. x 5 days), with the last menstrual period on December 30, 1965. [Exhibit 3] It also states that the pregnancy is "(a)ttributable to Clomid therapy." This unquestionably was a case involving conception during a treatment cycle. One would also question any claim that this erroneous statement was an oversight, in that Merrell's computer summary of the pre-market investigation also attributes this conception to the ingestion of Clomid.[99]

Although the next patient (208-033) did not conceive during a treatment cycle, her conception occurred only *one cycle* after last using Clomid. Her last treatment occurred from August 27 through August 31, 1965 (100 mg. x 5 days), with a conception date of October 6, 1965. Based upon the Boue study,[100] women who had conceived one cycle after last using fertility drugs had the same increased risk of abortuses with abnormal chromosomes (86%) as women who had conceived during a treatment cycle (83%). The two groups also had a similar incidence with regard to trisomy defects, namely 50.0% and 48.9%, respectively. It thus would not be appropriate to exclude this case from the original five.

If one is going to limit the cases of Down syndrome to those at risk from exposure to Clomid, then it might be appropriate to exclude the patient (069-014) who ceased using Clomid on September 12, 1963 and conceived on February 1, 1964. According to Merrell's argument, this would result in an incidence of 1.92 per 1000. Of course, this would still be *twice the expected frequency* of 0.93 per 1000. But Merrell's claimed incidence figure is factually inappropriate. If one is going to reduce the numerator because conception occurred two or more cycles after Clomid was last ingested, then one must also make a corresponding reduction in the denominator for all other cases falling into that category. But Merrell does not even make that suggestion, let alone provide the statatistics to make the calculation. This omission is even more surprising (perhaps not) in that during the hearing of July 18, 1975, Oakley specifically brought up this problem.

"The next possibility (of what caused the 5 cases of Down syndrome) seems to me that perhaps it could be due to (the) drug. There's one thing that argues against that: there were two patients[101] who did not take the drug during the cycle, two of the six, two of the five from Merrell. We're handicapped a little bit because *we don't have the denominator data, namely, of the 2000 other pregnancies*, we don't know how many of those women also became pregnant in the first cycle, in the cycle they were treated, *or whether they became pregnant some two or three cycles after that. It is not available.*" [Emphasis added, Hearing Transcript, pp.35-36.]

Merrell, of course, had the data; it simply chose not to provide it. Had it attempted to report the calculation, the FDA (and the Advisory Committee) would have learned that there were *242 pregnancies*[102] that had been reported in the investigational studies, during which conception occurred *two or more cycles after the last course of Clomid* and about which the pregnancy outcome was known. Of this number, 34 had spontaneous abortions. Removing those pregnancies from the denominator would result in an incidence rate of at least *2.38 per 1000* (4/1678); a 2.6-fold increase over the expected rate of 0.93 per 1000 – slightly more than the increase found by Oakley (2.3) when he included the subset. The increased rate could not be attributed to the underlying infertility condition.

The submission of March 30, 1976 also addressed the question of whether there was an increased incidence of other congenital anomalies as well. As might be expected, Merrell took this opportunity to challenge the uncomfortable issue of the excessive number of **anencephaly** DERs. This would be Merrell's response to my presentation on the subject during the July 18, 1975 meeting.

"The format presented in Table 14 also permits the analysis of reports to determine if a single anomaly or a general system of anomalies occurs in high frequency. *Anencephaly was reported for 10 offspring.* All were in Drug Experience Reports; none were in the investigational series. *Five of the reports were solicited after prior publication in a journal.* No Drug Experience Report of anencephaly has been received from the United States. Multiple anomalies within a system were reported in the cardiovascular system, but the percent of multiple anomalies is not unlike that previously reported (Tables 6 and 7). Both the cardiovascular system related data and anencephaly or central nervous system data are still *based on small numbers of anomalous offspring.* * * *

"Also, *the reports* (Table 16) *of anencephaly in* <u>The Lancet</u> *in 1973* (included without making any clinical judgment for exclusion), *contribute to the larger numbers of Drug Experience Reports of 1973 and 1974.* The absence of similar published case reports since 1974 is worthy of comment because the effect of publication of a letter in <u>The Lancet</u> *tends to stimulate publication of observations* (controlled and uncontrolled)." [Emphasis added, pp.18-19.]

Merrell was so preoccupied with convincing the FDA that half of the reported cases of anencephaly had been solicited that it overlooked the first report (#15252) it received on June 11, 1971. Thus, the total number received through the end of 1975 was *eleven* – not 10. This initial report of anencephaly was also striking because it involved one infant from a set of fraternal twins, again raising the question of whether there is a common mechanism that produces dizygotic twinning and anencephaly.

Aside from this oversight, Merrell's explanation for the flood of anencephaly cases is quite clear: five of *11* cases were reported because the physicians were stimulated to do so as a consequence of an earlier publication in *The Lancet*; and that the numbers are small and of little importance.

The suggestion that 5 cases of anencephaly were reported to Merrell as a consequence of an earlier publication in *The Lancet* is not only misleading but factually inaccurate. Although there is no question that adverse reaction reports can be stimulated by publication of similar abnormalities, a close look at the subject DER records discloses a different story.

The first report of anencephaly appearing in *The Lancet* occurred on June 2, 1973. This involved the histories of 2 cases (#21983 and #21984). These two cases, of course, were not reported because of reading about another case of anencephaly. Likewise, three *earlier* cases (#15252, #17685 and #19948) were not "solicited" because of a publication. The August 18, 1973 edition of *The Lancet* included a case report of a Clomid-related anencephalic birth, but this case had already been reported to Merrell on March 29, 1973 (#19948) and thus had not been stimulated by the June 1973 article.

The sixth case (#20901) was reported directly to Merrell on July 13, 1973, but did not appear in a journal and had not been solicited by the first article. In fact, it was received from the same individual (Sears) who had cared for case two (#21984) of the original *Lancet* publication; this was his second Clomid anencephalic baby. Case seven (#21915) was reported directly to Merrell on October 25, 1973, and the records make no reference to the doctor reading any publication, nor does the report appear in any medical journal. Case eight (#22796) appeared in *The Lancet*[103] on October 20, 1973 and is the *first* anencephalic case report that can be directly attributed to the June 12, 1973 edition of the same publication. Case nine (#23898) was reported to Merrell on or about June 12, 1974 and is unrelated to the publication appearing one year earlier – or for that matter, any other publication reporting an anencephalic birth. Case ten (#24550), reported on August 13, 1974, similarly was not stimulated to report by any earlier article. And, finally, case eleven (#25640)[104] would appear to be the second report that could be attributed to an earlier article involving the same anomaly.

According to Merrell's own records, only 2 out of the 11 cases of anencephaly reported were a direct result of the reporting physician reading an earlier article. Nine cases were spontaneously reported to Merrell uninfluenced by any earlier publication.

Were the numbers small and unimportant? Relative to the total number of pregnancies occurring world wide from initial marketing through December 1975, 11 case reports of anencephaly would be considered a small number. But their significance is not measured against total pregnancies. It is measured against the total number of Clomid DERs reporting birth defects. As stated by Merrell in its report, from May 1967 through 1975, "there were reports (Drug Experience Reports) received from 9 countries of 57 infants with 90 different birth anomalies from 57 pregnancies[105] of mothers who ingested Clomid (Tables 5 and 14)." [P.10.] Out of 90 different types of congenital anomalies reported, *one* type (e.g., anencephaly) was reported 11 times out of only 57 pregnancies (19.3%). Almost one out of every 5 DERs was an anencephalic infant.

Those numbers are neither small nor unimportant!

Consider also that if one included other neural tube defects (NTDs) as well, there would be three additional cases to add to the total. Neural tube closure defects were also reported for spina bifida (#17178),[106] myelomeningocele (#23896) and meningomyelocele (#25639). All three involved nonclosure of the spinal column. With these additions, NTDs represented 14 out of the 57 cases (24.6%) received during the subject period. Although these case reports may not have established a causal association between the ingestion of Clomid and NTDs, they certainly represented a "red flag" frantically waving at Merrell and the FDA, demanding appropriate epidemiological studies.

It is not surprising that the term, "neural tube defects," fails to appear anywhere in the entire submission, even in the 67 pages of tables. Although it lists each NTD individually (i.e., anencephaly, spina bifida, myelomeningocele, etc.) and discusses the anatomical system (e.g., central nervous system), it never identifies NTDs as a group. This is unfortunate because all NTDs share a common deficiency; they all involve nonclosure of the neural groove into the neural tube at approximately the same period of time during early gestation. Most scientific publications refer to them as a group, as do many studies. I personally mentioned them several times during my presentation on July 18. Yet Merrell chose not to do so in its report – for good reason.

First, it could avoid setting out any data from which one could calculate that *one out of every four* DERs involved an NTD (as demonstrated above). It was uncomfortable enough listing all of the cases of anencephaly. Why call greater attention to the problem by adding all NTDs?

The second reason is a little more subtle, but can still be drawn from Merrell's written submission. As has been discussed earlier, Dr. Godfrey Oakley from the CDC had been conducting an ongoing case-control study out of Atlanta, in which he interviewed mothers of Down syndrome cases to determine how many had been exposed to Clomid at the time of conception. These *cases* would then be compared to the *controls* of all other infants with congenital anomalies reporting to the same center. When Oakley testified at the July 18, 1975 hearing, he found no exposures of clomiphene to 109 Down syndrome cases and 9 exposures out of 621 controls. He suggested that if Clomid was causing Down syndrome, he would have expected at least a couple of exposures in the Down syndrome group. However, he added that "seeing a zero with the size of the sample we had doesn't necessarily rule out that particular hypothesis."[107]

Then, in further preparation of the written submission, Holtkamp and others from Merrell met with Oakley on March 12, 1976,[108] in order to add an update to the July 18, 1975 numbers. They had been following this further compilation over the prior 8 months. At the time of this meeting, Oakley gave the Merrell staff a four-page report on the update. It is dated March 11, 1976, and is attached as a supplement to the submission (pp.165-168). It then included zero exposures to 127 cases of Down syndrome and 11 Clomid exposures out of 738 controls with other congenital anomalies. Oakley also provided a list of the 11 other congenital anomalies that had been exposed to Clomid (p.168).

Guess what?

Of the 11 cases, *three of them involved neural tube defects*, including another case of anencephaly.[109] Out of this random set of Clomid congenital anomalies from Atlanta, Georgia, 27.3% of them were NTDs. And none were stimulated by an earlier publication of similar anomalies. In fact, they were compiled while looking at the association between Clomid and Down syndrome.

To include the recent numbers on Down syndrome from Atlanta, Merrell updated its January 16, 1976 report on March 22, 1976. It even went so far as to set out Oakley's chart under its *Comment on Down Syndrome* heading (p.22). Yet there is no comment on the 3 additional NTD cases or the additional case of anencephaly. Through March 22, 1976, Merrell had received 12 anencephaly DERs (17.1%) and 17 NTDs (24.3%) out of 70 case reports received through that date. But not once are those statistics cited or otherwise mentioned in the report.

As stated above, Merrell's effort to sell the FDA and advisory committee on the safety of Clomid also encompassed a discussion on the **combined incidence of all congenital anomalies** in association with use of the drug. The multiple deficiencies of the pre-market investigations (1960-1970), and how Merrell manipulated its numbers, have already been discussed. As might be expected, these design problems do not show up in its report. But the drug company did not stop there.

Another gross misstatement of statistics involved Merrell's recitation of data from the Clomid scientific literature. It cited "13 published papers having *original information without duplication of population*, having a sufficient number of patients, and in which there was a mention of one or more anomalies of offspring of Clomid associated pregnancies." [Emphasis added, p.20.] From this literature, Merrell quoted an incidence of birth defects of 4.1%.

However, when one reviews the 13 published papers cited in the report, it becomes apparent that the aforementioned representation is not true. The Goldfarb, Greenblatt and Karow papers were all from the investigational population, and *none* of those three publications contain any "original information without duplication of population." When the total number of pregnancies is deleted from these three, the remaining pregnancies total 406 (not 848). After a deduction for abortions, the delivered offspring (including multiple births) equal 367, from which there were 19 infants with congenital malformations (a 5.2% rate, not 4.1%).

I was never supplied with a copy of Merrell's report nor informed of its existence (prior to the hearing).

Although I was later notified by Gregoire of the upcoming hearing, I was not invited to participate during the oral presentation. I decided that it would serve no purpose to attend. In hindsight, it was a poor decision.

Hearing of May 6, 1976

On May 6, 1976, Merrell showed up with its contingent of experts, but this time without Terence Mix or anyone else to dispute the statements made to the Committee. Dr. Robert Brent again appeared on behalf of Merrell, as did Dr. Raymond Vande Weile. When I later reviewed a transcript of the hearing, I noted a number of statements made by both witnesses that could have been effectively challenged. Brent was the first one to step up to the podium.

"The attorney (Mix) proposed the hypothesis that clomiphene citrate is teratogenic, quote, 'by altering the chromosomes in the germ cells of the ova prior to conception,' end quote. The explanation for the chromosomal abnormalities is related to the attorney's hypothesis that clomiphene citrate produces alterations in the estrogen levels which in turn alters pH which in turn produces chromosomal abnormalities.

"Next the attorney *would have us believe that anencephaly and spina bifida and hydrocephaly can be associated with abnormal chromosomes*, and thirdly, he concluded that the five cases of Down syndrome reported in the 2,000 or so Merrell patients receiving clomiphene citrate represents a significant increase in the incidence of Down syndrome." [Emphasis added; transcript p.2.]

I could almost see the smirk when Brent commented on my suggestion that neural tube defects could be associated with abnormal chromosomes. Was it such an absurdity, as Brent suggested to the panel? Perhaps he should have reviewed the then-current literature, as I had done. If he had bothered to look at those papers, he would have seen numerous case reports of NTDs with associated chromosomal anomalies.[110] Then again, why should we presume that he hadn't? Every one of them had been cited in my written submission to the Advisory Committee in July 1975.

"Although, there was an increase in the expected incidence of Down syndrome, it was *not statistically significant* in (Oakley's) opinion, and he noted that *two* of the Down's cases' mothers had not received clomiphene for *many months* before conception. * * * The fact that *two* of the patients had not been exposed to clomiphene for *months* would further decrease the impact of the incidence of Down syndrome patients." [Emphasis added, transcript pp.3-5.]

When Oakley published his paper in 1972, and again when he made his presentation to the Advisory Committee on July 18, 1975, he combined 2,329 Clomid pregnancies with 255 Pergonal pregnancies, from which 6 infants were born with Down syndrome (5 from the clomiphene group). After an adjustment for maternal age, he concluded that 2.6 would have been expected from this population. *He found this number statistically significant* (P=.049) in his 1972 abstract. And his view didn't change in 1975: "based on this population with this maternal age distribution, 2.6 cases when six cases were seen, a two-fold increase with the probability around .05."[111] At no time in Oakley's oral testimony did he ever suggest that his numbers were not statistically significant.

Likewise, Oakley never stated that two of the Down syndrome mothers "had not received clomiphene for many months before conception." All he stated was that two of the patients had not taken Clomid during the cycle of conception, which was true. But one of the two mothers, as stated above, was treated only *one cycle* before she conceived, not "many months before conception."

Vande Weile's role was to undermine the Boue study, which no doubt was giving Merrell its biggest problem. He had, purportedly, met with the Boues in Paris and had a conversation with them about certain data and information that was not referred to in their published study. Vande Weile attacked the published paper and pointed to its many flaws, which he allegedly learned from his chat with the two authors.

"Actually, the *minority* of the patients included in this were *anovulatory* patients whose ovulation had been induced with gonadotropins and Clomid. The *majority* of the patients were patients who received medication *following conception*; here in the United States, we would consider completely unacceptable.

"As an example, a *significant part of these patients were repeated aborters who had normal ovarian function*, but were given Clomid or gonadotropin or combinations later on to induce better ovulation, whatever obvious figment of the imagination this is. Obviously, you all know that in patients of repeated abortions, the incidence of chromosomal abnormalities is much higher than in an average group. So this, already by itself, would probably invalidate the whole statistic.

"Another significant group in the study was patients with normal infertility, in other words, with infertility when work had been found to be normal. Everything was normal and so let's give some gonadotropins or Clomid or a combination of Clomid and gonadotropin and see what will happen. Again, obviously, this is an unacceptable indication.

"Perhaps more importantly, *at least one half* of the patients had been given actually, mainly chorionic gonadotropin and menopausal urinary gonadotropin *after ovulation* had occurred.

* * * * *

"It's an almost unbelievable study, but you can get out (information) when you actually talk to the investigators. They had no control of the clinical material. These are very distinguished geneticists who know chromosomes very well, but have no control over the material that was sent to them.

"When I asked the Boues whether *the treatment and the control group had been matched for the age at which the development had been arrested*; in other words, ovulating *earlier or later abortions*, they did not have the evidence there. And again, all of you know the earlier the abortion, the earlier (to) the point of conception, you're going to have a higher instance of malformation or chromosomal abnormality that you find. [Emphasis added, pp.17-19.]

According to the transcript of the hearing, Vande Wiele claimed that the majority had been given fertility drugs *after* ovulation had occurred, suggesting that they had not been induced to ovulate; that only a minority were anovulatory; that a significant number of the patients in the study were simply repeat aborters with normal ovarian function; that the two geneticists had no control over the aborted material they examined, which had been provided by others; and that they had no documentation matching the ages of the abortuses between the treated and control groups. Vande Wiele's pitch: this is nothing more than "trash in, trash out, junk science." If the data received is of no value, then the results of the study would likewise be valueless. In summary, the Boues had no control over what they got and did the best that they could, but the study is worthless.

Perhaps Vande Wiele should have looked closer at the Boue publications.

Not only did the study appear as a letter in *The Lancet* publication,[112] it also was reprinted as part of a *peer reviewed* study in *Teratology,*[113] and a noted French medical journal as well.[114] In other words, the quality of the study was scrutinized by other physicians and scientists before it was cleared for publication.

The text of those publications would also appear to be in conflict with a number of Vande Wiele's assertions. For example, Merrell's witness suggested that the study lacked validity because the Boues used "repeated aborters," which already had a higher than normal incidence of abnormal chromosomes. But the Boues looked at that question. "The results in groups 1 and 2 were *similar* whether therapy was given for amenorrhea (absence of menstruation) or *anovulation*, or for *recurrent abortion* in women of normal fertility."[115]

Were the Boues examining abortuses that had conceived prior to treatment? Vande Wiele conveyed the notion that the majority of the pregnancies during this part of the study had not been produced by ovulation-inducing therapy. Such a suggestion is absolutely false. Although some may have been exposed to ovulatory stimulating drugs after conception as well, every one of the 84 abortuses examined had received treatment *prior* to the date they were conceived. "We have collected 84 cases in which treatment with an ovulatory stimulant had been instituted *prior to conception* which led to a karyotyped abortion."[116]

Equally absurd is Vande Wiele's statement that the Boues had acknowledged to him that they had not matched the age of the abortuses in the treated and conrol groups; that they had not separated out early and late abortions. In truth, the Boues *only* looked at early abortions. "Only abortions in which the embryo was less than 12 weeks old were studied."[117] Examining abortuses following use of ovulatory stimulants was only part of a much larger study. In all, the Boues evaluated the chromosomes of almost 1,500 aborted embryos. By the design of the study, every one had occurred during the first trimester of each pregnancy. Accordingly, the treated and controls were all matched for embryonic age at the time of spontaneous abortion.

But, of course, I was not present to raise these points to the Advisory Committee. Every statement made at the hearing, not to mention the representations in the written report of January 16, 1975, went unchallenged. After one hour of testimony, the matter was concluded, and deliberations commenced later in the day.

Merrell never conducted either the retrospective or prospective studies.[118]

* * * * *

CHAPTER 8

Ancient Knowledge

The flight from Los Angeles to Cincinnatti had been a lot bumpier than I would have preferred. Actually, if my seatbelt had been any tighter, my legs would have turned blue. But now I was safely on the ground. I rented a car and drove to the Sheraton-Gibson Hotel on Walnut Street, only a mile from Merrell-National Laboratories. This had been the site of my two depositions in February 1974. I was anxiously looking forward to my first visit to Merrell's pharmaceutical facility and having a go at its voluminous IND and NDA files. My next Clomid trial was set in October 1977. I was not about to go into another trial without thoroughly viewing all of the Clomid records well in advance.

It was early spring, 1977.

The following morning I was up at the crack of dawn, ate breakfast and was on my way well before my scheduled appointment. The agreement with Merrell's defense counsel was that I would be provided with a conference room to inspect the records between 9:00 AM and 5:00 PM each day; not any earlier nor any later. I was to be inspecting records the entire week, Monday through noon on Friday, after which I would be returning to L.A.

At 8:30 AM I pulled into Merrell's parking lot at 2110 East Galbraith Road. In front of me loomed a large multi-storied building. Surrounded by green acreage, Merrell's facility was situated in a park-like setting. It was readily apparent that selling pharmaceutical products was a lucrative business.

The sun was out, but there was a definite bite in the air as I approached the entry to Merrell-National Laboratories. I entered the large mezzanined lobby and headed for the reception desk. After introducing myself to the receptionist and registering, I was provided with a badge and asked to be seated. Someone would shortly be out to direct me to the appropriate room.

A good half hour later, a young lady approached. She wore glasses and a dress suit, and had a professional – somewhat impersonal – presence about her. "Are you Mr. Mix?" she asked.

I immediately stood and grabbed my briefcase. "Yes, I am… I'm Terry Mix," I added, as I extended my hand. "I was to meet Jack Chewning to inspect some records."

She shook my hand firmly, as if to let me know that we stood on equal footing. She had yet to smile and apparently chose not to give me her name. "Yes. I work in legal," she said. "Dr. Chewning asked me to show you to your inspection room. We already have everything set up. So…why don't you follow me and we'll get you started."

With that, she turned and was off to the races, with me doing my best to keep up. Just beyond the lobby we entered through a door and into a labyrinth of hallways. After a number of left and right turns, I was totally lost and knew that I would need a guide if I had any hope of getting out at the end of the day.

Finally we arrived at my windowless workplace for the next 4½ days. Inside was a large conference table, surrounded by several chairs. At one end of the table sat another young lady, this one with a pleasant smile. In front of her was a stack of at least three magazines. She no doubt had been assigned the task of insuring that I behaved myself during the course of the day – maybe for the entire week. We were promptly introduced to one another.

At the other end of the room – behind my guard – sat a large number of labeled boxes, no doubt holding at least some of the Clomid IND and NDA records. "Those are the first set of your records," nodded my impersonal hostess. I was sure that someone had informed her that I was the enemy. "Dr. Chewning will be in shortly and explain how they are organized. There are boxes of paperclips and rubberbands for you on the table. Use them to mark anything you want copied. Coffee and water should be here within a few minutes. So…unless there's something else you need…?"

I just shook my head.

"Alright, I'll let Dr.Chewning know that you're here." With that she disappeared.

I first stepped over and looked at the dozens of boxes, pondering whether I should grab one of them and start my "document inspection." I judiciously decided to wait for Jack. The last thing I wanted to do was waste time. If I was to go through 80,000 pages of documents in four and a half days, I would have to be organized. And even then, I doubted that such a feat could be accomplished. There certainly was no way that I could *read* almost 20,000 pages a day. I couldn't even read a 500-page book in one day.

My plan was actually quite simple. Although I knew little about what I would be encountering, I was certain that the vast majority of the records had little to do with what

I was after. I wanted anything associated with birth defects – human or animal. I was also seeking proof of Merrell's culpability, including communications about the text of the drug's labeling. Everything else would be irrelevant to my goals. Some documents – hopefully most – I could exclude simply by their nature or form. They would be visually scanned, either individually or by group. Others I would read only a few lines, looking for "buzz words;" anything to give me a quick clue about its content. If it fell into a category I was after, I would mark it for copying. This way, most of my reading would be back in my office at my own leisure and pace. If it contained something of *real* interest, I would read it and make notes of its identity and content, insuring that the document would not get "lost" in the course of the agreed copying procedure.

Suddenly the door opened and in walked Jack Chewning.

"Well, hi, Terry," he said, with a broad smile. We shook hands, as he added, "I trust you had a nice flight?" John (Jack) Chewning, a physician/lawyer, had always been cordial – if not outright friendly – since the day I first met him on the Breimhorst case; a welcome change from Miss Personality.

"Slept most of the way," I responded. I was not about to give him the pleasure of knowing that the flight had been a "white knuckler" from the moment we approached the Rockies.

"Wonderful. Well, we'll do what we can to put you back to sleep," he winked. "We've got a mountain of records for you, so why don't I explain to you how they are organized and get you started."

Chewning then proceeded to explain the basic organization of the Clomid documents. Essentially they were identical to the file maintained by the FDA, with Merrell's set being the originals. The entire set of records was designated the "Drug Regulatory Affairs (DRA) file." It was comprised of approximately 200 bound volumes, each containing approximately 400 pages. Within the DRA were contained the IND and NDA. The IND dated back to 1963, when it was established pursuant to new federal law, but contained data and information back to 1960 and earlier. Its records primarily included the pre-market clinical investigations, animal studies and documents related to laboratory studies. The NDA had been filed on February 23, 1965. It initially contained 43 volumes and was given reference number 16-131. It likewise included investigational records, along with proposed labeling and additional information related to its expanding clinical studies. In addition to the IND and NDA, the DRA also contained post-marketing Drug Experience Reports (DERs). All records were pretty much maintained chronologically and were numbered sequentially. Also produced, pursuant to my request, were intracompany memoranda and correspondence between Merrell and the FDA, and other companies, related to Clomid.

"Jack, my preference is to get started on the clinical records, the pre-market investigations." My thinking was to look for transcription errors between the raw data from the investigators and the summaries appearing on the Analysis of Pregnancy forms. Were there references to congenital anomalies that did not appear on the forms? Were there omissions of critical information, such as the date of conception and dates of Clomid treatment? Had spontaneous abortions been omitted? These were some of my thoughts, but in truth I did not know what to expect once I started to read the documents. All I knew was that the clinical studies were Merrell's primary "proof" that Clomid was not teratogenic in humans. This was where I had to start.

"I'm way ahead of you, Terry. I anticipated as much, so that's what I have for you in these boxes. They're all there, all 2600 cases."

Chewning next explained Merrell's numbering system, pointing to the earliest cases and suggesting how I might want to proceed. After we had concluded our discussion, he gave me a playful wave of the hand and offered, "Have fun." And just like that he was gone and I was seated at the table reading the first volume of the clinical studies.

By the end of the first day, I had reviewed only 4 volumes of the IND.

Concealment of Pre-Market Cases

But the day was not a total loss. By chance I stumbled upon a record unlike any of the others I had been reviewing at the time. It was a summary prepared by a Dr. Gerhard Bettendorf from Hamburg, Germany. [Exhibit 4] All 364 investigators had been assigned a number. Bettendorf was identified as investigator number 157. The document summarized the results of *forty pregnancies*, out of which only 18 had been completed at the time. Out of the concluded pregnancies, 12 had resulted in spontaneous abortions

(SAs). But when I searched for the "Analysis of Pregnancy" forms, I could only locate *two* of them for this investigator!

To verify that only the two (rather than 40) cases were included in the 2,635 pregnancies that represented the official total from the study, I referred to the computer printout I had previously acquired from Merrell entitled, "Clomid Pregnancy Data as of January, 1970." [Exhibit 5] The document included a wealth of (purported) information on each pregnancy from the study that had been stored in Merrell's computers. I had also obtained all of the necessary legends, codes and other documents needed for its interpretation.

The first column sets forth the individual case numbers for each patient in the study. The first three digits of the case number represent the number of the investigator and the last three the number assigned to the patient. The comparison validated that Merrell had excluded 38 of Bettendorf's 40 pregnancies from its official data on the clinical studies. But what was particularly bothersome was that out of those 40 conceptions, *at least* 12 of them (30.0%) had resulted in SAs – and 11 of the twelve had been excluded from the already high statistics (20.4%) on the SA rate.

In one fashion or another, 38 of Bettendorf's clinical records had not found their way into the official set of documents of either the IND or NDA. Had they been pulled and destroyed? Set aside in some dusty boxes in a basement storage room? Sent back to Bettendorf? Never received from the German doctor to begin with? The last question would not seem to be a likely scenario. Why send the records on two, but withhold the balance of the remaining 38? Why send a summary of all forty if you haven't sent the records on all or, at least, a majority of them? It just didn't make sense.

For further assurance, I checked the literature upon my return from the inspection trip. And there it was. Bettendorf had published an abstract of an earlier stage of his Clomid investigations.[119] His brief summary was quite enlightening. "There were a total 29 pregnancies, 14 have delivered, 8 aborted and 7 are still pregnant."

How many other records had been discarded? Could I find them even if they had? Probably not. I had searched through more than 1,500 pages of records and had found this summary just by chance. It was also too easy to remove undesired reports and medical charts from the official documents – or never file them to begin with. After all, it was

Merrell that was preparing the summaries of the investigations, not the investigators. It would also not be the first time that Merrell had falsified official FDA records.[120]

After locating the Bettendorf publication following my return to California, I also did a random check on a number of other investigators who had published the results of their pre-market studies. My search was limited to papers reporting on pregnancies that could only have occurred prior to the date of initial marketing on May 15, 1967; and thus were not part of an independent post-market study. The effort was rewarding.

One paper had been published by a Karow and Payne.[121] Dr. Sheldon Payne was Merrell clinical investigator number 066. His publication reported on 180 pregnancies, including 140 on which the outcome was known at the time the paper was submitted for publication (1966). However, Merrell only reported on a total of 136 pregnancies for Dr. Payne.[122] What ever happened to the other 44 pregnancies? Why were they missing?

A second publication was by Kempers, Decker and Lee.[123] Dr. David Decker was Merrell clinical investigator number 271. This publication reported on *15 pregnancies*. "Nine of the 15 pregnancies (were) still in various stages of gestation. Of the remaining 6, five (had) ended in delivery of a single infant at term; 4 infants were normal and 1 had meningomyelocele and hydrocephalus. The sixth pregnancy ended in abortion at 6 weeks." Merrell only reported on 11 pregnancies.[124] Why were four missing?

Dr. Nathan Kase was from New Haven, Connecticut, and was assigned investigator number 118. His articles reported on 23 pregnancies,[125] but Merrell selected only eight to include in its composite list submitted to the FDA.[126] What happened to the other fifteen?

Yet another publication was authored by E. Rabau, et al., from Tel-Hashomer, Israel.[127] Dr Rabau (investigator number 238) reported on thirty-four pregnancies, which resulted in a spontaneous abortion rate of 20.6%. But *none* of the pregnancies were included in Merrell's official list of 2,635 reported to the FDA.[128] Why were they selectively excluded?

Then it got really interesting.

Dr. Naotaka Ishizuka was investigator number 250, from Nagoya, Japan. I was able to secure a translated copy of a published study by Ishizuka, et al. that reported on the results of their Clomid pre-market clinical investigations.[129] They detailed their then-current findings on 16 pregnancies. At the time, only seven had delivered: two resulted in spontaneous abortions and one female of a set of twins "had a visceral protrusion with umbilical hernia and died on the second day." The twins were delivered after 33 weeks of gestation and conception occurred during a treatment cycle with clomiphene. They acknowledged a possible causal relationship between the birth defect and clomiphene. "It may be presumptive to conclude that there was a cause-effect relationship with clomiphene administration in this case, but a possible effect of clomiphene in such a development must be taken into consideration in the future studies." Merrell only included one of the 16 pregnancies in its compilation, which, of course, *did not include the birth defect.*[130]

The final paper I located was authored by Curchod and Weihs.[131] Curchod was investigator number 264. His practice was located in Lausanne, Switzerland. Their article summarized the results of five pregnancies. One resulted in a spontaneous abortion. Of the remaining 4, one was delivered at 20 weeks, following 6 months of treatment, with "fetal malformations: evisceration of liver, intestine and stomach." This anomaly, also referred to as "exomphalos," involves the decribed organs protruding in a sac outside of the body cavity. Merrell did not include any of these five pregnancies within its clinical investigational data – and again, *another birth defect was excluded.*[132]

Stimulated by these disparities, I pursued yet another means of verifying the incompleteness of the pre-market clinical data. Clinical investigator Edward Tyler, M.D. (number 096) had testified during the Breimhorst trial that his clinic had reported on approximately 200 pregnancies induced by Clomid.[133] Yet the official records at Merrell only summarize 87 Tyler pregnancies.[134] Had Tyler exaggerated or misrecollected the number of Clomid pregnancies? As a means of determining which number was the correct one, I secured the official Correspondence File on Tyler that had been maintained by the pharmaceutical company. My effort again paid off. On December 11, 1967, Tyler had sent a telegram to A.H. MacGregor of the William S. Merrell Company in Cincinnati. The relevant language states, "Kindly send analysis of ovulation and pregnancies in 202 completed triplicates that you have as soon as possible." Tyler had previously sent pregnancy reports to Merrell in "triplicate forms." He now wanted Merrell's analysis of those reports to assist him in writing a paper for publication. So what ever happened to the other 115 pregnancies?

And how would Merrell Dow reconcile the discrepancy between its official set of records and the numbers from its clinical investigators? During the Gandy trial,[135] it was provided with such an opportunity. One of Merrell's expert witnesses was a James Goddard, M.D., the Commissioner of the FDA between January 11, 1966 and June 30, 1968, which included the year Clomid was initially marketed (1967). Now, 27 years later, he was coming to Merrell's rescue.[136] During my cross-examination, he was confronted with a number of these discrepancies. His half-hearted reply: "(Merrell) may have excluded others, because they didn't fulfill the criteria."[137] But what criteria and in what way was it not fulfilled? Certainly the investigators felt the cases qualified. In fact, they even chose to publish papers on them. Not only did Goddard fail to expand on this explanation, the subject was not even touched by Merrell's counsel on redirect examination. Bottom line; Merrell *had* no explanation.

Other than discovering the Bettendorf summary and a few errors in transcription, the first day had not been very productive. The method of inspection was also quite tedious, and I was feeling pressured by my self-imposed time limits. I had hoped to avoid a second trip, but now it seemed inevitable.

That evening I made a decision. I would bite the bullet and order the entire set of records covering the clinical studies. At 10 cents a page it would be expensive. But I had seen only 1,500 pages in my first full day, and at this pace would not even complete the investigational studies by the time I left on Friday. Not only would I save time during my inspection trip, by reading at my own pace back at the office, I would pick up detail I unquestionably would have missed in Cincinnatti. As it turned out, I found another important use for these records a few months later.

Upon returning to my cubby hole Tuesday morning, I quickly placed a rubber band around each volume of the investigational studies. I then requested what I considered to be the next most important documents: the intracompany memoranda and correspondence with the FDA. Now I would be doing some serious mining. And over the course of the day I came upon some real gems. In fact, some of my discoveries were quite stunning.

For a good part of the morning I found an occasional document worthy of note, but nothing earth-shaking. As I came upon each page of interest, I would make a notation of its identity on a tablet and paperclip the page or pages for later photocopying. Meanwhile, my week-long companion sat chewing pack after pack of gum and devouring a never-ending stream of magazines. Occasionally she would be spelled by a temporary replacement; then would return with a new supply of reading material.

Late morning I came upon my first important discovery.

My initial surprise was that the FDA was not as blamelessly ignorant of Clomid's teratogenic risk as I had originally assumed. Nor was this simply a matter of Merrell carelessly proceeding with a clinical study designed only to develop proof that its drug could stimulate ovulation – and ignoring what might occur to the products of the desired conceptions.

As it turned out, FDA staff members had expressed concern about a possible risk of birth defects as early as 1963. Not only did the FDA have the results of the 1962 Clomid teratology studies at this time, it was also a little dubious about anything coming from Merrell because of the Triparanol (MER 29) disaster – a drug chemically related to clomiphene citrate. Because of the animal studies, there had been a temporary interruption of the clinical investigations. It also prompted an FDA internal evaluation of Clomid by its own pharmacologists and other experts.

The Half-Life Concern

At the time, the medical officer assigned to the drug was A. Grace Pierce, M.D. She had recently suggested use of a double blind study with use of a placebo,[138] which was resisted by Merrell. On *October 11, 1963*, Dr. Pierce submitted to Merrell a summary of a pharmacological evaluation prepared by a Dr. Ernest Umberger, an endocrinologist, and requested data pertaining to absorption, excretion, and duration of activity after discontinuance of the drug. [Exhibit 6] Among other things, the summary stated:

> "Animal fertility studies are suggestive of prolonged action of the drug, perhaps due to deposition and sustained release from fat depots. The drug could therefore be effective longer than the duration of its administration. *It may carry over from the phase of induced ovulation into early pregnancy to interfere with the zygote and fetus.*" [Emphasis added.]

My theory at the Breimhorst trial had actually been suggested by the FDA over a decade earlier. I looked up from the summary at my silent companion. She sat at the end of the table, apparently absorbed in a story about her favorite movie star. Had I been so inclined, I could have easily removed the document from the binder with a cough and a slight tug. But, of course, a copy would serve the same purpose. To insure that it would not disappear, I made a note of all 13 names at Merrell who had received a copy – and continued to dig.

As it turned out, the suggestion that Clomid might carry over into early pregnancy had been run by the drug company more than once. Richardson-Merrell heard even more on the subject in the following months and years – a lot more.

A review of a July 27, 1964 Merrell internal memo, prepared by Hoekenga, revealed that a meeting took place on *July 24, 1964* between Drs. Pierce, Umberger, and two other FDA staffers, with Drs. Hoekenga, Johnson and Kuhn from Merrell. One of the topics covered at the time involved the metabolism of clomiphene citrate. Questions were posed by the FDA. Was there retention of the drug in fat or in other tissues? The FDA wanted measurements until there was zero retention. What was the status of the C_{14} studies? *"Is there an effect on the developing embryo as a result of retention of drug?"*

On *August 6, 1965*, another significant memorandum was prepared, this one by Dr. Victor Berliner of the FDA. It was submitted to Dr. Ridgley Bennett, who had taken over monitoring Clomid following the NDA filing in February 1965. The memo covered 9 pages and involved a comprehensive assessment of the drug, including the Merrell animal teratology studies of 1962. After noting the human half-life of Clomid at 5 days, Berliner made an astute observation. "The rather unexpectedly long persistence of part of Clomid-C_{14} in the system, even after single doses, *must be suspected of being able to produce adverse reactions, such as...a possible teratogenic action in instances of an initiated pregnancy."* [Emphasis added, Exhibit 7.]

In summarizing the animal studies, he also observed that at the highest dose, Clomid had caused a *limb reduction anomaly* in one of the rats (absence of a tibia). I was absolutely astonished. I had totally missed this observation when I had examined the same report before the Breimhorst trial. Another example of how thoroughly I was prepared for that one-month battle. Berliner then concluded (at p.7):

> "The test wherein the drug was administered as a single dose (during the animal studies) does not establish whether the teratogenic action got into play only at the time of administration, or if there was also a carry-over effect of retained drug. For this reason *it is difficult to deduct from these investigations if in human use the proposed schedule of five days would not involve the risk of a teratogenic effect if ovulation and conception take place at a stage that is still within the range of a residual drug action."* [Emphasis added.]

Twenty days later, *August 26, 1965*, Dr. Bennett had another discussion with Hoekenga, this time by phone. Hoekenga's memo[139] of the talk noted a familiar concern: *"Excretion pattern of drug may permit teratogenic effect, if drug stays in body."* Bennett suggested that therefore "should get conceptions in post-treatment cycle rather than treatment cycle." For the first time, the FDA had floated an idea about only allowing conception to take place during the first cycle *after* treatment.

I was now beginning to piece together a story.

For two years the FDA had been pressing Merrell for some proof that the prolonged retention of the drug did not present a risk to the developing embryo. So far, nothing had satisfied the governmental scientists. Merrell had also recently filed its NDA, seeking approval for marketing. This issue was becoming an obstacle to getting Clomid onto the shelves of your local pharmacy. It was even being suggested that patients be admonished not to conceive during a treatment cycle. If this occurred, the conception rate would drop dramatically – as would potential sales of the drug.

The next day, Hoekenga called Bennett and set up a meeting at the FDA for *September 8, 1965*. The FDA had also expressed reluctance about approving a dose level at 100 mg. a day, which it considered too high. Merrell would make a presentation with updated information from the Clomid clinical studies that would hopefully put both issues to rest.

The meeting took place as scheduled. Hoekenga, Bunde and Johnson appeared for Merrell. The FDA was represented by Dr. Ridgley Bennett, the NDA reviewing officer, Dr. John Winkler, the Acting Director of the Drug Evaluation Branch, and Dr. Victor Berliner, an FDA pharmacologist. Bennett also brought in a Dr. Robert Hodges, a review officer for the earlier Clomid IND. Hoekenga hand-carried a written presentation summarizing updated data on 564 pregnancies of anovulatory patients treated with Clomid.

A Merrell Interdepartment Memo[140] summarized the meeting. Among the topics discussed were the questions related to the safety and efficacy of Clomid at the 100 mg./day dose, the significance of the multiple births, the side effect of ovarian cysts and whether Clomid had any effect on the eyes.[141] Hoekenga's Memo also recorded:

> "Possible teratogenicity: *Bennett was concerned about possible teratogenic effect of the drug inasmuch as it (or the tag, at least) does remain in the body for some days.* We indicated that there simply was not any evidence at all on the basis of 564 completed pregnancies. Hodges thought that perhaps the 3 vascular anomalies[142] represented a pattern and suggested that the opinion of Wilson or Warkany be sought. We agreed to seek such an opinion as an easy way of settling the matter." [Emphasis added.]

As I read the Interdepartment Memo, I recalled the testimony from Hoekenga during his pretrial deposition in Breimorst. At the time, I was interested in discovering what efforts had been made to assess the risk to the embryo when conception occurred during the carry-over or half-life period.

> "Relative to the clinical investigations and all the investigative reports, was any analysis made or any conclusion formulated as to the possible teratogenic effect of Clomid when conception actually occurred during the half-life period?"

> "Not a specific analysis relating to half-life."[143]

As I could now see, this had been a major issue with the FDA for at least a couple of years. Notwithstanding the FDA's expressed concern, Merrell had avoided making such an assessment.

A solicitation of an opinion from James G. Wilson took place on September 22, 1965. Enclosed for his review were (1) the Physician's Drug Monograph on Clomid; (2) an updated *summary* of pregnancies occurring in patients treated with Clomid, including a table of congenital malformations observed; (3) a *summary* of metabolic data on Clomid; and (4) an updated Clomid bibliography. As one might guess, none of the deficiencies in the study were called to Wilson's attention.

As expected, and as we heard during the Breimhorst trial, Wilson concluded on October 4, 1965, that Clomid did not present a teratogenic risk and that he did not observe a pattern or increase in the incidence of congenital anomalies. This decision was based upon Merrell's summary of only 359 pregnancies. This did in fact turn out to be an "easy way of settling the matter."

Berliner later (December 13, 1965) summarized his position: "The *teratogenic hazard of Clomid is relatively low.* * * * Also, the evaluation by Dr. Wilson, submitted in the supplement of the clinical data that *may implicate Clomid as a teratogen*, seems to be adequate to eliminate this problem from further consideration as an obstacle to the use of Clomid." [144] [Emphasis added.] This was an interesting comment. Berliner did not view the teratogenic risk as *non-existent* after Wilson's report; he considered it "relatively low." He still held the opinion that there was some level of risk.

The lingering uncertainty about Clomid's teratogenic risk is also reflected in a couple of later memos as well. This came in the context of Merrell's desire to expand treatment beyond three cycles.

Following a meeting with Bennett, Hodges and Berliner on May 26, 1966, a memo[145] from John E. Johnson, Jr. to Bunde states: "(W)e shall have to expand our pregnancy file to provide further support for the *lack of effect on the fetus,* including more pregnancies occurring in the 4th to the 6th cycles of treatment." [Emphasis added.] Because of the prolonged carryover of the drug, any Clomid remaining after 30 days would build on the next treatment cycle. Thus, there existed some concern that continued treatment over a period of four to six months might expose the embryo/fetus to a larger quantity of the drug.

Another memo[146] related to the same meeting states: "They (Bennett, Hodges and Berliner) indicated that the type of additional evidence for 'safety' which would permit expansion of our claims or duration of treatment would be in the areas of information on: ...4. *Lack of effect on the fetus*, especially in pregnancies occurring in the fourth to sixth cycles of treatment." [Emphasis added.] The evaluation from Merrell's teratologist, however, was sufficient to set the issue aside and move on toward approval.

Clomid was approved for marketing by the FDA on February 1, 1967. Sales commenced on May 15, 1967.

For the next couple of years, Clomid's history with the FDA was relatively quiet. Merrell had placed a cutoff date of May 15, 1967, for its clinical investigations. Any undelivered pregnancies occurring prior to that date would be followed by the investigator until the patient delivered, and then would become part of the official pre-market investigations. Records trickled in on these pregnancies until early 1970. By that time, Merrell had compiled the clinical information on all 2,635 Clomid pregnancies, from which the outcome was known on 2,369 cases. This updated data was provided to the FDA in Periodic Reports, filed every three months during the first year and semi-anually during the second year. Thereafter, the PRs were to be filed annually. Also included with the Reports were DERs, suggested changes in the labeling, and an updated bibliography on all published literature involving the drug.

As the FDA staff continued to observe the tail end of the clinical investigations, someone must have noted a few of its deficiencies. The reports on the outcome of a number of delivered babies seemed sketchy and only reported their condition at the time of birth. Additionally, very few autopsies had been carried out on the stillbirths and neonatal deaths.

Correspondence of June 4, 1969

On June 4, 1969, Dr. Edwin M. Ortiz sent a letter to The William S. Merrell Company, Division of Richardson-Merrell, Inc. [Exhibit 8] In that correspondence he made three recommendations to the pharmaceutical company, two of which related to further efforts to detect the existence of congenital anomalies following Clomid-related pregnancies. Those recommendations were:

"1. That all living infants conceived in association with Clomid therapy be followed, if possible, by competent personnel for a period of at least two years, and a report submitted.

"2. That complete autopsies be performed, if possible, on all abortions, stillborns, deadborns, and neonatal deaths produced in association with Clomid therapy and the findings submitted. It is suggested that gross and microscopic anatomical studies be done and a search made for genetic and enzyme abnormalities."

Just two years after Clomid was initially marketed, the FDA was focusing on two major deficiencies in the pre-market clinical studies, namely, failure to conduct follow-up examinations and failure to perform autopsies on stillborns and neonatal deaths – both of which had been highlighted during the Breimhorst trial. Evidently Ortiz, or more likely one of his staff, had taken notice of these omissions and wanted to be satisfied that performing them would not have appreciably increased the rate of congenital anomalies.

Although acknowledging the feasibility of such studies, this request was met with immediate resistance. What prompted the FDA to make such a request? Merrell wanted to know what the FDA had seen in its submitted data that justified requesting additional investigations.

A meeting took place on *July 9, 1969* to discuss the issues. Another Interdepartment Memo,[147] prepared by Hoekenga, summarized the discussion. Dr. Ortiz and Dr. Leslie Dill were present on behalf of the FDA; Drs. Hoekenga and O'Dell for Merrell. Hoekenga noted that "apparently the June 4 FDA letter was mostly Dr. Dill's idea. He did most of the talking at the meeting." Dr. Dill called attention to the high abortion rate. As recorded by Hoekenga, Dill had a few other pertinent comments as well:

> "Dr. Dill has an impression that we should want to be able to show that *Clomid does not increase the abortion rate.* His thought is that chromosomal studies would clarify this point. It is well known, of course, that chromosomal aberrations are common in aborted human fetal material (XO aneuploidy, triploidy, tetraploidy, trisomics of Groups A, B, C, D, E, F and G, etc.). Dr. Dill thought that *if Clomid-related abortuses proved to have a 10% higher rate of chromosomal aberrations than non-Clomid ones, this would be significant."*
> [Emphasis added, Exhibit 9.]

As I read the last line, I am sure that my jaw must have dropped. Dill was actually expressing concern that Clomid might be increasing the spontaneous abortion rate by damaging chromosomes. In a sense, it was some form of vindication. Maybe my theories and hypothesis were not so far-fetched. I wondered what Dill would have thought of the Boue study where a *33% increase* was demonstrated following the use of fertility drugs, including clomiphene citrate.

The four doctors also discussed the request for follow-up examinations. Again, Dr. Dill took the lead in pushing the FDA's agenda. They were interested in reports from pediatricians that had examined the babies from the pre-market studies.

"Dr. Dill particularly had in mind the possibility of latent vascular defects.[148] The pediatricians would presumably be those in the same medical centers where Clomid was used most in its late investigative phase and any study would be a retrospective one. Dr. Dill further wondered whether it would be feasible to contact mothers directly regarding the health of Clomid-related offspring whose birth dated back to the investigative use of Clomid. We said that we would take the various comments under advisement, but that we would not want to initiate any review or study unless it would be known ahead of time that the design would yield statistically significant results."

I would agree that a study should not be pursued unless the number of offspring under investigation is large enough to make a meaningful statistical evaluation. But there were over 1,800 delivered pregnancies during the clinical investigations. Locating a sufficient number of them to make a valid study should not have been difficult.

And indeed it wasn't.

On *September 19, 1969*, Hoekenga wrote to Ortiz, addressing these two requests. As to the follow-up exams, Merrell was able to locate a number of physicians that were willing to participate in the study. One was a Dr. Rudolf Vollman, who was already conducting a larger study that also involved a number of Clomid patients. As stated by Hoekenga, "Although the number of women who took Clomid is relatively small, it is probable that enough of them did do so to make a statistical evaluation worthwhile." In addition, Merrell had also contacted several of its former clinical investigators.

"Seven of the physicians who had large pregnancy series during the years of Clomid's investigation have been contacted to ascertain whether they would be able to cooperate in a retrospective study. Five of them have indicated their willingness to participate; the other two have not yet replied. Participation would involve working with the pediatricians who have been supervising the care of infants born to the Clomid-treated mothers. Dr. James G. Wilson, Professor of Research Pediatrics and Anatomy at the University of Cincinnati, has aided in the drafting of a possible report form. *Because the mothers of Clomid-induced babies are an abnormal population to begin with, the question arises as to what population group could be used as a control.* Dr. Wilson has suggested that the pediatrician examining an infant born to a Clomid-treated mother be asked to also complete an identical case report form on the next well baby that he sees of similar age +/- 3 months, *but this procedure will still not ensure comparability among the two groups of mothers.* A number of other problems also will have to be worked out if this approach is to be considered a feasible one." [Emphasis added.]

According to Hoekenga, the second request would likely be even more difficult to complete. Discussing the suggestion about conducting chromosome studies on Clomid abortuses, he complained that "to show a meaningful incidence of (abnormal chromosomes) in fetal material from Clomid-treated women would require a very large number of cases."

As I sat reviewing the memoranda and correspondence related to the June 4, 1969 requests, I couldn't help but wonder where Merrell was going with this. At the outset, all the FDA was after were two-year follow-up examinations of all living Clomid-induced babies, and autopsies, and genetic and enzyme studies, of all abortions, stillborns and neonatal deaths from the same group.

Nothing was mentioned about using a control group. Indeed, when O'Dell first responded to the request on *June 19, 1969*, his reaction was that it would "probably be feasible to send a letter to many of our previous investigators, asking for a follow-up of all children over two years of age." As to the second request, he again indicated that "it probably would be feasible to send a letter to many of our previous investigators, asking for a report of all abortions, stillborns, deadborns, and neonatal deaths on whom autopsies were performed."

At the meeting of July 9, 1969, neither Dr. Ortiz nor Dr. Dill mentioned use of a control group for either recommendation. In fact, regarding request number 1, Hoekenga's memo states that "neither Dr. Ortiz nor Dr. Dill could suggest what kind of a specific follow-up might be considered for Clomid-related live babies." The discussion pertaining to request number 2 only centered on chromosome studies – not autopsies – and Dr. Dill's view that Merrell "should want to be able to show that Clomid does not increase the abortion rate."

In both instances it was *Merrell* that suggested that it would only be interested in conducting a study that "could be designed to be statistically significant." And it was *Merrell* that first suggested use of a control group for the follow-up examinations. As discussions about the two requested studies progressed, they became increasingly complex – and at the same time more difficult to conduct.

So why would Merrell want to make the two studies more complicated and difficult? This was a question that I posed to myself as I sat, surrounded by stacks of Clomid records, staring at a page I had already read two or three times. The answer, of course, was that the more difficult the study – the closer it got to impossible – the less likely it would ever be conducted. Aside from the question of chromosome studies, O'Dell had already acknowledged that they could round up enough pre-market offspring to do the follow-up exams and easily secure the requested autopsy reports.

Conducting a chromosome study on abortuses of Clomid-induced pregnancies likewise would not have been an insurmountable problem, as suggested by Hoekenga. It certainly wasn't for the Boues, who had designed and executed their study between 1965 and 1972. Their numbers were also statistically significant, even though they had only used 84 abortuses from pregnancies following ovulatory stimulation by fertility drugs. As I read Hoekenga's lament about how such a study "would require a *very large number of cases*," I could not help but chuckle out loud.

My amusement broke the silence and captured the attention of my companion for the first time in a day and a half. She immediately pulled herself away from her third magazine of the day and stared inquisitively at me at the opposite end of the table.

I shook my head with a broad smile. "It's nothing," I said. "Just thought of something funny."

She just smiled, shrugged her shoulders, and returned to her reading.

Hoekenga's final statement in his letter of September 19, 1969: "At such time as we have any further information on these subjects we will make a further report to you." He should have added, "Oh, by the way, don't hold your breath."

On May 1, 1970, Ortiz sent a brief letter to Merrell related to the subject. It stated: "Reference is made to your communication of September 19, 1969, pertaining to your new drug application for Clomid (clomiphene citrate) Tablets. Your communication is in response to our letter of June 4, 1969, which made certain recommendations on Clomid therapy studies. The material submitted is being retained as part of your application for this article."

And there the trail ends.

The reference to "material submitted" was mystifying, since I could find no further memoranda, correspondence or other documents related to the requested studies, even though I scanned every file and Periodic Report between June 1969 and the spring of 1977. The problem? As will become clear throughout the course of this book, Merrell dragged its feet about conducting the studies until the FDA, with its built-in short-term memory, shrugged its shoulders and forgot about it.

Years later, I inquired of Merrell whether it had ever initiated the requested studies. Its response: "By reply of June 19, 1969, Merrell-National replied and requested reasons why these recommendations were made. The FDA *did not pursue the matter* except to acknowledge the reply by letter of May 1, 1970, from Dr. Ortiz."[149] [Emphasis added.] Omitted in the answer is any reference to the meeting of July 9, 1969 and Hoekenga's letter of September 19, 1969. The ball, of course, was in Merrell's court. But suffice to say, the requested studies were never conducted and the FDA "did not pursue the matter."

Correspondence of January 22, 1970

During this same period of time, the FDA focused on another subject I had recently addressed, namely the increased incidence of Down syndrome. On *January 22, 1970*, a Marvin Seife, M.D. of the FDA, requested the following information as part its review of congenital malformations:

209

"1. The maternal age of all the women who have taken Clomid and become pregnant.

"2. Case histories of the five mongoloid births and of the mothers, and in particular the age of the mother.

"3. Whether any of the multiple abnormalities reported in the package insert have involved chromonsal (sic) abnormalities (trisomy, translocation etc., and if so the details).

"A search of the data submitted with your original new drug application has revealed *incomplete information on a great many of the individual patient reporting sheets* submitted by the investigators, namely *no age is stated for the patient*. We feel that you may have this age data and the other desired information in a readily available form. We would greatly appreciate any assistance that you can provide in securing the information requested above." [Emphasis added.]

So, why did the FDA suddenly become interested in the 5 Down syndrome cases? The timing would suggest that it may have had something to do with Oakley's study at the CDC. From his testimony at the July 18, 1975 hearing, I knew that he "became interested in the problem of chromosome anomalies and ovulatory drugs back in 1969 when (he) saw a child born with Trisomy D from a young mother." He then looked at the pre-marketing data from Clomid and Pergonal. This no doubt came from the FDA, another agency of the federal government. But when Oakley looked for the important statistics on maternal age, the FDA could not deliver. The Analysis of Pregnancy forms did not include a space for maternal age. The letter of January 22, 1970 followed.

The desired information was supplied by Merrell on March 17, 1970. Of course, none of the records on the infants with multiple abnormalities contained reports of chromosomal anlysis. This should not have been surprising since only two of the 5 cases of Down syndrome included records of such studies. [One additional report was obtained in December 1975, well after the July hearing.]

Two years later Oakley published his study, which concluded that there was more than twice the expected frequency of Down syndrome following use of fertility drugs.

To me, this request reflected awareness among members of the FDA of the excess number of cases of Down syndrome in the Clomid clinical investigations. Yet Merrell's need to follow-up on this information did not occur until after the July 18, 1975 hearing. From there, of course, it disappeared into a twilight zone known as the "federal bureaucracy."

* * * * *

CHAPTER 9

Feathering the Nest

The morning of day three was spent completing my review of the FDA correspondence and memoranda. I was about midway through my week-long task and my enthusiasm still seemed to override my developing fatigue. The discoveries of the previous day served to fuel my interest. Reward is a powerful incentive for continued hard work.

My next find involved no less than the commissioner of the FDA, Dr. James L. Goddard, who headed the agency between January 11, 1966 and June 30, 1968. Since Goddard had been in charge during the period leading up to and including approval and initial marketing of Clomid, his communications with Merrell took on added importance.

The first contact of significance related to an article by Morton Mintz that appeared in the Washington Post on February 19, 1967. The piece began:

"A ruling by the Food and Drug Administration that a new antisterility drug may do more good than harm is being questioned on Capitol Hill. The drug is Clomid. It was cleared for the prescription market on Feb.1, but is not expected to be generally available to physicians until April. In a letter dated Tuesday, Rep. L.H. Fountain (D-N.C.) asked Commissioner James L. Goddard to explain FDA's reasoning in deciding to release Clomid. Fountain heads the House Intergovernmental Relations Subcommittee, which monitors the agency's performance. His letter was prompted in part by deaths among infants born to women who had multiple pregnancies after taking antisterility drugs."

The article went on to summarize the text of the package insert, including the statistics involving the pre-market investigations. Discussed are reports of birth defects following use of Clomid and the animal teratology studies. Mintz pointed out that the product labeling admonishes the physician and patient to avoid use of the drug after conception (because of the animal studies), but discloses that 6% of the patients in the clinical investigations "inadvertently received (clomiphene citrate) during early pregnancy." Individual cases of multiple births and the deaths of some of the newborns are also detailed. Reference is even made to the drug's chemical relationship with Triparanol, which had caused cataracts in its users.

On February 21, 1967, J.K. Lindsay, the president of Richardson-Merrell, called Goddard to speak with him about the Mintz piece.[150] Lindsay advised the Commissioner that the purpose of the call was to assure Goddard that Merrell would make available all of its research help and medical staff to assist the FDA in replying to the article. Lindsay's memorandum on the call states:

> "At this point Dr. Goddard explained very emphatically that the problem of the reply was theirs - - that the FDA knew all about the drug - - that they had made a decision to approve the drug for marketing - - that they would stand by that decision - - that *clomiphene was one of the most important drugs to be approved this year, if not the most important, that there might be some risk in its use but that the drug was so important.* He was very clear that the question of Fountain and Mintz was their problem." [Emphasis added.]

As I read the memo, it seemed a little odd that the Commissioner of the FDA would be touting Clomid to Merrell as possibly the most important drug to be approved that year. His enthusiasm for the product appeared to go beyond what one would expect from a professional overseeing a regulatory agency. Rather than being objective and impartial, Goddard seemed unduly preoccupied with the "importance" of Clomid.

The two men also spoke about methods of promotion and the target audience of advertising for the drug, in order to insure that Clomid would reach the hands of those qualified to prescribe it. This portion of the discussion appeared appropriate. But when their dialogue turned to Merrell's frustration about updating the data on its labeling, I observed assurances from Goddard that smacked of favoritism. [One day earlier (February 20, 1967), the Chief of the FDA's Medical Advertising Branch had advised Merrell that the Clomid brochure would not be approved unless and until the clinical information had been updated.[151] This position was taken in reaction to the Mintz article and Fountain letter to the FDA.] Lindsay's memo continued:

> "I said that what we were concerned about is a supplement - - that the rules are quite clear as to supplements and that then *we could run into a question of some months' delay*, whereas our intention had been to go on the market at the beginning of April. Dr. Goddard interrupted and said that *he could handle that very quickly if we would bring the material directly to him.* He said that if there

213

were no significant changes on efficacy, dosage, etc., *he could clear a supplement (with the Bureau of Medicine organization) in 24 to 48 hours.* I expressed my delight and said that I thought this would be most helpful to proper use of the drug." [Emphasis added.]

Bringing "delight" to the president of Richardson-Merrell was not a bad move. One day Goddard would no longer be parking his car in the FDA parking lot, and would need a little more security than a governmental pension could provide. In fact, that day was only 16 months away. A little favor here, a little favor there; drug companies have long memories and know how to demonstrate their appreciation.

Was this improper? Many years later I had the opportunity to take Goddard's deposition. At the time, he either did not recall the event nor had knowledge that I possessed the Merrell memorandum documenting the subject conversation.

"Did you ever make any suggestions to members of the personnel of Richardson-Merrell that you could do any favors for them with regard to Clomid?"

"Never."

"Would that have been an improper act on your part?"

"Of course."

"Did you ever suggest to Richardson-Merrell that you could get changes in labeling more quickly if it was brought directly to you?"

"I don't recall ever having done that."[152]

On March 10, 1967, Hoekenga forwarded to Goddard an updated and revised package insert. The current data included "twenty-eight reports of defects at birth from 1450 completed pregnancies," compared to the report of 12 birth defects from 672 pregnancies from the labeling approved on February 1, 1967. Ten days later a meeting was held at Goddard's office during which the new language and data were approved, with the exception of a couple minor changes – all quickly agreed upon. With the help of Goddard, Merrell met its targeted deadline of April, although marketing did not commence until the following month.

Settling Into the Nest

I was provided with an opportunity to trace Goddard's post-FDA history when I took his deposition on a later Clomid lawsuit on April 22, 1994.[153] At the time, I was gearing up for trial on the case in the Los Angeles Superior Court. Goddard had been designated as one of the expert witnesses to testify on behalf of Merrell Dow Pharmaceuticals. Typically, I would explore issues that might reflect some reason for bias. Financial ties to a defendant or its industry can often distort an expert's objectivity.

Following his departure from the FDA on June 30, 1968 (at the age of 45), Goddard spent three and a half years in upper management positions outside the industry. Upon his return in February 1972, he took over as chairman of the board of Ormont Drug and Chemical, a manufacturer of generic pharmaceutical agents. He remained at Ormant until May 1977, at which time he resigned and became a full-time consultant to the pharmaceutical industry.[154] This consulting work extended right up to the date of his deposition and involved several different pharmaceutical companies.

Goddard's connection with drug companies, however, became more lucrative in 1979, when for the first time he was requested to be an expert witness for Merrell. *The National Enquirer* had just released a story involving David Mekdeci and his lawsuit against Merrell, alleging that his limb-reduction defect was attributed to his mother's use of *Bendectin*. This publicity spawned over a thousand lawsuits nation wide. Merrell's counsel quickly sought out Goddard to help with the litigation.

The association between Merrell and Goddard was a perfect fit. With lawsuits coming out of the woodwork, the drug company needed someone with impressive credentials to sanctify its testing methods and compliance with industry standards. What better person to attest to Merrell meeting all of the requirements established by the FDA than a former commissioner of the agency itself?

From Goddard's perspective, it was a win-win situation. Expert witnesses get paid a premium stipend. This becomes especially beneficial when the witness works out of his home or otherwise has low overhead. He can also bill at his own pace and justify almost any amount – which will never be questioned. "So you want me to express an opinion on whether you have complied with those demanding standards set down by the FDA? Be glad to, but you understand that I will have to review most of the NDA and IND. Better give me at least a month; that's a lot of reading, you know?"

Then there's the preparation time needed before testimony, meetings and discussions with counsel, reading the current literature on the drug, and any number of other items only limited by the creative mind of the expert. Bottom line: the total number won't bother the drug company as long as the expert can deliver on the witness stand and the final bill can be justified to the jury.

Goddard's intial bill on the Mekdici case was $20,000 – and that was in 1979 dollars. When I cross-examined him on May 13, 1994, during the Gandy trial, he admitted to charges of $28,800 for the current case.[155] However, I had no way to challenge this number. During Goddard's deposition I sought to discover the actual amount he would be receiving from Merrell. Among other documents, I inquired whether he had generated any invoices or billings on the case.

"No. None so far."

"Do you intend to bill the company?"

"Yes. I do after the trial."

"Okay. Is there some reason you're waiting until after the trial?"

"That's my customary practice."

"Is there some reason that that's your customary practice?"

"I just felt it was fair to wait until the trial was over and then submit the bill."

"Is your bill in any way dependent upon the result of the trial?"

"It's not at all."

"How much time have you...you must keep records of the time."

"Oh, I keep time records. Sure."

"Do you have any of those time records here with you today?"

"No. I simply just jot down in my office how many hours I've spent."

When I requested that these notes be produced for my inspection, Goddard balked at the idea because the time was jotted down on a log with all of the other cases he was currently involved with, including the name of the attorney, the venue and the expected date of trial.[156] Although it was ultimately agreed that I would receive a copy of the time log with the other cases redacted, I never saw the document at any time before or during trial.

I was convinced back then – and still am now – that Goddard's billings were never generated before trial because neither the witness nor Merrell wanted the jury to know exactly how much was being paid for the testimony. Although the former commissioner was on record as charging $300 per hour (at the time) and $2,400 per day,[157] there was no way to verify the total number of hours or days actually billed to Merrell. In any event, rest assured that Goddard was generously paid for his time.

But that wasn't all.

Between 1979 and Goddard's testimony in 1994, he had been retained as an expert for Merrell on approximately two dozen Bendectin cases. Out of that number, he eventually testified in trial about 13 to 15 times (his estimate).[158] His minimum fee was $5,000 per case and, excluding his first case (Mekdici), his billings on the lawsuits that went to trial averaged $12,000.[159] Using Goddard's own numbers, by mid-1994 he had received in excess of $250,000 from Merrell in expert witness fees.

But there was more.

In addition to Merrell, Goddard also acted as an expert witness for several other pharmaceutical manufacturers. That list included such giants as Wyeth, Lederle, Pfizer, Dupont and Upjohn. In fact, during the 15 years between 1979 and 1994, no less than 40% of Goddard's income was derived from acting as an expert witness for drug companies.[160] And this was supplemental to income generated from his services as a "full-time consultant" to the same industry.

The circumstance involving Goddard and Merrell is but one example of how the drug industry and its regulatory agency are tethered together in a "back scratching" relationship. It is not unusual for FDA personnel to migrate over to the industry that they have been overseeing. After years of experience in the agency, they have inside knowledge on how to effectively negotiate a drug through all of the hoops toward approval of its NDA. They are also highly skilled professionals in fields of chemistry, pharmacology, epidemiology, endocrinology and other specialties that are needed by pharmaceutical companies. Thus, it is only natural that many would seek higher paying positions in the private sector.

On its face, there is nothing wrong with moving on to advance one's career. But many have developed friendships and other ties with those remaining at the FDA. Problems arise when one tries to take advantage of those relationships. It could be as subtle as an ex-FDA staffer calling upon a friend and inquiring about the status of his employer's "important" drug – or more overt, such as encouraging an overworked medical review officer to expedite the processing of an application. This might be unfair to other pharmaceutical companies if the application is simply placed in a priority position. But it might be tragic if the review is rushed and serious side effects are overlooked or minimized.

Catering to the interests of potential future employers is an even bigger problem. Some might think it was harmless for Goddard to process Merrell's revised labeling in 24 to 48 hours, rather than the anticipated "some months' delay," expressed by Lindsay in his memorandum. However, the wording of labeling on a drug is of critical importance and by federal law must be approved by the FDA. As has already been pointed out, the choice of even a single word can have a major influence on how a prescribing physician might view a drug.

But under the circumstances that existed in the early spring of 1967, it was not just the choice of the words or statements in the labeling that was at issue; it was whether they were backed up by the new clinical data being supplied by Merrell. Recall that the language contained within the package insert that was approved on February 1, 1967, was based upon data from only 672 completed pregnancies. The updated information involved reports and statistics on 1450 completed pregnancies. The number had *more than doubled.* Although the FDA could have reviewed the statistics, summaries and conclusions from Merrell during this expedited timetable, it would have been impossible for its staff to have validated the accuracy of the submitted data within 24 to 48 hours.

The FDA simply accepted Merrell's numbers at face value and gave the labeling its stamp of approval.

* * * * *

CHAPTER 10

Controlling the Controls

Day four finally arrived, and by early afternoon I was beginning to experience a few of the anticipated symptoms from my venture. My back was aching and my right hand cramping from all of the note-taking. Scanning through the multitude of medical and scientific terms was tough enough, but the words were now tending to blend together and I found myself re-reading some of the pages. My companion at the other end of the table was probably as tired of seeing me as I was of seeing her – and if she popped her gum one more time, I would be tempted to physically remove it from her mouth. Was this a designed distraction? Was I getting paranoid?

I had been reviewing published papers on Clomid for several hours now – and still was getting an education. Earlier I had found four published studies confirming that clomiphene citrate was teratogenic in the rat and rabbit. Diener and Hsu[161] were able to produce hydronephrosis (enlarged kidney), hydroureters (enlarged ureter), deformed tails, missing phalanges (toes), *exencephaly*, fused kidneys and severe growth retardation in the offspring of rats. Exencephaly is a *neural tube defect* involving partial absence of the cranial vault and exposure of a portion of the brain. Eneroth and others[162] were able to induce hydramnion (excess amniotic fluid), cataracts and palatoschisis (cleft palate), likewise in rats. Lopez-Escobar[163] found clomiphene to be teratogenic in the rabbit (protrusion of bowels and liver through abdominal wall and *absence of cranial vault*), as did Morris, who produced *cranioschisis* (external opening of the skull), absence of eyelids, stunted limbs, cleft palate and hydrocephalus.[164] There were now published studies demonstrating that Clomid could cause neural tube defects in the rat and the rabbit.

It was at this point that a familiar title caught my eye, as I continued to rapidly view the publications, paperclipping those I wanted copied for a later read. The paper was by Charles, Turner and Redmond, and it was entitled, "The Endometrial Karyotypic Profiles of Women after Clomiphene Citrate Therapy." This was the same study I had seen a couple of years earlier, in which the authors looked at the chromosomes of the endometrium before and after Clomid treatment. I started to go on to the next paper – I had read the Charles article several times before – but instinct prompted me to hesitate. There was something I wanted to check before I moved on.

I pulled my list of clinical investigators from my briefcase and quickly scanned the names. And there it was; David Charles had participated in Merrell's pre-market investigations. This meant that Richardson-Merrell would have a file on him. His records would also fall within the description of documents to be produced by Merrell. I ordered the entire file on Charles.

Within an hour it was sitting in a box next to me on the floor. I pulled out a volume and started reading. My digging was worth the effort. Not only did Charles have a history with Merrell, the subject study had a track record that went all the way back to the sixties.

The story that unfolded was quite interesting – and revealing.

On January 7, 1972,[165] Charles called Merrell and spoke with Dorsey Holtkamp to inform him about a study he had conducted years earlier with Clomid. He had found a *change in chromosomes* when he compared pre-treatment and post-treatment biopsies of endometrial (lining of the uterus) tissue from users of clomiphene. Although he had initiated the study during the clinical investigations, he was just now completing his evaluation of the data. He was considering submission of a paper for publication and was working on a draft of the manuscript.

As a former and current[166] investigator for Merrell, Charles no doubt felt duty-bound to inform Holtkamp of his results and his intention to publish the findings. He was currently the Director of the Department of Obstetrics and Gynecology at Boston University School of Medicine.

You can imagine Holtkamp's reaction. The Merrell employee had never even heard a rumor of the study. Yet one of its carefully selected investigators was about to go public with it in front of the worldwide medical community. I could almost hear the conversation.

"Come again? You found what?"

"Changes in the chromosomes…structurally altered, Dorsey. I know this probably comes as a surprise…"

"Surprise! You're damn right, surprise. I never *heard* about this thing. When did you take these tissues?"

"Back in the investigations, mid-sixties, I guess. But I doubt that anyone there would know about it. It's something I did on my own, not part of your protocol."

Holtkamp must have realized that dealing with this important physician about a potentially damaging paper would require some finesse and diplomacy. He immediately scheduled a meeting in Boston. The two of them would spend the entire day together reviewing and discussing the results of the study. This would be Merrell's first stab at damage control.

That meeting took place during the evening of January 13, 1972 and the entire following day.[167] Most of the time was spent reviewing and discussing drafts of various tables related to the karyotype (photo of arranged chromosomes) studies on the biopsies. They had been performed by a Dr. J. Howard Turner back in Pittsburgh in early 1965. Turner was a geneticist working out of the University of Pittsburgh. The discussion between the two men eventually turned to the issue of *controls*.

Holtkamp and Charles both agreed that there would be a need for controls: tissue biopsies taken from women who had not been using Clomid. Perhaps normally ovulating and menstruating women had changes in endometrial chromosomes during the course of their menstrual cycle. The only way to establish with certainty that the chromosomal anomalies were resulting from treatment with clomiphene – and not from hormonal changes during the cycle – was to compare karyotyping between the two groups.

Their views became divergent, however, on the type of controls to be used. Charles was of the opinion that they could use the results from tissue previously taken from women participating in another study in which they had not been exposed to drugs during their menstrual cycle. "(Turner) is sending further information concerning control studies to me, specifically cytogenetic (cell) data and karyotypic patterns derived from skin biopsies from the same site of an individual taken at weekly interval over a three week period. He and I also discussed (the) endometrium…and he feels that he has control data from individuals where no drugs have been prescribed."[168] He and Turner would also be looking at the literature for any karyotyping studies done on the subject.

Conversely, it was Holtkamp's thought that the controls should be part of the same original study, conducted at the same time, and with the same type of patients. He suggested that Charles seek a grant from the National Institutes of Health (NIH) and referred him to Dr. Arthur Heming, a former colleague of Holtkamp's who was in charge of grants. A letter was shot off to Heming the same day, along with a plan of the proposed study.[169]

Holtkamp began to document his multiple criticisms with the study and forwarded a letter to Charles on January 26, 1972, itemizing all of them. The list ranged from lack of information on the "total number of cells evaluated pre-treatment and post-treatment" to absence of "sequential biopsies in infertility or other patients that received placebo or no drug." Perhaps he might be able to dissuade Charles from going ahead with the paper.

On the same date, a strategy meeting was held between Drs.R. H. Levin (Corporate Vice President), M. T. Hoekenga (Vice President – Research, Medical and Regulatory Affairs), W. L. Kuhn (Director – Research Planning & Coordination), J. W. Newberne (Director – Drug Safety & Metabolism) and Holtkamp (Group Director, Endocrine & Metabolic Clinical Research). The game plan included securing input from Merrell's consultant, Dr. James G. Wilson, and to submit everything to the FDA with the Annual Periodic Report on Clomid, which was due the following week.[170]

The concern at Merrell, of course, went beyond any thought that its drug might change the structure of chromosomes in the endometrium of its users. The potential implications might well extend to the embryo residing in the same environment. Not to take any chances, the following day a letter was hand-delivered to Wilson, Merrell's local teratologist.

> "Your appraisal of whether the attached information is sufficient for even an initial evaluation of importance or meaning would be appreciated, bearing in mind that additional information on this investigation has been promised for delivery to me in February, 1972. Your prompt aide in this evaluation is appreciated."

That letter was taken by Holtkamp, who was accompanied by Newberne. The three men met at Wilson's office on January 27, 1972. Holtkamp noted all of Wilson's criticisms,[171] and then requested him to prepare a report, which would be submitted to the FDA. Even before Merrell had received all of the data (some of which may have addressed a number of the criticisms), Holtkamp was securing a report from its longtime consultant. He no doubt wanted it to accompany Merrell's submission to take any sting out of Charles and Turner's preliminary data.

Wilson's report a few days later echoed the complaint about no controls as well a number of other technical problems he had with the study. Merrell was already accumulating its ammunition for a full broadside.

Everything was presented to the FDA on February 3, 1972.

But there was still concern and uncertainty at Merrell. Five of the top brass in Cincinnati did not have a meeting to laugh off a meaningless study. If Charles and Turners' findings had validity, they could create all kinds of problems in Rockville. Hoekenga was even in favor of Merrell conducting a study of its own. If the data from 1965 ever reached the quality to qualify for a peer-reviewed publication, it might be necessary to back Merrell's position with a study reaching a different conclusion. Hoekenga's memo of February 15, 1972 to Newberne and Holtkamp provides some insight into his thinking.

"I'm increasingly concerned that we not wait very long in *getting a pilot study underway* to check on the chromosome changes reported to us by Dr. David Charles. Although we may be sure in our own minds that the 1965 observations are meaningless, *we have no scientific support for our position*. Might an animal study be feasible and meaningful?" [Emphasis added.]

The first full draft of the paper was forwarded to Holtkamp on February 18, 1972, along with a letter soliciting any conclusions and suggestions. Not surprisingly, it contained references to literature where chromosome samples had been taken from women who had not been using Clomid. *They were all normal.*

One week after Hoekenga's interdepartment memo, Holtkamp responded to the vice president's query. He also informed him of receipt of Charles and Turner's first draft.

"In follow-up of the January report from Charles, Dr. Newberne and I have been discussing the possibility of starting a pilot study for trying to evaluate the effect of Clomid (clomiphene citrate) on chromosome pattern. In response to your question, we feel that it is too early to try to start a laboratory approach in vitro or in animals and that the literature be reviewed first.

"We have reviewed the Clomid bibliography. *One in vitro test was reported with the use of Clomid and at high concentrations, chromosome changes were induced.* On the other hand, reproduction tests using the methodology employed currently, were conducted at Merrell with the isomers and these tests failed to show problems." [Exhibit 10, emphasis added][172]

The memo then acknowledges receipt of a copy of the first draft of the Charles and Turner paper. It had been prepared by Turner and sent to Charles for his additions and editing, including a description of the methods he used in securing the tissue samples. Once the next draft was complete, "(r)eferences to methodology in this report will be pursued." The memo concluded:

"Dr. Newberne and I feel that a more critical and objective type of pilot study could be designed after more opportunity to review the literature and receipt of the more detailed report. *Methodology, per se, will be especially important and since so many approaches could be tried, we need time for selections.*" [Emphasis added.]

Not only did Merrell have to address the potential impact of the Charles and Turner study, a search of Merrell's own bibliography on Clomid turned up yet another study – this one an in-vitro (test tube) publication which had induced chromosome changes with "high concentrations" of the drug. If they were going to conduct a useful pilot study, great care would have to be made in the selection of the methodology.

Although they had previously spoken over the phone, the first meeting between Holtkamp and Turner took place in Pittsburgh on March 7, 1972. A second draft of the paper was handed to Holtkamp at that time, along with a second copy for Charles, who would be seen later in the day in Boston. Other than discussing the study and its needed refinements, Turner made his position quite clear to the man from Merrell. He considered his data "technically clean," assuring that it was accurate and dependable.[173] The geneticist was also unequivocal in his position that the study should be published.

Holtkamp next flew to Boston and met with Charles in the evening. Most of the time was spent with Charles addressing – and eliminating – a number of the earlier

224

concerns expressed by Holtkamp back in January. Like his study partner, Charles was increasingly convinced with the quality of their study and the need for its publication.

As Holtkamp flew back to Cincinnati he could not have been very happy. Each time he and his team would come up with a potential problem with the study, Charles and Turner would provide data that would resolve the issue. The end effect – and I doubt the desired one – was to improve the quality of the paper and enhance the likelihood of its publication. When Holtkamp went back to the issue of the lack of controls within the study itself, *Charles requested the opportunity to submit a grant proposal to Merrell.* If this is Merrell's major criticism, then it should be willing to fund such a study. Charles had still not heard back from NIH.

This request no doubt presented Holtkamp with a quandry. For the past two months, he had been working closely with Charles and Turner, purportedly to "help" them tackle technical and substantive issues related to the study. How could he now reject a grant application without revealing a more devious motive? On March 16, 1972, Holtkamp prepared another Interdepartment Memo to the Files.

> "I called Dr. Charles today. I told him that Dr. Hoekenga had verbally approved that he submit a grant proposal for control studies but that this would need other approvals here."

The implication: Holtkamp and Hoekenga were in favor of the grant, but the final approval was out of their hands. Even as I read this memo, I knew exactly where it was going. The lack of first-hand control data was Merrell's ace-in-the-hole. It was not about to take any chance with a new study by Charles that could strengthen the findings and eliminate a major criticism.

By early April 1972, the Charles and Turner paper was in its final stages of refinement. Turner was also pushing for publication, even without added control studies. He was satisfied that the data from the literature would establish a sufficient base line for comparison; women who had not been exposed to Clomid had normal chromosomes throughout their cycles.

But Charles was still seeking a study funded by Merrell. On April 10, 1972, he submitted his protocols to Holtkamp for a simple study involving 6 patients with anovulation. On May 5, 1972, Holtkamp forwarded the proposal to Hoekenga with his *recommendation for approval* of the grant application. *The total cost for the study: only $15,000.*

At first, I was surprised to see that Holtkamp had recommended approval of the grant application. After all, he had criticized every facet of the study from the beginning. But after further thought, it made sense. Throughout his remaining discussions with Charles and Turner, he could remain honest with the researchers; he had attempted to assist them to overcome his major complaint with the study. Holtkamp's forwarding memo, however, contained language that no doubt dictated rejection of the application: "These (control studies) are *necessary for the appropriate evaluation* of the endometrial studies conducted by D. Charles in clomiphene treated patients...." [Emphasis added.] Upper management at Merrell would never approve a grant for a study that could potentially add merit to the Charles and Turner findings.

In the meantime, the NIH informed Charles that his application for a grant would need to be more detailed and on one of its own forms. On June 14, 1972, Charles submitted a 31-page grant application to the NIH. The estimated cost for the more comprehensive study was $167,724. The objective of the study was "to ascertain whether steroidal and non-steroidal fertility agents produce chromosomal aberrations in the endometrium." The design included use of fertility drugs *and* oral contraceptives, as well as controls for each group. A copy, of course, was forwarded to Holtkamp.

As to Charles' grant application to Merrell, on June 26, 1972, Holtkamp informed him of the response he did not want to hear – but should have expected. Their conversation was set out in Holtkamp's letter of July 7, 1972.

"This letter confirms my discussion with you on the night of June 26, 1972, in which I told you that there was *general agreement here at Merrell that we would not at this time financially support control studies as back-up for your original observations* on endometrial chromosomes in patients that had received Clomid (clomiphene citrate). Such consideration has been deferred until after you have received judgment on the application you now have pending at NIH. Any studies that we might be able to support at this time would fail to provide sufficient control data *because each of the various patient and treatment types proposed for study in your NIH grant application should be included.* We do not see any

singular group among those proposed which would be an adequate control."
[Emphasis added.]

Merrell was critical of the study because it lacked controls, but was unwilling to spend $15,000 to verify whether or not its own drug product was damaging chromosomes in the endometrium. There were two justifications for this decision. First, if the NIH was going to fund the study, there would be no reason the approve Charles' application with Merrell. Second, if the study was going to be funded by Merrell, then it should be properly designed and should include "each of the various patient and treatment types proposed for study in (the) NIH grant application." If the study is going to be done at all, it should be done right.

The fallacy of the second justification was that the application submitted to the NIH included a comprehensive study design that looked not only at Clomid, but other steroidal and non-steroidal compounds as well. That list included patients exposed to diethylstilbestrol (DES), exogenous (external) estrogen and 5 different birth control pills. Whereas the use of anovulatory patients, unexposed to Clomid or other hormones, would constitute a meaningful control population, incorporating all of these other patients would be absolutely unnecessary if one was only studying the affect of clomiphene on the endometrium. The first justification was likewise meaningless – or soon would be.

Four days after Holtkamp's "kiss-off" letter to Charles, the Merrell employee met with Dr. Arthur Heming, Chief of the Research Grants Branch of the NIH. Holtkamp's letter to Heming of July 13, 1972, suggests that the occasion was strictly social.

"Dear Art: It was indeed a pleasure to see you, to visit with you and have lunch with you on Tuesday, July 11, 1972. I was happy to be able to compare experiences with you of government vs. industry. I hope you will stop to visit us in Cincinnati if your travels take you to this part of the country. I apologize again for coming in unannounced."

To anyone viewing this letter, it would seem that an old friend had been in town and had simply stopped by for a social visit. There are three facts, however, that put a more sinister spin on the meeting. First, of course, is that it would take place only four days after informing Charles that his Merrell grant application had been declined. Second, the letter itself had been filed with Merrell's records maintained for Dr. David

Charles. Further, a letter from Holtkamp to Charles, dated July 28, 1972, confirms that Holtkamp and Heming spoke about Charles' NIH grant application, although suggesting that it was being reviewed by another department. Third, and most importantly, shortly after the meeting the NIH grant application was *denied*.[174]

Merrell never reconsidered its initial decision to deny Charles' grant request.

Whatever became of the proposed "pilot study" remains a mystery. No further reference was made of it throughout the remainder of the Charles' file. Nor did it ever show up in the published literature. If it was ever conducted by Merrell, the drug company was not sufficiently motivated to share its findings with the medical profession – or with yours truly.

The Charles and Turner paper, however, was published in 1973 in *The Journal of Obstetrics and Gynaecology of the British Commonwealth*.[175] The authors cite no less than 6 different published studies in which chromosomes from endometrial tissue were examined for abnormalities. None of the subjects of the studies had used fertility drugs and all had normal chromosomes.[176] The issue of controls obviously survived the scrutiny of peer review.

* * * * *

CHAPTER 11

A Homemade Study

The flight back from Cincinnati was a welcome relief – even though I had to pass over the Rockies again. Four and a half days of sitting in one location reviewing tens of thousands of records was about my limit. Physically and mentally I was spent. In the final hours on Friday, I had reached a point of diminishing return. Due to mental fatigue, my comprehension level had dropped so low that I found myself reading the same lines two and three times. I thus was paperclipping more and more documents, including many that otherwise would have been disregarded. I was not looking forward to the photocopy bill.

About two months later I received delivery of several boxes of photocopied records from Merrell. My first task was to compare my notes with the records to insure that everything had been produced. To my surprise and relief, every designated document had been delivered, including all 2,635 case histories from the pre-market clinical investigations. I actually had possession of my own set of Merrell's pre-market studies.

Over the next several weeks I reviewed, analyzed, noted and organized each document that had been produced – every one, that is, except the clinical investigations. That would be my most tedious and time-consuming effort. So, as was my custom, I procrastinated. Every day I would enter my office, take a long look at the stack of boxes sitting against the wall, then shrug my shoulders and announce to myself, "Not today." This was easy, because I always had something more important to deal with. After all, my 3 pending Clomid cases[177] were not the only lawsuits in my office. I had 75 other cases and my practice was beginning to blossom.

Then one day an idea struck me. And from that day forward the records would become an obsession. I would create my own study design to test the *Mix Hypothesis*.

If Clomid can cause abnormally high levels of estrogen; if high levels of estrogen can alter the pH in the oviduct (fallopian tube) at around the time of ovulation and damage the chromosomes of ova; if the abnormal chromosomes in the ova and subsequent embryo can lead to spontaneous abortions; and if abnormally high levels of estrogen can at the same time produce ovarian hyperstimulation syndrome (OHSS),[178] then there should be an increased rate of first trimester spontaneous abortions following OHSS compared to conceptions during a treatment cycle without OHSS.

To test this theory, I would first set up my own *protocols* for the study. [Exhibit 11] This would be of critical importance. Because of my obvious bias, I doubted that there was anyone at the FDA who would give the results any credibility. For the same reason, members of the medical profession would likely scoff at any meaningful statistics derived from my effort. But there was someone else I had to satisfy – myself.

Just two years earlier I had stood in front of an FDA advisory committee and attempted to sell a theory of how Clomid was causing Down syndrome and other congenital anomalies. Was I now prepared to back up my position? If I truly believed Clomid to be a human teratogen, was I willing to devote the time and energy to prove it? Self-sacrifice is the truest test of one's convictions. I would put myself to that test.

I then created a log. I would review each case history from the produced records and enter all of the relevant information into the log (Exhibit 12) as prescribed by the protocol. Once I had completed the log, I would divide the cases into four groups. Group one would be patients who conceived two or more cycles after their last Clomid treatment; group two would be patients who conceived one cycle after their last treatment; group three would be patients who conceived during a treatment cycle *without* OHSS; and group four would be patients who conceived during a treatment cycle *with* OHSS.

Although I would initially record *all* spontaneous abortions (SAs) from the clinical records, in the final phase of my study I would only be looking for *first trimester* SAs. This was for three reasons. First, whereas late abortions can be associated with an inability to maintain the growing fetus, first trimester abortions are associated with a high incidence of abnormal chromosomes and other anomalies of the embryo and fetus. Second, the Boues had only looked at the chromosomes of first trimester SAs and I wanted to compare my study with theirs. Similar to the Boues, I would have subgroups that included patients who conceived during a treatment cycle, patients who conceived one cycle after treatment, and patients who conceived two or more cycles after treatment.[179] Finally, first trimester SAs were the most accurately recorded statistic on the outcome of pregnancies in the clinical investigations. All of the investigators followed each pregnancy for at least the first three months, after which many sent the patients back to referring physicians.

At the outset, I had no idea what I was getting myself into. If I relied exclusively on the Analysis of Pregnancy forms (Exhibit 3), the procedure would have gone much quicker. However, many of the records included other forms that had been typed or hand-written, as well as charts, reports and, in many instances, lab studies. I wanted to insure that my log contained accurate data. I also wanted to eliminate any possibility that there were any errors in transposing the information from the original records to the Analysis of Pregnancy forms – inadvertent or otherwise.[180] As expected, the work was indeed tedius and time-consumming. All entries were made by hand.

Completing the log extended for almost 18 months.

During that period, I reviewed in excess of 10,000 pages of documents. Most of the work took place at the office, but many times I would bring the records home and work at my dining room table. As one might imagine, that did not go over well with my wife. When I started the study, my daughter was five years of age; when I completed it, she was six and a half. I also had a son born on March 25, 1978, and a second one, shortly after completing my analysis, on March 1, 1979. With a small child and two new babies in the house, Janet was in need of help. I contributed, but my obsession with the Clomid study intruded on my responsibilities at home. Our marriage was strained as it had never been before.

But stubbornly I pressed on to complete my project.

As I worked my way through the individual cases, I noted a number of problems with the data. For example, each Analysis of Pregnancy form had a line requiring a description for "Congenital anomalies." Whenever an infant was born with birth defects, they were either described on this line or a statement made to "see attached," when a more detailed report accompanied the form. But how was a blank line to be interpreted? Since many investigators entered "none," "normal," or words to that effect, would the absence of any entry mean that the outcome was unknown? This would seem to be a reasonable interpretation when the *same* clinical investigator entered "none" on one patient's form, but left the same line blank on another's. This was usually the case.

A good example of this ambiguity involved investigator, William Barfield, a physician out of Augusta, Georgia. For patient no.005-042, he entered, "None – entirely normal female infant." However, the line reserved for "congenital anomalies" was left blank for patient no.005-041. Had it been left blank because the outcome of the pregnancy was unknown? It would seem so. A letter received by Barfield *four years later* from the referring physician states, "Dr. Barfield, we did not see this patient after May 18, 1962 as she moved out of state. *By word of mouth from another patient* we heard she has a normal female." [Emphasis added.] In other words, another patient of the referring doctor informed him that the baby was normal; and he in turn so informed the clinical investigator. Since the estimated date of delivery was December 3, 1962, this would suggest that the patient was still pregnant when she "moved out of state." Thus, the line had been left blank because Barfield did not know the outcome of the pregnancy at the time the form was completed and sent to the pharmaceutical company.

This pregnancy was recorded by Merrell as resulting in a *normal* infant.[181]

I could only shake my head as I recalled Tyler's testimony during the Breimhorst trial, when he described relying upon letters and birth announcements from his patients to determine whether they had delivered normal offspring. This, of course, went one better. The information did not even come from the patient in question, but from someone else who allegedly knew the patient and the outcome.

To address this uncertainty, I would enter "L" (live) or "S" (stillborn) in my log, rather than "N" (normal), when the investigator failed to make an entry on the line after "Congenital anomalies." Thus, "LPF" would identify a live premature female and "STM" would describe a stillborn term male. Neither would be considered a normal infant (by me), even though Merrell had designated each as such in its IND and NDA. These entries were not inconsequential. Out of 1,886 delivered pregnancies where the outcome was known, I made 510 "L" or "S" (27.0%) designations due to the investigator's omission. *One out of every four case histories failed to note whether or not the baby was born without congenital anomalies.*

Even when the investigator identified a "normal" infant resulting from a Clomid pregnancy, the records often reflected equivocation. The following are just some of the examples:

"Delivered an *apparently* normal infant" (019-011); "Delivered of an *apparently* normal baby" (019-034); "This patient ovulated within two weeks and conceived twins which have since been delivered and *apparently* are entirely normal" (019-035); "Delivered elsewhere – *apparently* normal infant at term" (019-045); "I am *advised* that she delivered 'at term' a normal baby of about seven pounds in early 1965" (019-069); "full term delivery of an *apparently* normal infant on December 7, 1964" (019-072); "She was delivered in August, 1965 an *apparently* normal infant" (019-074). [Emphasis added.]

"Congenital anomalies: None noted" (026-016); "Delivered by another physician" (029-037); "Congenital anomalies: None known" (035-098); "Per letter of 4/11/63 'delivered 5# 2 oz. girl at term" (036-001); "could identify no *definite* evidence of birth defects in any of the infants" (038-036) [emphasis added]; "The following day an infant weighing 7lb. 6oz. was delivered" (041-031) [identified as "normal term baby" *prior* to delivery]; "No *obvious* congenital abnormalities" (041-054) [emphasis added]; "Delivered of a *healthy* living male infant 8' 3½" on September 1, 1965" (041-093) [emphasis added]; "Congenital anomalies: None noted" (041-164); "Congenital anomalies: None known" (042-173).

The above uncertainties derive from an inherent deficiency in the design of the pre-market studies; namely, that the investigators were not delivering the majority of the infants. Instead, they relied upon others to make the assessment and supply them with this critical information.

The log was completed in early 1979.

My next step was to compile the resulting data. I would first need to break out the spontaneous abortions and make a determination of the relationship between the dates of treatment and the date of conception. Because Merrell included ectopic (tubal) pregnancies in its spontaneous abortion statistics and coding, I would eliminate all such terminations. I only wanted pregnancies that were naturally expelled. I likewise excluded all spontaneous abortions that exceeded 3 months of gestation or where the length of gestation was unknown. I then made my calculations.

The Results Are In

1. Last treatment two or more (2+) cycles prior to conception:

Total number of cases:	278
Outcome of pregnancies unknown:	36

	242
Abortions:	34 (34/242 = 14.0%)
Less ectopic pregnancies:	4
	30 (30/242 = 12.4%)
Less gestation period unknown:	6
	24
Less gestation period over 3 months:	13
First trimester spontaneous abortions:	*11 (11/236 = 4.7%)*

2. Last treatment one (1) cycle prior to conception:

Total number of cases:	236
Outcome of pregnancies unknown:	31
	205
Abortions:	40 (40/205 = 19.5%)
Less ectopic pregnancies:	2
	38 (38/205 = 18.5%)
Less gestation period unknown:	6
	32
Less gestation period over 3 months:	5
First trimester spontaneous abortions:	*27 (27/199 = 13.6%)*

3. Treatment during cycle of conception/before conception only (*without* hyperstimulation of the ovaries):

Total number of cases:	1,712
Outcome of pregnancies unknown:	155
	1,557
Abortions:	348 (348/1,557 = 22.3%)
Less ectopic pregnancies:	15
	333 (333/1,557 = 21.4%)
Less gestation period unknown:	38
	295
Less gestation period over 3 months:	71
First trimester spontaneous abortions:	*224 (224/1,519 = 14.7%)*

4. Treatment during cycle of conception/before conception only
   (*with* hyperstimulation of the ovaries):

Total number of cases:	119
Outcome of pregnancies unknown:	8
	111
Abortions:	38 (38/111 = 34.2%)
Less ectopic pregnancies:	5
	33 (33/111 = 29.7%)
Less gestation period unknown:	2
	31
Less gestation period over 3 months:	6
First trimester spontaneous abortions:	*25 (25/109 = 22.9%)*

The results were stunning, but not surprising. I had been taking sample statistics throughout the study. [A year and a half wait for the answer was unthinkable.] Group one (conception 2 or more cycles after treatment) had a first trimester spontaneous abortion rate of only *4.7%* (11/236); group two (conception 1 cycle after treatment) had a rate of *13.6%* (27/199); group three (conception during a treatment cycle *without* OHSS) had a rate of *14.7%* (224/1,519);[182] and group four (conception during a treatment cycle *with* OHSS) had a rate of *22.9%* (25/109). [Exhibit 13]

As the date of conception approached the date of treatment, the first trimester spontaneous abortion rate rose. Then when conception occurred one cycle after treatment, the rate was approximately the same as when conception occurred during a treatment cycle without OHSS. This was quite significant because it was consistent with the Boue findings that both groups had spontaneous abortions with approximately the same percentage of abnormal chromosomes (86% and 83%, respectively). Finally, when hyperstimulation occurred during a treatment cycle – *when estrogen levels were at their highest* – the rate jumped still another 56 percent.

The day I put those final numbers together and made the calculations, I was absolutely elated. I was on an emotional high matched only by the Breimhorst verdict. True, the FDA bureaucrats would shrug their shoulders at my effort – and I'm certain the Obstetrics and Gynecolgy Advisory Committee would find considerable amusement at my latest foray into the field of science. But for one special moment in my life it made absolutely no difference. Regardless of who might buy the results, I had satisfied myself. Whatever lingering doubt may have existed, it had been purged forever. I was now absolutely convinced that Clomid had the capacity of damaging chromosomes in the human ovum and subsequent embryo. Clomiphene citrate was a human clastogen that could induce spontaneous abortions.

Next question: could I find the literature to back me up?

Supporting Literature

It was time to return to the UCLA medical library. [As a former Trojan, this was always painful.] Over the past few years I had made a number of trips to the stacks in Westwood and was becoming quite adept at medical research. Okay, I was a little on the slow side, but I would inevitably find what I was after. After two days I discovered several papers that added strength and meaning to my study.

Garcia and others conducted a ten-year study[183] that involved 255 women who had used clomiphene citrate. Out of a subgroup of 199 infertility patients, 63 became pregnant as a result of using Clomid. From that number, 16 (25.4%) spontaneously aborted. In contrast, only four of the 38 (10.5%) infertility patients who later conceived without the aid of fertility drugs spontaneously aborted. Infertility patients who conceived with the use of Clomid had two and a half times the abortion rate than those who later spontaneously ovulated and became pregnant. The authors only looked at total spontaneous abortions and made no note whether they were early (first trimester) or late. Although mentioning the above disparity, Garcia et al. failed to explain it.

A paper by Toshinobu et al.[184] looked specifically at the question of whether Clomid was causing spontaneous abortions. They first investigated the timing of clomiphene ingestion in relation to the date of conception.

"Ninety-three pregnancies have been confirmed in our sterility clinic after ovulation-inducing therapy and (22) cases out of them resulted in abortion within the 16th gestational week. Therefore, the abortion rate was 23.6%. On the other hand, there were 270 pregnancies between January 1964 and December 1977 after various kinds of treatments excluding Clomid therapy, and out of them 24 cases resulted in abortion within the same gestational week (abortion rate, 8.9%). *The abortion rate in Clomid-induced pregnancy was significantly higher (P<0.005)."* [Emphasis added, pp.193-194.] The likelihood of these numbers occurring by chance was only 5 out of a thousand. Statistically, this was highly significant. These numbers were also strikingly similar to those from the Garcia study.

Additional issues were similarly explored. Although the researchers failed to find a relationship between the *dose levels* and the spontaneous abortion rate, they did discover a relationship between the *number of cycles* treated with Clomid and abortions occurring through the 16th week of gestation.

"Correlation between Clomid-related cycles and abortion rate was investigated by a classification into three groups. The mean maternal age was the same in each group. Independent of Clomid dosages, the abortion rate of pregnany in the first cycle was 28.1% (9/32), that of pregnancy after two to six consecutive administrations was 9.3% (4/43), and that of pregnancy after seven to 15 continuous cycles was 70.0% (7/10). *A significant correlation between cycles treated by Clomid and the abortion rate was observed (P<0.001)."* [Emphasis added, p.194.]

These numbers were even more significant. The odds were less than one in a thousand that these statistics occurred by chance. Toshinobu and his colleagues discussed several potential causes, including delayed ovulation (because of infertility), atrophy (deterioration) of the endometrium and chromosomal abnormalities. They suggested that the high rate after the first course might be due to the "overripeness" of the ova. The difference between groups two and three was explained as possibly due to atrophy of the endometrium from prolonged exposure to the drug. "The causes for a high abortion rate in Clomid-induced pregnancy can be thought of as the atrophy of the uterine endometrium and the *increased frequency of chromosomal abnormalities."* [Emphasis added, p.195.]

I had my own thoughts. A reasonable explanation for the higher incidence of abortions following longer usage might be the Clomid half-life factor. If Clomid can be around for as long as 6 weeks, perhaps the drug was accumulating after several months of treatment. Perhaps the levels of estrogen produced by the ovaries became progressively higher with prolonged use.

An explanation for the high abortion rate for conceptions following the intial course of treatment, as distinguished from pregnancies after two to six courses, might have something to do with the body's ability to acclimate. The intial sudden jolt of Clomid may have a more profound effect on the ovaries than after two to five more courses. Clomid can produce a surge of estrogen, at around the time of ovulation, which is *four to five hundred percent higher* than women unexposed to the drug.[185] After an extended period without ovulation, the surge might be more dramatic than after a couple more exposures. If the culprit is the pH level in the ovaries, fallopian tubes and/or endometrium, its ability to adjust to the normal swing in estrogen levels throughout the cycle might be more likely compromised with an initial dose of Clomid.

In any event, I found two published studies in which the spontaneous abortion rate of *infertility* patients was significantly lower following non-stimulated conceptions than pregnancies induced by Clomid. Our three studies would represent a firm rebuttal to those that suggest infertility patients have a higher abortion rate because of the underlying pathology which made them infertile.

I also found a couple of papers that specifically dealt with estrogen levels in relation to spontaneous abortions. Oelsner and others found a statistically significant association between spontaneous abortions and *higher estrogen levels* prior to treatment with hMG (Pergonal) and hCG.[186] The patients were divided into two groups. Group I had *negligible* estrogen activity prior to treatment; Group II had *distinct* pre-treatment estrogen activity. Treatment with fertility drugs, of course, would further elevate those levels. Their numbers were quite impressive.

SPONTANEOUS ABORTION RATE

Group	Preg.	1st Trmstr SAs	2nd Trmstr SAs	Total
Group I	184	**26 (14.1%)**	16 (8.7%)	42 (22.8%)
Group II	72	**21 (29.2%)**	9 (12.5%)	30 (41.7%)
Total	256	47 (18.6%)	25 (9.8%)	72 (28.1%)

The difference in the total SA rate between Group I (22.8%) and Group II (41.7%) was highly significant ($P<0.005$). The odds were less than 5 out of a thousand that the numbers occurred by chance. As can be seen, the primary reason for the difference was the high rate of first trimester spontaneous abortions. Oelsner and his associates could not account for this phenomenon. Jewelewicz and colleagues found a similar association with higher pre-ovulatory estrogen levels.[187]

Of greater interest was a study conducted by Caspi and others.[188] Although Pergonal and chorionic gonadotrophin were used (instead of Clomid), they reported an incidence of spontaneous abortions at 35.0% and 33.3 % for pregnancies associated with mild hyperstimulation and severe hyperstimulation of the ovaries (OHSS), respectively, compared to an incidence of 17.5% where pregnancies occurred without OHSS. Although they did not break out statistics for first trimester spontaneous abortions, most of them (83%) were early. The differences were not due to maternal age. The comment about a possible explanation suggested a hormonal etiology (cause).

"The causes of the high rate of abortion is (sic) not understood. Brown *et al* (1969) suggested that *abnormal ovarian steroid patterns might be responsible* and though the differences did not attain statistical significance, it is interesting to note that *patients with hyperstimulation had the highest abortion rate* and those with corpus luteum[189] deficiency (and hence the least disturbance of ovarian steroidogenesis) the lowest." [Emphasis added, pp.971-972.]

Steroid hormones include estrogen and progesterone. The authors are suggesting that the abnormal estrogen patterns that produce OHSS may be responsible for the increased spontaneous abortion rate when that adverse reaction is produced by fertility drugs.

An additional paper by Schenker and Polishuk[190] also caught my interest. They reported on 14 cases of OHSS, five of which were associated with conception. From the 5 OHSS pregnancies, there was 1 quintuplet delivery, 1 *early* quintuplet *abortion*, 1 twin *abortion*, 1 normal delivery, and 1 *missed abortion*.Out of five cases, 3 (60%) resulted in spontaneous abortions, including 2 (40%) early abortions. The authors also point to the correlation between high levels of estrogen, OHSS and multiple births.

I also looked at animal studies. Although the results in teratology studies cannot be directly extrapolated to humans, they are of considerable value when assessing biological feasibility and investigating a possible mechanism of action. For example, is it biologically possible for fertility drugs to induce chromosomal abnormalities in fertilized eggs? The answer appeared to be in the affirmative.

The first paper I located was entitled, "Chromosome Abnormalities in Rabbit Preimplantation Blastocysts Induced by Superovulation."[191] Fujimoto and his colleagues exposed 9 rabbits to human chorionic gonadotrophin (hCG), a commonly used fertility drug, in an effort to produce superovulation. A total of 6 rabbits were used as controls. Approximately four times as many ova (eggs) were produced in the treated group over the controls. Blastocysts (actively dividing fertilized eggs) were recovered from both sets of rabbits prior to implantation in the uterus. They found 9.7% in the superovulation group had abnormal chromosomes compared to none in the controls. As a further effort to establish a baseline for controls, the scientists cited two other published studies. The incidences of chromosomally abnormal blastocysts of rabbits mated without fertility drugs were reported as 1.7% (1/58) and 1.4% (1/72). They concluded, "The results of the present study indicate the need to consider the possible genetic effects of superovulation on ovum maturation, fertilization and early growth of embryos."

I was able to locate two additional studies[192] involving superovulation with *mice*. In both instances, chromosomal abnormalities were produced by the use of fertility drugs.

Follow-up question: what was I going to do with the results?

Communicating the Results

Actually, this was not a difficult question. Step one was to send off my findings to Merrell. Not that I thought this would prompt it to run off to the printer and redraft the Clomid labeling. But the lawyer in me was intent upon establishing *corporate knowledge* about the results of my study. On March 23, 1979, I sent a letter to Frederick Lamb, corporate legal counsel for Merrell-National Laboratories Division of Richardson-Merrell, Inc. Enclosed was an early summary of my study.[193]

I was a little slower in my communication with the FDA. I was disappointed and frustrated with my effort four years earlier. With all of the expended time, energy and money, in the end I had accomplished little or nothing. I realized that I would again be butting my head against the wall, but the last time I had at least seen a small crack. Maybe this time I could bring down a little plaster. So one more time I decided to give it a shot.

A letter was sent to A.T. Gregoire, Executive Secretary of the Obstetrics and Gynecology Advisory Committee, on October 8, 1979. Included was my paper entitled,

"Ovarian Hyperstimulation/Abortion Relationship Study." To give the FDA a little more to think about, I also enclosed the published study by Charles et al. related to inducing abnormal chromosomes in the human endometrium. The text of my correspondence did not hold anything back – subtlety is not exactly my style.

"How many women presently using Clomid are aware that the drug can damage chromosomes within their uterus? If Clomid can cause structural damage to chromosomes within the endometrium at about time of ovulation, is it so unlikely that it could also cause damage to the ovum at the same point in time? Further, considering the higher abortion rate…when Clomid is stimulating higher levels of estrogen by the ovaries, it would seem that the FDA should take a closer look at this drug than it has in the past. It also seems grossly unjust that physicians and patients are not warned of these risks, instead of the present assertion that "no causative evidence of a deleterious effect of Clomid (clomiphene citrate) therapy on the human fetus has been seen." After reviewing the enclosed material, can the FDA honestly say that there is not even a *possibility* that Clomid can cause birth defects in the human fetus?" [Emphasis in the original.]

This time I received a response after just one letter. [Now that's progress.] Dr. Franz Rosa, of the FDA, telephoned me at my office on November 1, 1979. He acknowledged receiving and reviewing my recent correspondence and enclosures. My memorandum of that date sets out the substance of our conversation.

"He stated that he was very interested in my statistics involving hyperstimulation of the ovaries in relation to abortions and wanted to know where I obtained my data. I advised him that I obtained it from Merrell's own records and that in a pending lawsuit they had essentially admitted the accuracy of the summaries.[194] He stated he wanted to talk to Merrell about these statistics. I advised him that if I could be of any further assistance, to give me a call at his own convenience."

A Surprise Proposal

What followed next set me back on my heels – temporarily. Within a week of the Rosa phone call, I was approached by counsel for Merrell while at a routine court appearance in the downtown Los Angeles courthouse. I had already settled two of the four post-Breimhorst Clomid cases and was going through the customary obstacle course of trying to get the remaining cases to trial. As I exited the courtroom into the hallway, Robert Dickson called out to me.

"Hey, Terry!"

I stopped and turned. "Yeah, Bob."

"Got a moment?"

"Sure. What's up?"

Dickson was a senior partner with Haight, Dickson, Brown & Bonesteel, a firm that specialized in the defense of pharmaceutical product cases. He was a slender, rangey man with sandy-colored hair, maybe 5 years my senior. His voice was somewhat raspy, with a slight southern drawl. We had been on the opposite sides of other cases as well and now had a history going back four years. In addition to being a highly-skilled trial attorney, I had found Dickson to be a man of his word and straight forward in his approach to a case. You always knew were he stood.

"I've got a proposal for you, straight from Cincinnati."

That got my interest. Drug product cases are risky business, even with the best of them. But up until now Merrell had not thrown any meaningful money my way on either of the remaining Clomid cases. "I'm listening," I said.

I expected a straight forward offer on one or both of the cases. Instead, it came with a major curve. "Merrell wants to buy you out of the Clomid business. Two hundred and fifty thousand dollars. That's for both cases and you walking away from Clomid.

I stared at Dickson, pondering the offer, not knowing quite what to say. It was not major money, but not inconsequential either for 1979.[195] Both of the cases had problems and both sets of parents were in need of funds to care for their deformed children. It was also an opening number and I was sure Merrell could be pushed for more money. Perhaps my study had hit some corporate nerves.

"How do those numbers break out?" I asked.

"That's up to you," said Dickson.

This created an immediate conflict of interest. The numbers were not allocated between the two cases. Who would determine how the sums should be split in the event that my clients expressed an interest in settling? That I could possibly work out with their equal involvement. But the biggest problem was the condition that I could no longer

242

litigate Clomid cases. That put me directly at odds with my clients for two reasons. First, I would be giving up the right to earn additional fees on possible future cases. How would we divide up the pie? The second conflict involved my desire to at least bring about some form of a warning in the labeling, something I could only achieve through the use of litigation and the records I would not otherwise have access to.[196]

I shook my head. "Bob, I'm going to need to have this broken down."

He shrugged his shoulders. "I'm sorry, Terry. I know what this does, but this is the way Merrell wanted it presented."

I pensively nodded my head. "Let me give it some thought. I'll get back to you within a week."

A couple of days later I had both sets of clients in my office and explained the offer and its myriad of conflicts. I suggested that as between the two of them, I did not have a problem suggesting an allocation, although they may want to consult with another attorney to advise them on the reasonableness of the split. Both rejected this idea and eventually agreed on an equal split, whatever the number we might mutually agree upon.

The next issue was a lot more significant: the conflict between my clients and their lawyer. I strongly urged that they retain independent counsel. I would even pay the fees; it would not cost them anything and would be in their best interests. Again they refused. "We trust that you will be fair with us," said one of them.

When it was clear that both sets of parents were resolute in their intent to move forward without independent counsel, I prepared a detailed statement setting forth their acknowledgements of the various conflicts and waiving their rights to an outside attorney. Each signed the agreement, which also set out the numbers on the split.

They also agreed on one added condition – an important one. There would be no settlement involving my "retirement" from Clomid litigation unless Merrell included a warning about the potential risk of birth defects. I explained that although we might have a reasonable shot at our bottom-line numbers, this last condition would likely be a deal breaker. "We're with you all the way on this, Terry," said one of them. "There are other potential parents out there just like we were. Maybe we can help them avoid what we have gone through." The other three nodded their agreement.

I could not have been prouder of my clients.

On November 12, 1979, I shot off my counter proposal to Bob Dickson. Our combined number totaled $450,000,[197] which I considered to be quite reasonable; even conservative, when one considered what was included in the package. Aside from the condition related to the labeling, I felt that Merrell would have considered this amount to be a reasonable price to get rid of that pesty lawyer from Torrance, California. But then came the kicker: also included would be "(a)n agreement by Richardson-Merrell to set forth a warning in its product information that there is a *possibility* that Clomid may cause birth defects when ingested during a conception cycle." [Emphasis in the original.] I also proposed that the exact wording would be the subject of further negotiation.

As expected, it was a deal breaker. Merrell was not about to add language that might impact sales. But never again did it attempted to buy me out of Clomid litigation.

An Evidentiary Challenge

As it turned out, less than a year later one of the two cases settled at the exact number I had suggested in my letter of November 12, 1979. The remaining lawsuit (Manzo vs. Richardson-Merrell, Inc.), however, appeared destined for trial. All settlement negotiations had broken down. *Try your winners* is an adage that most trial lawyers attempt to follow. Merrell's attorneys were apparently convinced that I could be beaten on this case and were intent on testing the waters.

My challenge: how to get my study into evidence at the trial. Over objection, I could not be a witness and the trial attorney for my client in the same case; nor would I want to be. Since I was working under a contingent fee agreement, my credibility would be seriously compromised by the fact that I had a vested interest in the outcome of the trial. Testifying would also be a major distraction. To succeed at trial, a lawyer must remain focused on every aspect of the case and be aware of what is going on in every corner of the courtroom. Such awareness would be impossible while contemplating an answer to a probing question. These and other reasons dictated that I would have to find some other method to introduce the results of my study into evidence.

The easiest, quickest and least-costly approach was to request Merrell to admit the accuracy of my numbers. This would be done through a set of request for admissions of fact, a procedure allowed in California and most other states. When a relevant fact exists in a case about which there is no dispute, a party can request other parties to admit the

244

accuracy of such facts. When so admitted, they become *conclusively established* for the purpose of that lawsuit. Such an admission can then be introduced into evidence during the trial without the necessity of offering traditional proof on the same fact or facts.

On March 13, 1981, I served a set of request for admissions of fact on Merrell, requesting that it admit the accuracy of each of 292 attached summaries of patients experiencing OHSS in asscociation with pregnancy during the pre-market clinical investigations. Each summary included the age of the patient, history of prior spontaneous abortions, the dates and dose of last Clomid treatment, the date of ovarian enlargement, the date of conception, and the outcome of pregnancy. Included were 119 cases where OHSS occurred during a treatment cycle.

One month later, April 13, 1981, Merrell admitted the accuracy of the OHSS summaries.[198] I had thus conclusively established all of the facts set forth within my summaries, including a *first trimester* spontaneous abortion rate of 22.9% (25/109) where hyperstimulation occurred during a conception cycle.

But I was only part way home. For comparison, I still needed to establish the abortion rate for the other three categories of Clomid patients. And Merrell was not about to cooperate on my further request for it to admit the accuracy of the balance of my summaries on 2,635 case histories. Additional requests for admissions were met with multiple objections, which were followed by my motions to overrule the objections and compel responses. I was determined to force Merrell to either admit or deny the accuracy of each summary. Although it could simply choose to deny each one, a denial would obligate the company to set out all factual bases for its denial. I could then introduce the records on each such case to establish that Merrell's factual bases were erroneous. The pharmaceutical company did not want to be cornered and aggressively fought being placed there.

Statistical Significance

Merrell had a very good reason to resist admitting my study into evidence. I had previously retained the services of a biostatistician to calculate the statistical significance of the data from my study. Dr. Alan B. Forsythe received his Ph.D. from the Biometry Division, Department of Epidemiology and Public Health, at Yale University. He made his statistical calculations derived from my data and four different questions I had posed to him, looking only at first trimester spontaneous abortions. All were recited in a report, dated February 10, 1982, which included:

Question one: "Does the spontaneous abortion rate differ with timing of treatment to conception cycle?"

Answer: "Yes. Highly significant. (Chi square = 25.178 on 3 degrees of freedom, P< 0.00001)." The odds of these numbers occurring by chance were less than 1 in 100,000.

Question two: "Is there a statistically significant difference in the spontaneous abortion rate between pregnancies with conception two or more cycles post treatment and those with conception during the treatment cycle (with hyperstimulation)?"

Answer: "Yes. Highly significant. (Chi square = 26.644 on 1 degree of freedom, P< 0.00001)." Again, the odds of these numbers occurring by chance were less than 1 in 100,000.

Question three: "Is there a statistically significant difference in the spontaneous abortion rate between pregnancies with conception two or more cycles post treatment and those with conception during the treatment cycle (without hyperstimulation)?"

Answer: "Yes. Highly significant. (Chi square = 17.916 on 1 degree of freedom, P< 0.00005)." Odds of 5 in 100,000.

Question four: "Is there a statistically significant difference in the spontaneous abortion rate between pregnancies with conception two or more cycles post treatment and those with conception one cycle after treatment?"

Answer: "Yes. Highly significant. (Chi square = 10.743 on 1 degree of freedom, P= 0.0010)." Odds of 1 in 1,000.

In a field of science where statistical significance is reached at 0.05 (odds of 5 out of 100), no one could reasonably pass these numbers off to chance. Dr. Forsythe also backed up his report with testimony when he was deposed by counsel for Merrell on March 10, 1982.

Expert Testimony

Merrell was also no doubt concerned about one of my expert witnesses. In December 1981, I had retained the services of Gerald F. Chernoff, Ph.D. Dr. Chernoff was a teratologist with a doctorate in medical genetics. Along with Kenneth Jones, M.D., he had established and ran the California Teratogen Registry, which offered free advice to the public about possible teratogens and collected data about birth defects. The registry operated out of the Department of Pediatrics of the University of California San Diego's medical school. In addition to doing extensive literature research in the field of teratology, he had also done original studies with animals involving fetal alcohol syndrome and neural tube closure defects.

Dr. Chernoff was currently participating in a study involving *behavioral teratology* under a grant supplied by the National Institute of Environmental Health Sciences.[199] "Behavioral teratology" involves the study of functional anomalies of the brain, rather than structural malformations. This expertise was of critical importance because my client, who had severe mental retardation, did not have any structural malformations of the brain that could be detected using standard procedures at the time (i.e., x-rays, CAT scans, etc.). This, of course, was one of the big challenges of the case; my client did not have a demonstrable birth defect.

My teratologist, however, was of the opinion that there was a "good probability" that Clomid had caused a genetic mutation in the brain, "most likely prior to fertilization."[200] His opinion was based substantially on the Boue study published in 1973 and Dr. Alan Forsythe's statistical analysis and report of February 10, 1982 – calculated from my study.[201] Dr. Chernoff was of the view that Clomid was a probable clastogen that could damage chromosomes and produce genetic mutations. Under no circumstances did Merrell want to admit to the accuracy of my data.

After a series of legal skirmishes that went all the way to the Court of Appeals, the case ultimately settled in 1982 for *three times* the proposed amount set forth in my letter of November 12, 1979.

And just like that, I was out of Clomid cases.

* * * * *

CHAPTER 12

The Evidence Grows

Prior to the marketing of Clomid, and during the early post-marketing years, the only published studies on the drug were authored by clinical investigators procured by Merrell. The company also sponsored most of the studies and/or supplied the clomiphene citrate. Eventually truly independent studies began to emerge, as did case reports by physicians concerned about the possible association between the use of Clomid by their patients and birth defects in the offspring.

While preparing for the Manzo trial in 1982, I again found myself isolated at the UCLA medical library. Inspired by the post-Breimhorst discoveries in my medical research, I began to spend more and more time researching the medical and scientific literature on fertility drugs. Since the pre-market Clomid studies were worthless in assessing the drug's teratogenic risk, any hope of strengthing the evidence would have to come from studies published by truly independent researchers.

But when Manzo settled in mid-1982, all research stopped. It was my last case and the barrel was empty. My Clomid career appeared at an end. So was the motivation to spend endless hours in a library with a notepad and a stack of medical journals. It had been over 7 years since I had last been retained on a case involving clomiphene citrate and for all intents and purposes the book was closed. Clomid was history.

Then came my sixth Clomid case.

No sooner had the smoke cleared on Manzo, when another Clomid client walked through my door. On January 20, 1983, I signed a retainer agreement with the parents of two daughters who had both delivered with severe congenital anomalies. One had died in the neonatal period from her malformations, and the other had survived. The first daughter was born on March 2, 1974 and the second on July 31, 1975. Both pregnancies had been induced by Clomid.

To me this was truly astounding. The most recent delivery had occurred about the last time I had been retained on a fertility drug case – over seven years earlier. Yet within 6 months after I had concluded my last case, the clients showed up at my door. It was as if unseen forces were playing some kind of role in insuring that I would continue my involvement with Clomid – that I would continue carrying the torch.

And so my research continued.

In 1985 I made a series of visits to UCLA to update my 1982 research effort. The time was well spent. Meaningful studies were beginning to appear in the literature. Medical science often moves at an agonizingly slow pace – I had expected something at least a decade earlier. But researchers were beginning to take a closer look at the potential teratogenic risks presented by fertility drugs. This was demonstrated at several levels: in vitro and in vivo studies; animal studies; and in human epidemiology studies.

Limb Reduction Anomalies

The most striking paper that I found appeared in the *International Journal of Epidemiology*, authored by Dr. Andrew Czeizel and colleagues.[202] Following a significant increase in the incidence of congenital limb reduction abnormalities (CLRA) in Hungary between 1975 and 1978, the researchers were intent on discovering the cause or causes of the increase. This was done by designing and implementing a *case-control* epidemiology study.

A case-control design is the quickest, easiest and least expensive of the epidemiology studies. It is also of considerable benefit when looking at a specific anomaly, rather than the incidence of a total birth defect rate.

Not that it doesn't have its drawbacks. First, it is a *retrospective* study, meaning that the investigators are reviewing events that have already occurred. It is thus dependent upon the accuracy of recorded histories and memories of the patients being studied. The problem: when the histories were being recorded and the relevant events occurring, the patient and the treating physician did not know that they were going to be part of a study. Thus, their motives for recalling and recording were not optimum at the time.

Another problem is *recall bias*. This can best be explained by describing how the study is designed. In this instance, the "cases" were 274 infants born with CLRA in Hungary between 1975 and 1978. The "controls" were 274 other infants born during the same period of time *without* CRLA. "The control cases were matched for sex, week of birth and residence of (case) patients after ascertainment from medical files of the same hospital in which (case) patients had been born." The cause or causes of the anomalies are determined by counting the *exposures* to potential teratogens in both groups. If the case group has a higher incidence of exposures than the control group, and it is statistically significant, it is considered scientific proof of causation. The concern about recall bias originates from the belief that a patient who delivered an infant with congenital anomalies is more likely to remember events occurring before and during pregnancy than a patient delivering a normal infant.

What was interesting about the study was that the researchers were looking at *all* potential causes, and were not particularly fixated on fertility drugs. Among the factors considered were heredity, maternal and paternal age, threatened abortion, x-rays, abdominal trauma, psychological stress, drug ingestion, alcohol consumption, smoking, maternal illness, method of family planning and occupational data. Yet out of all these factors, only four came to the surface as potentially related to the increase in CLRA defects.

Exposure to ovulatory stimulating drugs was one of four different risk factors found to involve a statistically significant increase (P< 0.05). Six of the 274 cases (2.2%) had been exposed to fertility drugs, compared to no exposures in the controls. Three cases involved clomiphene citrate, 2 patients were exposed to human menopausal gonadotropin (Pergonal), and one had used chorionic gonadotropin. All "were used according to the usual protocol and dosage in order to induce ovulation." In other words, the authors had good evidence that the pregnancies had in fact been induced by ovulatory stimulating drugs.

It would also seem that recall bias would not be an issue with the use of fertility drugs. Unlike exposures to other prescription and over-the-counter medications in utero, a woman is more likely to accurately recall that her pregnancy was induced by a fertility drug, and the use more likely documented in medical charts - regardless of whether the infant was born normal or abnormal.

Because the fertility drugs had been ingested prior to conception, Czeizel et al. excluded a direct teratogenic influence.[203] Instead, they focused on the drugs' impact on the maternal hormonal system.

"The origin of these (causal) factors may be a *maternal effect* including an endocrine dysfunction as a predisposition and some environmental, mainly hormonal factors as the triggering impact. The final common pathway of these different hormonal influences may be a disturbance in implantation, after the 'all-

or-nothing effect' of the zygotic phase, may cause an insufficient blood supply in one of the limb buds and consequently unimelic CLRA." [Emphasis in the original.]

They theorized that the fertility drugs may have triggered hormonal action in the mothers which, in conjunction with their underlying endocrine (ovarian) dysfunction, disturbed implantation on the uterine wall in such a way as to deny adequate blood supply to one or more of the limb buds. The fertility drugs were an *indirect* cause of the anomalies as a result of stimulating abnormal hormonal action by the ovaries.

Although coming nine years too late, this 1983 study added validation to the Breimhorst verdict. It took 16 years after Clomid was marketed before anyone published an epidemiology study assessing its potential for causing limb reduction defects. Even then, the discovery was by chance. Fertility drugs were just one of many risk factors examined as part of the study.

Adding support to the causal association between fertility drugs and CLRAs was an older animal teratology study published by Elbling in 1973.[204] The author induced ovulation in mice with the use of gonadotropins, including hCG. There was a statistically significant increase in the incidence of *limb reduction defects* in the offsring of treated mothers over controls. Anomalies involved absence of digits and reduction of front limbs. This study is useful in establishing *biological plausibility*; that it is biologically plausible to induce limb reduction defects by stimulating ovulation, as distinguished from administering the drug during pregnancy. Conventional animal teratology studies had produced limb reduction defects as well. Administering clomiphene during organogenesis in rats had resulted in missing phalanges (toes) in the offspring;[205] and similar treatment in rabbits had produced stunted limbs.[206]

Spontaneous Abortions

Two other studies that caught my eye did not involve Clomid, but instead human menopausal gondaotropin (hMG aka Pergonal) and human chorionic gonadotropin (hCG). The first paper, authored by Ben-Rafael (1981), et al., appeared in the medical journal, *Fertilty and Sterility.*[207] It was of interest because the researchers were specifically looking at the spontaneous abortion (SA) rate following pregnancies induced by hMG and hCG and comparing it to the abortion rate of the same patients who later conceived without the use of fertility drugs. I considered it relevant because, as I have expressed before, all of these drugs have similar actions on the ovaries and produce a similar set of side effects, including excess estrogen, ovarian hyperstimulation syndrome and multiple births.

Ten out of 34 pregnancies (29.4%) induced by the hMG/hCG combination resulted in SAs, whereas the same infertility patients who later conceived spontaneously (without inducing ovulation) had an abortion rate of only 8.8% (3 out of 34). When multiple pregnancies were removed from the data, the difference was still significant: seven out of 29 (24.1%) of the treated group and three out of 34 (8.8%) of the unassisted pregnancies resulted in SAs. The likelihood of these numbers occurring by chance was less than four percent ($P<0.04$).

Reference was made to different theories proposed in the literature to explain the high incidence of SAs following hMG/hCG induced pregnancies. Included were "early diagnosis of pregnancy and abortion, *chromosomal abnormality due to treatment*, hyperstimulation of the ovary, and a high multiple pregnancy rate." [Emphasis added.]

Multiple pregnancies often result in late abortions because of the physical dynamics of two or more fetuses co-existing in the same uterus. However, when this potential cause was eliminated from the study, there still remained a statistically significant difference. Early ascertainment of pregnancy and abortion following use of fertility drugs would not have been a factor in this study either. Both groups were part of the same protocol and subjected to the same examinations. This leaves hyperstimulation of the ovaries and/or chromosomal abnormalities due to fertility drug treatment; both of which implicate fertility drugs – and fall under the Mix Hypothesis.

This study further strengthened the argument that, excluding habitual aborters, patients with ovulatory dysfunction did not have a higher incidence of SAs than those in the general population. In fact, along with two earlier studies, there was an amazing consistency in the ratio of the SA rates between spontaneous and induced pregnancies, respectively: Garcia (10.5%-25.4%); Toshinobu (8.9%-23.6%); and Ben-Rafael (8.8%-29.4%).

The second study also involved Ben-Rafael and his colleagues, and was published two years later (1983).[208] Not only did they update their data, they also evaluated three important factors not considered in their earlier study, namely pretreatment estrogen levels, hyperstimulation of the ovaries and first trimester SAs.

The patients were divided into two groups. Group I had *negligible* endogenous (internally produced) estrogen activity; Group II had *distinct* estrogen activity. This classification was important because, among other things, it reflected on the patient's capacity to produce significant estrogen levels in response to ovulatory-stimulating drugs. Hyperstimulation of the ovaries, of course, results in even higher levels of estrogen activity. And first trimester SAs are associated with a high incidence of embryonic and fetal abnormalities.

In this context, the authors looked at the incidence of SAs following (1) the first pregnancy induced by the hMG/hCG treatment; and (2) the second pregnancy induced by hMG/hCG treatment involving the same patients. They also calculated separate incidence rates for both first and second trimester SAs. Indeed, by looking at both sets of numbers, the causal association between pre-treatment estrogen levels and the incidence of first trimester SAs becomes dramatically clear:

FIRST INDUCED PREGNANCIES

Group	Preg.	1st Trmstr SAs	2nd Trmstr SAs	Total
Group I	119	**19 (16.0%)**	12 (10.1%)	31 (26.1%)
Group II	84	**24 (28.6%)**	3 (3.6%)	27 (32.1%)
Total	203	43 (21.2%)	15 (7.4%)	58 (28.6%)

SECOND INDUCED PREGNANCIES

Group	Preg.	1st Trmstr SAs	2nd Trmstr SAs	Total
Group I	60	**4 (6.7%)**	3 (5.0%)	7 (11.7%)
Group II	24	**3 (12.5%)**	0 (0.0%)	3 (12.5%)
Total	84	7 (8.3%)	3 (3.6%)	10 (11.9%)

When one looked at the *total* abortion rate, there was not an appreciable difference between Group I and Group II. Following the first induced pregnancies, the percentages were 26.1% and 32.1%, respectively. Following the second induced pregnancies, the percentages were 11.7% and 12.5%, respectively. But when one screened out the second trimester SAs, the group with active estrogen levels prior to treatment had *almost twice the frequency* of SAs. The ratio also remained the same whether the SA rate was calculated from the first induced pregnancies or the subsequent ones.

The researchers noted that there was a significant difference in the SA rate following the first induced pregnancy (28.6%) compared to the second induced pregnancy (11.9%). [P< 0.01.] Yet they had no explanation for the disparity between the two pregnancies.

They did, however, dispel the "overripeness" of ova theory. Toshinobu[209] and others had suggested that a high incidence of SAs following a first induced pregnancy might be the result of defective ova that developed after a lengthy term without ovulation (e.g., an "overripe" ova or egg). But Ben-Rafael et al. noted that their "findings would appear to contradict Toshinobu's (theory), because (they) found that the abortion rate remained unchanged irrespective of the number of ovulatory cycles prior to conception." In other words, the high abortion rate remained even when the theoretical "overripe" ova had been purged by earlier treatment cycles.

In my view there were probably higher levels of estrogen produced by the fertility drugs with the first induced pregnancies than there were with the second induced pregnancies. Without measurements, of course, we cannot know with any degree of certainty. Yet some of the data from the study would suggest that this might be the case. Out of the total number of patients who delivered the first induced pregnancies, 41.4% (84/203) had active estrogen levels prior to treatment, whereas their counterparts with second induced pregnancies had 28.6% (24/84). First induced pregnancies also experienced hyperstimulation of the ovaries 19.2% (39/203) of the time, and fourteen of the 39 had SAs (35.9%). But second induced pregnancies experienced this side effect only 11.9% (10/84) of the time, and only two of the 10 experienced SAs (20.0%). If one removed the hyperstimulation cases from the statistics, the SA rates between the two sets of pregnancies become significantly closer: 17.7% (29/164) and 10.8% (8/74), for the first and second pregnancies, respectively.

But the data on hyperstimulation of the ovaries and its influence on the SA rate was the real prize.

"Nevertheless, the degree of hyperstimulation had significant influence on the outcome of pregnancy. In the hMG-pregnancy 1 group, grade 1 hyperstimulation had 17 complicated pregnancies, 4 of which aborted (23.5%), whereas that with grade 2 and grade 3 hyperstimulation had 18 pregnancies with complications, of which 10 were aborted (55.5%). This difference was statistically significant (P< 0.05). The influence of grade 2 and grade 3 hyperstimulation on the abortion rate is even more prominent when one considers all pregnancies after hMG/hCG-induced ovulation. In the first and second pregnancies taken together, 5 of 27 women (18.5%) with grade 1 hyperstimulation aborted, while 11 of 22 women (50%) with grade 2 or grade 3 hyperstimulation aborted. This abortion rate was found to be highly significant (P< 0.01)."

When the ovaries were experiencing severe stimulation – *when estrogen levels were at their highest* – one out of every two pregnancies resulted in a SA. Although the authors did not break the numbers down for first trimester SAs, the vast majority (73.5%) of the SAs for the combined first and second pregnancies involved early abortions. Earlier, Caspi, et al.[210] had found a SA rate of 35.0% and 33.3% following grade 2 and grade 3 hyperstimulation, respectively, compared to 17.5% in pregnancies without hyperstimulation. I now had two published studies to back up my hyperstimulation data from the pre-market clinical investigations.

Chemical Similarity to Diethylstilbestrol

The chemical composition of Clomid is structurally similar to diethylstilbestrol (DES), a known human teratogen. DES causes congenital anomalies and cancer in the reproductive organs of the female and male offspring of women exposed to that drug during a specific period of gestation.

Two researchers out of Houston, James Clark and Shirley McCormack, authored a series of papers in which they compared the action of clomiphene citrate with DES on neonatal (newborn) and embryonic rats.

The first paper I reviewed was published in 1979.[211] Pregnant rats were injected with Clomid on either days 0 (date of mating), 5 or 12 of gestation. Rats injected on day zero did not become pregnant; the other two groups successfully conceived. When the female pups exposed on days 5 and 12 were examined fifteen weeks after delivery, they had a number of abnormalities of the reproductive tract.

"The incidence of disorganized and vacuolated epithelium in the vagina and cervix of the offspring is reminiscent of the vaginal adenosis that has been observed in young girls whose mothers received diethylstilbestrol during pregnancy."

Interpretation: When examined microscopically, the researchers found that the cells of the membrane-type lining (epithelium) of the vagina and cervix to be abnormal. The cells were disrupted and contained cavities (e.g., vacuoles). This appeared similar to the vaginal adenosis seen in daughters exposed to DES during gestation. In its broadest sense, "vaginal adenosis" exists when the epithelium fails to complete its development throughout the vagina. These and other abnormalities were found, and also extended to the uterus and oviduct (fallopian tube) – and were even seen in the mothers.

McCormack and Clark expressed their concern. "These results indicate the potential danger which may be inherent in the use of this drug in women."

Their 1980 article[212] expanded on the earlier study. This time they compared neonatal uterine stimulation by estrogen, DES, Clomid and two other triphenylethylene derivatives, namely Tamoxifen and Nafoxidine. They also evaluated the long-term effects of Clomid and Nafoxidine when administered to neonates.

In terms of uterine stimulation, Clark and McCormack discovered that estrogen, DES and Clomid had a similar effect on the cells of the epithelium. In fact, Clomid was even more potent than the other two compounds. Exposure of Clomid and Nafoxidine to rat neonates on day one of life resulted in a large array of abnormalities of the reproductive tract when examined two to three months later. Included in the abnormalities were *uterine tumors*.

"These results indicate that a single injection of Clomid or Nafoxidine during fetal or neonatal life will cause a wide number of abnormalities of the reproductive tract. These abnormalities may arise from the intense and sustained estrogenic stimulation of the epithelial lining of these organs. *Continuous exposure to high levels of estrogen during fetal and/or neonatal life is known to increase the incidence of preneoplastic and neoplastic changes in the reproductive tract.*" [Emphasis added.]

A "neoplastic" change refers to the development of a tumor, which can be either benign or malignant. The authors are cautioning about the possible risks of tumors as a consequence of use of these drugs.

"The eventual effects of such stimulation may remain unknown for many years. We have recently demonstrated that Clomid stimulates epithelial hypertrophy (swelling of cells) in the baboon uterus and hence the possibility exists that Clomid and othet triphenylethylene derivatives could cause hyperestrogenization of certain cell types in humans."

A third animal study of interest involved the use of mice. In 1982, Gorwill et al. published a paper[213] in which *clomiphene citrate and DES* were injected into neonatal (newborn) mice on days one through five post-delivery. The development and evolution of the mouse vagina during this period corresponds to a similar transformation in humans during the late first and early second trimesters. Neonatal mice were thus considered a good model to determine what might happen to humans when exposed to a drug chemically similar to DES during that critical period of gestation. Not surprisingly, they found similar abnormalities in the epithelial cells produced by both drugs. "In many animals in both the diethylstilbestrol and clomiphene citrate groups, the columnar cells had assumed an adenosis configuration."

The "adenosis configuration," of course, is what was seen in DES daughters resulting from in utero exposure to that synthetic estrogen. Gorwill and his associates offered their perspective on the study.

"If, indeed, the mouse is a model of the human, what then is the significance of this adenosis? In the human, adenosis is a prominent diethylstilbestrol-related vaginal finding, and a small percentage of diethylstilbestrol daughters develop malignant tumors in the vagina. In older mice which have developed tumors after neonatal diethylstilbestrol, there seems to be a relationship to adenosis."

They caution that Clomid exposure which reaches the fetus in the late first or early second trimesters might lead to adenosis of the vagina, and on rare occasions result in vaginal cancer. Fortunately, even with its long half-life, the chance of an appreciable amount of clomiphene reaching the fetus in the late first trimester (e.g., 75-90 days post-conception) would seem remote; although it is conceivable where the patient has received multiple courses in high doses over an extended period.

A more likely risk, however, would exist where there is inadvertent exposure during pregnancy. The authors of the paper expressed their concern.

"This effect of diethylstilbestrol and clomiphene citrate appears to be similar to the biologic response to transplacental diethylstilbestrol in the human. After transplacental diethylstilbestrol, malignant vaginal tumors rarely develop. If clomiphene citrate, given to the human prior to pregnancy to induce ovulation or by inadvertence during pregnancy, *were to circulate into the critical time of vaginal differentiation, a similar biologic potential may exist.* The first situation seems to be unlikely. The second is of more concern." [Emphasis added.]

The focus of this book is on birth defects and the adverse effects on the human embryo/fetus that can be produced by clomiphene citrate and other fertility drugs. However, I would be remiss if I did not make passing mention about the possible carcinogenic risk from the use of Clomid. Since I have not researched the literature on the subject, nor reviewed corporate records involving the subject matter, I cannot speak from any position of knowledge or expertise. But I would caution the reader that the current (2005) product information makes the following statement under *Adverse Reactions*. "Ovarian cancer has been infrequently reported in patients who have received fertility drugs. Infertility is a primary risk factor for ovarian cancer; however, epidemiology data suggest that prolonged use of clomiphene may increase the risk of a borderline or invasive ovarian tumor." I would thus suggest that anyone who has a family history of carcinoma of the reproductive organs, or has taken large doses of fertility drugs over a prolonged period of time, explore this issue with an expert in the field.

In Vitro and In Vivo Animal Studies

In vitro (test tube) and in vivo (in the body) studies also have their place in the field of teratology. They are intended to supplement human epidemiology studies, not replace them. However, they play an important role in demonstrating *how* a teratogen can produce congenital anomalies, and exploring a possible *mechanism of action*. As previously explained, such an assessment – along with animal teratology studies – can demonstrate a drug's pharmacologic capability of producing a specific type of anomaly.

By 1985, I had substantial data on how fertility drugs could influence the rate of spontaneous abortions (SAs). I could present statistics establishing an increased incidence of first trimester SAs: (1) when conception occurred during a treatment cycle verses conception two or more cycles after use of fertility drugs; (2) when infertility patients had a higher pre-treatment level of endogenous estrogen; and (3) when infertility patients experienced OHSS while conceiving with fertility drugs. These statistics represented evidence that high levels of estrogen produced by Clomid, and other ovulatory-stimulating drugs, caused first trimester SAs. In conjunction with the Boue paper, I could further argue that these SAs were a result of abnormal chromosomes and other anomalies of the embryo and fetus produced by the elevated estrogen.

To further establish Clomid as a clastogen – capable of inducing chromosomal abnormalities – I could point to the Charles paper, a study on the capacity of Clomid to alter chromosomes in the endometrium of the uterus. And, of course, Oakley had presented epidemiological evidence of the capability of ovulation induction to increase the risk of Down syndrome, a birth defect one hundred percent associated with abnormal chromosomes.

With discovery of the 1983 paper by Czeizel, et al., I had epidemiologic support that ovulation induction could likewise produce a congenital anomaly unassociated with abnormal chromosomes, namely limb-reduction defects. By now, there were also numerous teratology studies effectively demonstrating that Clomid and other fertility drugs were capable of inducing a wide variety of congenital abnormalities in several different species of animal.

Yet all of this evidence was *circumstantial*. Of course, in the field of teratology, this is often all that we have. Even animal teratology studies are not *direct* evidence of what a drug can do in humans.

Direct proof of what a fertility drug was capable of doing to a human ovum/egg might be presented via an in vitro observation of such gametes following ovulatory stimulation and comparing them to human control ova/eggs produced naturally. As of 1985, such studies had yet to be performed – at least, that I could find. There were, however, a couple of articles involving in vitro and in vivo tests on the oocytes (eggs) and early embryos of mice.

Laufer, et al. evaluated the effects of clomiphene citrate on mice ova when exposed to the drug both in vivo and in vitro.[214] Female mice were injected with clomiphene on days one through three after ovulatory stimulation (by another drug), using progressively higher doses. The treated mice were then mated with their male counterparts on day four. They found that "when the drug was administered in the late follicular phase, a dose-dependent decrease was seen in the rate of successful copulation, ovulation, and embryo development." When administered closer to the time the ova were expelled from the ovarian follicle, there was a dose-dependent decrease in ovulation, conception and *growth of the embryo*. "A short in vitro treatment of oocytes with clomiphene prior to in vitro fertilization resulted in an increased proportion of degenerated and unfertilized ova. Moreover, this treatment caused a dose-dependent decrease in blastocyst formation." A "blastocyst" is the egg after it has been fertilized by the sperm and has evolved to multiple cells through the cleavage process. It is a blastocyst that attaches to the uterine wall.

The second paper was authored by Schmidt, et al.[215] Mice ova were exposed to clomiphene via two methods: through in vitro fertilization by placing the ova into a clomiphene medium with mice sperm; and a standard in vivo procedure by securing fertilized eggs after mating and placing them in a similar clomiphene medium. Progressively higher concentrations of Clomid were used in both methods. When measured against controls, the researchers found that in both methods there was a dose-dependent effect on the rate of fertilization and blastocyst formation. "It appears that clomiphene citrate-exposed embryos may undergo subtle changes that later manifest themselves in the form of decreased embryo growth rates and increased embryo degeneration rates." Schmidt and his associates also offered an interesting suggestion.

"The findings reported here suggest that fertilization, embryo growth, and embryo degeneration rates are affected by exposure of the mouse oocyte-early embryo to clomiphene citrate and that these results *may occur several days after actual exposure.* The implication from these data is that these effects may be responsible, in part, for the differences between ovulation and conception rates and for the *increased spontaneous abortion rates reported in women treated with clomiphene.*" [Emphasis added.]

If Clomid can inhibit the growth and development of early embryonic mice, is it such a stretch to suggest that it might have a similar action on early human embryos? Schmidt and his colleagues didn't seem to think so. Whether by chromosomal abnormalities induced via elevated estrogen levels and/or a direct action of the drug on the early human embryo, the elevated rates of first trimester SAs would seem to support such a relationship. The evidence in support of Clomid and other fertility drugs being human teratogens was beginning to build.

At least, the Canadians were starting to take notice.

The 1985 edition of the Canadian publication, *Compendium of Pharmaceuticals and Specialties* (CPS)[216] reflects an initial awareness that – at least with our northern neighbors – there may be a risk factor involving the use of clomiphene citrate and the development of congenital abnormalities. Listed under *Adverse Effects* for Clomid are multiple births, ovarian enlargement and "birth defects." With reference to precautions, it states that "(t)he patient should be advised of the frequency and potential hazards of multiple pregnancies as well as the incidence of abnormal infants being born."

Drug Experience Reports

In late 1985, I decided to take another scenic tour of Merrell's Cincinnati plant – and, of course, kick back and do a little reading while I was at it. It had been eight years since my last visit and I needed to update my records.

One area of interest was the pattern of birth defects being reported by the medical profession. Of particular concern was the incidence of case reports on neural tube defects. Had the ratio dropped off? Clomid had now been on the market for 18 years. Perhaps the surge of NTDs in the 1970s was nothing more than a temporary spike. The last time I had checked the Drug Experience Reports (DERs) was in the spring of 1976. Through March 22, 1976, Merrell and the FDA had received 17 DERs involving neural tube defects out of a total of seventy (24.3%) reports on congenital anomalies.

As I had expected, the ratio had remained somewhat consistent. At the time of my inspection, I was able to locate 135 DERs, received through June 30, 1985, that provided a sufficiently accurate description of the congenital anomalies from which I could ascertain whether or not they included NTDs. Out of that number, 30 (22.2%) of them were neural tube defects. There had not been a meaningful drop. More than one out of every 5 case reports involved closure defects of the neural tube.

The "red flag" was still waving.

Although not as dramatic, another congenital anomaly seemed to be surfacing as well. I also found a considerable number of limb reduction defects (LRDs). These included absence or shortening of the fingers, toes, hands, arms and/or legs. Sixteen cases were reported out of 135 (11.9%). Three of the DERs[217] were of phocomelia, the anomaly that brought attention to thalidomide. This is a rare type of LRD where one might see a hand protruding from a shoulder or a foot or toes from a hip. For example, one report described bilateral absence of the radius and ulna (lower arm) and missing thumbs. The hands (absent thumbs) were present at the elbows.

Along with the above Czeizel study, in my view another flag was waving.

* * * * *

CHAPTER 13

The Check is in the Mail

Another goal of my 1985 venture to Merrell's facility was to track the recent history of the language used in the product labeling (e.g., package insert). Once a drug has been approved for marketing, delay plays a significant role in maximizing sales – and is another means by which a pharmaceutical company can work the system. New and more-severe adverse reactions can have a major impact on sales. When such reports are received by the company, the longer the FDA takes to act on them the longer the drug remains on the market without added warnings or removal. Delay thus equates to an economic benefit.

One important opportunity to postpone changes in the labeling exists with the slow and archaic back and forth procedure to obtain final approval of modifications to the relevant language. My effort to secure labeling changes with Clomid would be no exception. Proposed language and drafts were exchanged between the regulatory agency and the pharmaceutical company, but at an incredibly slow pace. Picture a tennis match with the ball traveling at super-slow speed – say, at about a foot an hour.

Think I'm exaggerating?

Following the request of the FDA on August 15, 1975 that "further prospective and retrospective data be collected by (Merrell) regarding the occurrence of congenital anomalies," the company responded in the form of two submissions. A one-volume presentation was submitted on March 30, 1976. A nine-volume set was dated November 14, 1980. The 1976 edition has already been discussed; the 1980 version will be addressed in Chapter 16. There were also multiple meetings.

Apparently, neither the submissions nor the meetings sold the FDA.

Five years after my presentation to the advisory committee, the Mix Hypothesis was still giving Merrell problems. A letter from Thomas O'Dell to Dr. A.T. Gregoire of the FDA, dated April 15, 1980, confirmed a request for a meeting between Merrell and the agency. Among the four proposed agenda items was the following topic:

"Discussion of the hypothesis set forth by Mr. Terence Mix and a critique of this hypothesis by Drs. R.L. Van de Wiele and G.M. Jaguello of Columbia University, New York."

The meeting eventually took place on June 24, 1980.[218] The Merrell team consisted of Mark Hoekenga, M.D., James Newberne, DVM, J.G. Page, M.D., F. Shubeck, M.D., two legal representatives – all from Merrell – and Dr. Van de Wiele, James Wilson, Ph.D. (teratologist) and W. Leavitt, Ph.D. This was a full attack team intent on protecting Merrell's product. Although I could never locate a memo outlining the meeting, subsequent events would suggest that neither the meeting nor the November 1980 package were successful in dissuading the FDA from adding incriminating warnings to the package insert. The original draft was dated August 12, 1980. Important revisions were added on February 6, 1981.

On March 19, 1981, Merrell submitted a draft of its proposed revised labeling for approval. The cover letter assured that "all suggested modifications (had) been incorporated in the text." Those modifications included some important changes:

"Some Clomid and/or its metabolites (here measured only as $_{14}C$) may, therefore, *remain in the body during early pregnancy* in every woman who conceives in the menstrual cycle of Clomid treatment.

Under the general heading "PRECAUTIONS," and subheading "Patient Counseling," the following language was added:

"The physician should counsel the patient with special regard to the following *potential adverse reactions* that may be encountered.

* * *

"4. Pregnancy Wastage and Birth Anomalies

* * *

"Among the birth anomalies spontaneously reported as individual cases since commercial availability of Clomid, *the proportion of neural tube defects has been high* among pregnancies associated with ovulation induced by Clomid, but this has not been supported by data from population-based studies.

* * *

"Population-based reports have been published on *possible elevation of risk of Down Syndrome* in ovulation induction cases and of *increase in trisomy defects among spontaneously aborted fetuses* from subfertile women receiving ovulation inducing drugs (no women with Clomid alone and without additional inducing drug)." [Emphasis added, Exhibits 14a and 14b]

Further, the representation that "no causative evidence of a deleterious effect of Clomid therapy on the human fetus has been seen," was deleted in its entirety.

Think about it. At least as early as February 6, 1981, the FDA was of the mindset that patients should be cautioned that birth anomalies were a "potential adverse reaction" from the use of Clomid. In support of this statement, it makes reference to the high proportion of neural tube defects among the DERs of congenital anomalies, the population-based elevated risk of Down syndrome reported by Oakley in 1972 and 1979, and the increase in chromosomal trisomy defects among spontaneous abortions from the 1973 Boue study – and proposes that this evidence be discussed with the patients.

Responding at its customary pace, *over two and one half years later* (November 30, 1983), Dr. Solomon Sobel, the then-current Director of the Division of Metabolism and Endocrine Drug Products, requested final print labeling and advised Merrell that it would be approved if it was "identical in content to the draft copy except that a HOW SUPPLIED section should be added and inclusion of the prescription caution statement (was) also recommended."

When I read the draft of the proposed changes, I was absolutely elated. All three cautionary items had been argued by me in 1975. True, they were not exactly leaping onto the shelves of local pharmacies around the country, but something was actually happening. Although Merrell may have avoided conducting additional studies, the system was actually working – albeit, at a pace that would embarrass a snail.

Or so I thought.

Rather than present a "final print labeling," Merrell thought it might be desirable to update its product information.[219] So on February 1, 1984, it instead submitted a second draft – and bought itself *another two and a half years*.

[Note that the following history was acquired over the subsequent years in stages, through various production requests to both Merrell and the FDA. Only after multiple efforts over the following decade did a picture emerge on how a drug company sidesteps documented mandates for changes in its labeling.]

Still moving in slow motion, on November 3, 1986, Dr. Sobel approved the second draft of the labeling and requested that it be resubmitted in final form. He advised Merrell that the "labeling should be identical in content to the draft copy," except for a couple minor revisions including use of Pregnancy Category X language.

The response of Merrell Dow Pharmaceuticals seemed justified. Because of the reformatted labeling requirements dictated by the Code of Federal Regulations (21 CFR 201.57), on December 11, 1986 Merrell argued that the suggested language under Pregnancy Category X, which contraindicated use in women who are or *may become pregnant*, was inappropriate because the drug was intended for use by women desiring pregnancy. The language of the contraindication would be confusing. But the March 5, 1987 change suggested by Sobel, I am sure, was neither anticipated nor acceptable by Merrell:

> "CONTRAINDICATIONS: Clomid is contraindicated in pregnant women. Clomid *may cause fetal harm when administered to pregnant women.* Since there is a reasonable likelihood of the patient becoming pregnant while receiving Clomid, *the patient should be apprised of the potential hazard to the fetus.*" [Emphasis added.]

But, then, Merrell could now submit another *draft*. And just maybe it could slip by without Sobel's suggested contraindication language. In late 1987, Merrell's August draft of the reformatted labeling was submitted to the FDA for approval. Not surprisingly, although it contained all of the previously approved changes in the submission of March 19, 1981, Sobel's proposed language was missing. Instead, it simply stated that "Clomid is not indicated and should not be administered during pregnancy." I, of course, preferred Sobel's version – and presumably so did Dr. Sobel.

Why wasn't it caught? A better question would be: Whatever happened to the 1987 reformatted labeling?

Based upon language set out in the *Federal Register*[220] on June 26, 1979, new regulations had been established to reformat the labeling for prescription drugs. As explained in its summary, "(t)his rule designates a required format for the physician labeling of prescription drugs for human use and provides standards for the kind of information that must appear in each section of the required format." The pertinent regulations were contained within 21 CFR 201.57. They were to become effective December 26, 1979.

The language set out in the *Federal Register* related to "Warnings" is worth reviewing, as it expresses the standards – at least through April 1, 2001[221] – that dictated when physicians and patients should be apprised of a risk. It would also appear that the new regulations provided the impetus for including the three pieces of evidence referred to in the draft of the reformatted insert above.

> "A serious hazard *must* be included in the 'Warnings' section of the labeling of a drug when evidence exists on the basis of which experts qualified by scientific training and experience can reasonably conclude that the hazard is *associated* with the use of the drug. *A causal relationship need not be proved.* As discussed fully in the preamble to the proposed revision…, the act requires labeling to include warnings about both *potential* and verified hazards. Accordingly, when medical information justifies a warning, the act *requires* that it be included in drug labeling. Although FDA often refers questions of whether a warning should be included in the labeling of a drug to its standing advisory committees, the decision as to whether a warning is legally required for the labeling of a drug must rest with the agency." [Emphasis added, p.37447.]

There it is. A warning was required, effective December 26, 1979, when experts qualified by scientific training and experience could reasonably conclude that a *potential* hazard was *associated* with use of a drug, even though a causal relationship had not yet been proven.

The term "associated," as used by scientists to describe a potential adverse reaction to a drug, means that the adverse condition is occurring following use of the drug with such frequency as to suggest that the two might be related. For example, Oakley found that Down syndrome was associated with use of Clomid and Pergonal, but initially speculated that it might be attributed to the underlying infertility condition – a position he appeared to back away from when he updated his studies in 1979.

However, after a close review of the May 1991 Clomid insert (#J014K), it was evident that the above changes had yet to find their way into the labeling, even by the early 1990s. Indeed, over the years there had been very little change in the text used.

Except for deleting "(clomiphene citrate)" after "Clomid," the language in the 1991 insert, under the headings for Indications, Contraindications, Warnings, Precautions, Adverse Reactions (except for reference to one paper), Dosage and Administration, and Animal Pharmacology and Toxicology, was *identical* to that contained in the labeling in use in July 1972 (#3798). Thus, for over 19 years, physicians and pharmacists were essentially using the same package insert – and for over twelve years the reformatted labeling had yet to be put to use for Clomid.

An Unfortunate Change of Pace: the 1995 Labeling

But even glaciers have movement, and in 1994 the FDA finally pressed Merrell to update its product labeling. On May 31, 1994, Dr. Solomon Sobel sent a letter to Merrell requesting changes to the Clomid prescribing information. Included was a list of desired modifications.

Merrell was happy to accommodate; along with a few "minor" revisions to the existing insert. Just three months later (August 23, 1994) it had a draft ready for review and approval. Its cover letter to Dr. Solomon Sobel explained its desired changes – already incorporated in the draft, of course.

"In addition to the changes you requested, we propose the following wording for the Precautions Section.

- Precautions Section, Pregnancy subsection, paragraph one, page 5.

    – Delete the sentence, 'Clomid may cause fetal harm when administered to a pregnant woman.'

    – Add the wording stated below in place of the deleted sentence.

    'Clomid should not be administered during pregnancy. Clomid *may* cause fetal harm in animals (see Animal Fetotoxicity). Although no causative evidence of a deleterious effect of Clomid therapy on the human fetus has been *established*, there have been reports of birth anomalies which, during clinical studies, occurred at an incidence within the normal range range reported for the general population (see Fetal/Neonatal Anomalies and Mortality; ADVERSE REACTIONS).'" [Emphasis added.]

These suggested changes had far-reaching implications. First, Sobel's proposed warning was to be eliminated. Second, whereas the replaced labeling stated in clear language that

Clomid was teratogenic in the rat and the rabbit, the advocated change introduced uncertainty about the question. Even in the face of numerous published studies establishing clomiphene as a teratogen in animals, Merrell was intent on pressing the FDA to convey equivocation.

Finally, Merrell was also intent on pressing the FDA for a version that replaced the word "seen" with "established" – which had its own ramifications. Consider the earlier paragraph in the May 1991 insert.

"Although *no* causative evidence of a deleterious effect of Clomid therapy on the human fetus has been *seen*, such evidence in regard to the rat and the rabbit has been presented (see Animal Pharmacology and Toxicology). Therefore, Clomid should not be administered during pregnancy." [Emphasis added.]

From May 15, 1967 through 1994, the product labeling for Clomid carried the above statement. For almost three decades, Merrell represented to every prescribing physician that there was absolutely no evidence that Clomid was a human teratogen; no epidemiology studies, no in-vivo studies, no in-vitro studies; not one study – nothing. Actually, this absolute assurance of safety extended to *any* deleterious effect on the human fetus (i.e., including growth retardation, spontaneous abortion, etc.).

Yet, as has been previously detailed, there had been incriminating evidence as far back as the original pre-market studies that have implicated Clomid with having a "deleterious effect...on the human fetus." Although Merrell may have wanted to challenge the studies, or even term them as only "suggestive" or "questionable," they still represented evidence, to be weighed, analyzed and considered. In the early 1970s there were published studies suggesting that Clomid and other fertility drugs were "clastogens" capable of *damaging chromosomes* in the human body. Into the late seventies and early eighties, additional papers were published, including human epidemiology studies, animal studies, and even laboratory studies assessing clomiphene's action at the cellular level, all adding further support for the contention that Clomid and other fertility drugs were human teratogens. .

Then, as will be discussed in the next chapter, in the late 1980s a series of human epidemiology studies began appearing in published medical journals demonstrating a statistically significant increase in neural tube defects and other congenital anomalies following exposure to clomiphene and other fertility drugs. Serono Laboratories recognized the need to say *something*. Its July 1992 labeling for Serophene (clomiphene citrate) expressed a watered-down warning to prescribing doctors to address these recent studies:

> "Some medical literature reports have implied an increased occurrence of neural tube defects, while others indicate that an increased incidence over that found in the general population does not exist."[222]

By 1994, not even Merrell could justify an assurance that there was "no causative evidence of a deleterious effect of Clomid therapy on the human fetus." But that was an easy fix. Simply modify one word by changing "seen" to "established." In Merrell's view, perhaps causative evidence of a deleterious effect on the human fetus had been *seen*, but it had not been *established*. Rather than delete the sentence in its entirety – as had been required in the two earlier drafts – Merrell urged the use of language that continued to convey that Clomid did not pose a teratogenic risk.

But what was the justification for the presence of the paragraph?

As stated in the *Federal Register* as far back as 1979, even *potential* risks were to be included as warnings. To state that causation had not been established, without making reference to studies supporting a potential risk, conveys the lack of *any* evidence that Clomid could cause human congenital anomalies. As will be seen, by 1994 there was a substantial body of scientific data supporting the position that Clomid, and other fertility drugs, were *probable* human teratogens. Yet not only did the presented draft lack the three warnings approved in 1981, nowhere within the four corners of the document was there a reference to *anything* that might implicate the drug as a cause of human birth defects.

The reason for the paragraph? To deceive prescribing physicians into believing that by 1994 there was still a lack of evidence that Clomid could cause birth defects in humans. Merrell was not about to take the slightest chance that the results of recent studies might reach unknowing physicians or – worse yet – their patients.

Even the earlier approved warning that Clomid could carry over into early pregnancy was watered down. Compare the two passages. The language approved in 1981 stated:

"Some Clomid and/or its metabolites (here measured only as 14C) may, therefore, remain in the body during early pregnancy in *every woman* who conceives in the menstrual cycle of Clomid treatment." [Emphasis added.]

The updated version in the 1994 draft read:

"Thus, it is *possible* that some active drug may remain in the body during early pregnancy in women who conceive in the menstrual cycle during CLOMID therapy." [Emphasis added.]

Notice the subtle change. The 1981 language conveys that the drug may remain during early pregnancy in every woman who conceived during a treatment cycle. By 1994, this became only a possibility.

But there was more – a lot more.

Examine the paragraph again. The words are quite reassuring. "Although no causative evidence of a deleterious effect of CLOMID therapy on the human fetus has been established, there have been reports of birth anomalies which, during clinical studies, *occurred at an incidence within the range reported for the general population* (see Fetal/Neonatal Anomalies and Mortality; ADVERSE REACTIONS)." [Emphasis added.] This assurance of safety is repeated under the subheading *Fetal/Neonatal Anomalies and Mortality*. "The overall incidence of reported birth anomalies from pregnancies associated with maternal CLOMID ingestion during clinical studies was *within the range of that reported for the general population*." [Emphasis added.] Then, to insure that this representation reaches each patient, it is repeated again under the additional subheading, *Information for Patients*. "The overall incidence of reported birth anomalies from pregnancies associated with maternal CLOMID ingestion during the investigational studies was *within the range of that reported in published references for the general population*." [Emphasis added.]

The above language from the proposed draft had never been included in the package insert over the prior 27 years. The references to "clinical studies" and "investigational studies" pertain to the *pre-market* clinical investigations (with humans) conducted by Merrell's predecessor entity (Richardson-Merrell, Inc.) between 1960 and 1967.[223] The words assure the prescribing doctor and patient that the incidence of birth defects during the Clomid pre-market investigations was no greater than seen in the general population. They seem to say, "Hey, there have been a few reports of birth defects, but it's no big deal." The inference is that there was a design to the pre-market investigations that allowed a meaningful comparison with birth defect rates "in published references for the general population." The words are comforting to anyone with lingering doubts about the possible risk of the drug to the resulting fetus.

But the tragic truth is that no one *knows* the incidence of congenital anomalies that occurred during the pre-market investigations. The above representations serve no purpose other than to deceive readers into believing that Clomid is not a human teratogen.

Merrell reported a total of 58 birth defects from 54 pregnancies (two each from four multiple births)[224] from a total of 2,635 pregnancies, about which the outcome was known in 2,369.[225] When one deducts the 483 cases of spontaneous abortions, he is left with 1,886 delivered pregnancies. The incidence rate would thus equate to 3.1% if one counted total birth defects (58) or 2.9% if one used instead the number of pregnancies resulting in a congenital anomaly (54). But as previously demonstrated, the pre-market investigations were *never designed to assess the risk of birth defects*. The "clinical studies" used to assure that Clomid lacks any form of a teratogenic risk for its users were never intended to make such an assessment.

On March 3, 1979, I took the deposition of Carl A. Bunde, M.D. at Merrell's pharmaceutical plant in Cincinnati. Bunde had been the Director of Medical Research from 1960 to 1970, and had supervised the Clomid pre-market investigations during the entire period they were conducted.[226] He also personally participated in setting up most of the protocols for the studies.[227] During the course of my examination, the following testimony was given:

> "Well, doctor, was there any formal protocol set up to evaluate the drug during the clinical studies to determine whether or not it might cause birth defects?"
>
> "I doubt if that was an objective of any protocol."
>
> "So if I understand correctly, at no time prior to marketing of Clomid was there any protocol specifically designed or set up to evaluate whether or not Clomid could cause birth defects; is that correct?"
>
> "I believe that's correct."[228]

There can be little question that Bunde was well-acquainted with the type of design necessary to evaluate the potential teratogenicity of a drug, including the need for a control group. Two years prior to the marketing of Clomid, Bunde and H. M. Leyland co-authored a paper entitled "A Controlled Retrospective Survey in Evaluation of Teratogenicity."[229] At the time, their focus was on Bendectin and Tenuate; both drugs having been manufactured by their employer, Richardson-Merrell. They controlled for such factors as race, religion, ethnicity, time and location of delivery, and even the same physician. Yet, notwithstanding its involvement in the thalidomide tragedy and the positive animal teratology studies with Clomid, Merrell made a conscious decision not to design a study to evaluate whether its drug could cause birth defects.

A meaningful *epidemiological study* to assess the risk of congenital anomalies would require the use of a control group. Such studies are conducted by comparing the incidence of birth defects of a population exposed to the drug with the incidence of birth defects in another population not exposed to the drug (e.g., a control group). The desire is to have all factors that might cause or contribute to congenital anomalies equal in both groups (i.e., age, race, geographical location, etc.), so that the only difference between the two groups is the drug. If an increase occurs in the exposed group, and it is statistically significant, it is considered scientific evidence that the drug is the cause. The pre-market clinical investigations did *not include any control group* with which to compare the incidence of congenital abnormalities. This is why the above language compares the rate of birth defects from the clinical studies with rates "in published references for the general population."

Bunde's view was echoed by Mark T. Hoekenga, M.D. Hoekenga was the Associate Director of Clinical Research for Merrell from 1961 to 1964 and Director of Medical & Scientific Coordination from 1964 to 1968,[230] and likewise participated in the Clomid investigations. I examined him at a deposition on the Breimhorst case on March 1, 1974.

"Was Clomid ever investigated as to any possible teratogenic effects, in the clinical investigation?

"No, Clomid was not specifically evaluated to see if it would have a teratogenic effect. The outcome of every pregnancy that was temporally related with Clomid was assiduously searched for and tabulated and evaluated."[231]

Although acknowledging that the Clomid study was never designed to determine the teratogenic risk of the drug, Hoekenga wanted to make a point that they had documented and evaluated "the outcome of every pregnancy." As previously seen, this did not happen either. The study was never designed to make an *accurate count* of Clomid-related birth defects.

It would seem self-evident that to make a correct count of all infants born with congenital anomalies, one must examine all such babies for that purpose. Just as important, the physician conducting the exam must have an obligation to report the results of his examination to Merrell – and at the very least, be aware that the baby is part of a study group.

The numerous deficiencies in the design of these studies have already been covered at length. They include delivery and examination of offspring at outside medical facilities; lack of knowledge of the names of many of the delivering physicians and facilities; reliance upon patient letters and birth announcements to determine the condition of the babies at birth; failure to conduct follow-up examinations of the delivered infants; failure to request that autopsies be performed on all stillborns and neonatal deaths; failure to include a definition of "birth defects;" failure to note the existence or non-existence of congenital abnormalities on up to one quarter of the case histories; and outright concealment of records on a significant number of the pregnancies. As a measuring stick for assessing its teratogenic risk, the Clomid pre-market clinical studies are absolutely worthless.

But over the years, the manufacturer of Clomid has become quite skilled at the art of deception. Whether to sell more drug products, pass muster with the FDA or to have a fallback position in later civil litigation, Merrell has practiced that art with the skill of a barker at a carnival sideshow. One way to defend its language in the product labeling is to play the game of semantics. Another is to play the numbers game. This "gamesmanship" is evident in the previously-cited language. But one must look more closely at the words and do a little digging to appreciate the deceit.

First, take a look at the semantics. Notice the choice of a very key word in the following three quotes. "Although no causative evidence of a deleterious effect of

CLOMID therapy on the human fetus has been established, there have been *reports* of birth anomalies which, during clinical studies, occurred at an incidence within the range reported for the general population...." "The overall incidence of *reported* birth anomalies from pregnancies associated with maternal CLOMID ingestion during clinical studies was within the range of that reported for the general population." "The overall incidence of *reported* birth anomalies from pregnancies associated with maternal CLOMID ingestion during the investigational studies was within the range of that reported in published references for the general population." [Emphasis added.]

How can one compare the incidence of birth defects from the Clomid population if one does not have a clue about how many infants were born with congenital anomalies? Simple; use only the "reported" ones. Merrell "reported" 58 infants born with congenital anomalies from the pre-market clinical studies. From that number, one comes up with an incidence of 3.1% (58 out of 1,886 delivered pregnancies) of "reported" birth defects. Thus, even though the inference from the above quotes is that the *incidence* of birth defects following use of Clomid is the same as the incidence in the general population, technically Merrell is not really stating that. Even though the *actual* incidence is unquestionably higher, the manufacturer of Clomid can justifiably state that the "reported" incidence in the pre-market investigations was 3.1%.

Now, the numbers game. Where this language is really deceptive is in the suggestion that the 3.1% rate is no higher than seen in the general population. Without question there are incidence rates from the general population that are equal to, and even exceed, 3%. The critical question, however, is not just what those rates are, but *how they are calculated*. Otherwise, one is comparing those proverbial apples and oranges.

As pointed out above, there are many factors which can directly affect the number of birth defects one finds in a given population of offspring. Are the statistics calculated from examinations conducted at time of birth, or at one year post-delivery or even at two years of age? Are autopsies conducted on all stillbirths and neonatal deaths? How thorough are the examinations? What is the definition of "birth defects"? Does the study include minor abnormalities, or is it only reporting on major anomalies? Birth defect rates can vary depending upon the race and/or geographical location of the study population. Where was the study conducted? What is the ethnicity composition of the study group?

Age can affect rates because older women tend to have more children with abnormalities. What is the average or median age of the population being studied?

Although the above list is not exhaustive, one starts to get an idea why rates can be all over the board. We are also dealing with small percentages. If a *similar* study from the general population is at 1%, then a rate of 3% would reflect a tripled risk. Rather than one out of a hundred it is 1 out of every 33. It is thus all the more critical that we be comparing "apples with apples." Unless one compares the Clomid pre-market clinical studies with another study from the general population with the same design, such a comparison is *meaningless*. It is for this very reason that epidemiologists use control groups to make an accurate assessment of whether there is a true increased risk.

But since Merrell never used a control group for the Clomid pre-market studies, it has chosen to compare its "reported" birth defect rate against incidence figures for the general population. Given this circumstance, the next logical question would be whether the pre-market study was patterned or designed after another study on the rates of birth defects in the general population. Again, the answer is an unequivocal "no." Merrell has formally acknowledged that the protocol and guidelines for the pre-market studies were not patterned after another study on malformation rates in the general population.[232]

So how did Merrell expect to convince the FDA that the reported incidence of birth anomalies from the pre-market studies (3.1%) was "within the range of that reported in published references for the general population"? As previously discussed, the answer is buried in the text of the two Merrell submissions of March 30, 1976 and November 14, 1980. Both presentations cite the same references on the incidence of birth defects in the general population. Myrianthopoulos reported an incidence rate of 15.56%; McIntosh a rate of 7.5%; and Shapiro a rate of 7.1%. Conversely, Clomid only had a birth defect rate of 2.4% (58 birth defects out of 2,369 pregnancies), according to both submissions.

But those reference populations used a birth defect rate based upon total deliveries, not total pregnancies; performed follow-up examinations on all infants at one year (Myrianthopoulos), one year (McIntosh) and two years (Shapiro) post-delivery; used very specific and inclusive definitions for "birth defects;" conducted comprehensive and thorough examinations of the infants; and performed autopsies on over 85% of the stillborns and neonatal deaths.

Technically, again, Merrell's incidence of "reported" birth defects did in fact fall within the range of that reported for the general population. A rate of 3.1% is certainly less than 15.56%, 7.5% or 7.1%; it is "within the range of that reported for the general population." But the *inference* from the statement is that there is a justifiable basis for making a comparison. It is also the interpretation that any prescribing doctor would reasonably give to the language, *because that is the only meaning that would justify its presence in the package insert.* As the assumption no doubt goes, the FDA would never approve the statement if a meaningful comparison could not be made. What is not disclosed is that Merrell is comparing "apples" from its clinical studies with "oranges" from published references. Indeed, it has made a science of it.

But for now, why be concerned? Surely we had another two-and-a-half year wait. After all, that was the pattern. We also had yet to hear from Sobel about his assessment of the recent draft.

"Hey, Sol. Did you notice that they tossed out your suggested warning? How about the omission regarding neural tube defects, Down syndrome and chromosomal anomalies in spontaneous abortions? You know, the ones you wanted back in 1983 and 1987. Then there's the language about the pre-market studies. What a joke, right? Oh, and catch what they did to the warning about Clomid hanging around in early pregnancy. Guess you're gonna kick it back, huh?"

Not a chance.

In the world record time of 37 days, on September 30, 1994, Sobel approved the text of the draft as submitted, save for a few minor typos and errors. In his letter of the same date back to Merrell, Sobel requested the company to submit fifteen copies of the final print labeling "as soon as available." By the time they caught a few more errors – no doubt initially missed in their haste – final labeling dated June 1995 (#J014M) was off to pharmacies across the country in the fall of the same year.

Welcome to the new FDA, circa 1994.

* * * * *

CHAPTER 14

A Prophesy Validated

It had been eight long years since I had set my eyes on a medical article that had anything to do with fertility drugs. But here I was again, relentlessly scanning the pages of the *Index Medicus* and searching the stacks of the multi-leveled UCLA Biomed Library. The year was 1993, and at the moment I was sitting at one of the many conference tables reading what turned out to be a major discovery. I was beginning preparation for my next Clomid trial, Gandy vs. Merrell Dow Pharmaceuticals. The trial was scheduled for the spring of 1994.

My sixth clomiphene case had settled in September 1988. But sixteen months earlier I had been retained by Linda and Curtis Gandy to represent their infant son, Brandon. Following an induced pregnancy, he had delivered on May 7, 1986 with multiple congenital malformations, including absence of the left kidney, imperforate anus, rectourethral fistula, hypospadias, undescended testicles, bilateral hip dysplasia and club feet. An *imperforate anus* is the absence of an anal opening; a *rectourethral fistula* is an opening or passage between the rectum and urethra; *hypospadias* exists when the urethral opening is at a location other than the tip of the penis (usually beneath the shaft); and *bilateral hip dysplasia* is present when both hip joints are shallow and underdeveloped. By the time he was seven, Brandon had undergone over a dozen surgeries; some with successful results, others not.

When I had earlier scanned my reference source, one title had caught my attention: "Congenital Malformations after In-Vitro Fertilisation." I was aware that fertility drugs were used to produce the eggs. Maybe there would be something of interest, perhaps a description of one or more of the anomalies suffered by Brandon.

I had no idea – not a clue – that a huge door was about to open.

Neural Tube Defects

The paper had been written by Dr. Paul Lancaster, of the National Perinatal Statistics Unit in Sydney, Australia. The publication was the December 12, 1987 edition of *The Lancet* (pp.1392-93). [Exhibit 16] Lancaster and his staff had conducted a cohort analysis of 1,697 deliveries resulting from in-vitro fertilization (IVF) and gamete intrafallopian transfer (GIFT) pregnancies in Australia and New Zealand for the period between 1979 and 1986. Thirty-seven of the fetuses and infants had major congenital malformations. National data were used to calculate the expected frequency of major malformations diagnosed at birth or in the first week. Two types of anomalies were excessively high.

"6 infants had *spina bifida* compared to an expected number of 1.2 (p = 0.0015; one-sided Poisson). 2 of these infants had other malformations. 1 had *trisomy 18* and an absent left auditory canal, renal dysplasia, absent urethra, and imperforate anus. *There is a well-recognised association between trisomy 18 and spina bifida* but even if this infant is excluded, the probability of 5 cases is 0.0075. The other infant with multiple malformations had sirenomelia, renal agenesis, colonic atresia, and ventricular septal defect. 1 of the infants with isolated spina bifida *had a twin with trisomy 18*. The spinal lesion was in the lumbosacral region in all 6 infants." [Emphasis added.]

Three of the 6 infants with spina bifida were from *multiple births*. Two of the 6 pregnancies resulted in infants with trisomy 18; one of the infants with spina bifida and the twin of another similarly-afflicted baby. Not only was this almost a six-fold increase in the expected rate of spina bifida, at a minimum it was suggestive of a possible tie between the use of fertility drugs, trisomy 18 and a neural tube defect. Two of the described abnormalities (renal agenesis and imperforate anus) were also included in Brandon's array of anomalies.

Lancaster also found that there were four infants born with transposition of the great vessels (TGV), when statistically only 0.6 would have been expected (P = 0.0034). TGV is a congenital heart defect where the ventricle that supplies the pulmonary artery is reversed (left rather than right). Two of the 4 were from multiple births. Thus, fifty percent of both types of congenital abnormalities were associated with multiple conceptions.

I read the article again, and then a third time. I was overcome with excitement. One would have thought I had just won the lottery as I enthusiastically looked up, wanting to grab the nearest person to share my discovery. There it was – validation. It had taken 12 years, but I was actually holding a study that had shown a statistically significant increase in the incidence of a neural tube defect when exposed to fertility drugs. I could almost recall my words verbatim.

"Ladies and gentlemen, there is very strong evidence with this clinical summary on neural tube defects, and with the mechanism of action that I have indicated, that there is a probability, and certainly a reasonable medical probability, that clomiphene citrate and other ovulatory-stimulating drugs are actually causing neural tube defects by altering chromosomes."

This was a statement that I made to the Obstetrics and Gynecology Advisory Committee to the FDA on *July 18, 1975*. I also pointed to a study[233] that found a direct correlation between dizygotic (multiple-egg) twinning and neural tube defects, and suggested that there was a common mechanism causing both. This was an important observation since no one disputed that fertility drugs could cause fraternal twins. All present had also been reminded that nine of the first 34 Drug Experience Reports on Clomid were neural tube defects, eight of them anencephaly. A red flag was being waved that needed to be addressed. But while the FDA and Merrell sat on their collective hands, someone in Australia had taken a look at the problem.

So had others, as I would soon learn.

Within minutes, I was back at the reference source digging for more papers. It didn't take long. I quickly discovered a second study on neural tube defects, this one out of the Netherlands.[234] The article had been published on June 17, 1989, and was authored by Martina Cornel and others. It was a case-control study in which the researchers looked at the records from a local registry of 94 infants born with neural tube defects (49 with anencephaly and 45 with spina bifida) and found that 3 (3.2%) had been exposed to ovulation inducing drugs, including clomiphene citrate. *One of the three was from a quadruplet pregnancy.* Control data from 970 live births without NTDs were used, and it was found that only eight (0.8%) had been exposed to fertility drugs. There were four times as many exposures in the case group than there were in the controls. The resulting odds ratio (OR) was 3.96. An "odds ratio" is the ratio of the odds of an event occurring in one group to the odds of it occurring in another group. These data were statistically significant (95% CI, 1.03-15.2), since the bottom of the confidence interval was above 1.0. There was a 95% likelihood that the real OR was as low as 1.03 or as high as 15.2.

They also reported on another Dutch case of anencephaly, but outside of their region of study. *It was one of a set of fraternal twins.*

After noting the above Lancaster study, Cornel et al. commented, "These data suggest once more an enlarged risk of NTD defects in pregnancies established with the aid of ovulation stimulating drugs." Addressing the issue of causation, they concluded, "James[235] suggests that subfertility may be a risk factor for NTD, but a teratogenic influence from ovulation-stimulating drugs cannot be excluded."

One more time I went to the well. This time I came back with a handful. I was like a child in a candy store.

On July 15, 1989, yet another case-control study involving NTDs was reported, this one by a Dr. Andrew Czeizel out of Budapest, Hungary.[236] Czeizel reported from the Hungarian case-control surveillance system of congenital anomalies. He found that out of 825 children born with NTDs, three (.36%) had been exposed to clomiphene citrate, whereas only 12 out of 18,904 matched controls (.06%) had been similarly exposed. Again, the study was statistically significant (OR 5.75; CI, 1.62-20.4). His concern was also reflected in the paper. "A relation between ovulation induction and some congenital anomalies cannot be excluded. My purpose in writing is to stimulate collaborative epidemiological studies for the assessment of risk of ovulation-stimulating drugs."

Then on December 30, 1989, Cornel et al. reported a fourth NTD study,[237] this time looking at a cohort of several combined IVF centers from the United States, the Netherlands and Australia. Against a baseline incidence rate of 1.3-1.4 per thousand, they found a total of 12 NTD cases out of 4,385 children following in-vitro fertilization. And one more time it was significant (2.7 per 1,000; 95% CI, 1.6-4.8 per 1,000). The bottom of the confidence interval was above the baseline NTD rate. Included in their data were current numbers from Lancaster's National Perinatal Statistics Unit for Australia for 1988. After pointing to the fact that one of the steps of IVF was ovulation stimulation, the authors summarized their view. "We conclude that, apart from the case reports, there are three lines of inconclusive evidence on an association between disturbed fertility and NTD, all three suggestive of a relative risk of at least 2."

A fifth study on NTDs was reported by Elisabeth Robert and others from Lyon, France in 1991.[238] This case-control study drew its statistics from a local registry of congenital malformations. Infants with non-NTD malformations were used as controls. Out of 180 babies born with NTDs, 11 (6.11%) had been exposed to ovulatory-stimulating drugs. But from 4,247 controls, only 114 (2.68%) had a history of ovulation induction. For the fifth time, the difference was again statistically significant (OR 2.36; 95% CI, 1.25-4.46; P = 0.013). The comment by the authors had a familiar ring to it. "These data, combined with those previously published, indicate an association between stimulation of ovulation and increased rate of NTD. This association, if real, *could be the result* either *of the drugs used in the treatment of fertility problems* or of the subfertility itself, as previously suggested." [Emphasis added.]

A couple years after his intitial paper on the subject, Lancaster updated his observations from the same pool of IVF and GIFT pregnancies in Australia and New Zealand.[239] This time he drew from more than 3,000 births. And again he found a significant increase in the expected incidence of spina bifida, along with tracheo-esophageal fistula (abnormal pathway between the trachea/windpipe and esophagus), urinary tract malformations and vertebral abnormalities (P<0.01). Even though he had compiled his data from almost twice the original number of pregnancies, there was still an increased risk of developing spina bifida. Still later, when the same pool of infants had grown to 5,011, he reported on higher rates for spina bifida, anencephalus, TGV, esophageal atresia (closure or absence of the esophagus), imperforate anus, exomphalos (extrusion of the intestine), and prune belly syndrome (partial or complete absence of abdominal muscles).[240]

Although not reaching a level of statistical significance, four other NTD studies – each demonstrating an increased risk – were reported about the same period of time. One was by Cuckle and Wald;[241] another by Aubrey Milunsky and others;[242] a third by Karabacak, et al.;[243] and a fourth by Goujard, et al.[244]

Cuckle and Wald secured their case-control data from a local hospital in Oxford, England. They cited 107 NTD cases (48 with anencephaly and 59 with spina bifida) from which 4 (3.7%) had been exposed to clomiphene citrate. This compared with 214 controls from which 5 (2.3%) had been exposed to the same drug. The odds ratio was

1.62; there was approximately a 60% increased risk with exposure to clomiphene. However, because the study lacked a sufficient number of cases, the results were not statistically significant (95% CI, 0.43-6.0). As part of their paper, the two authors attempted to do a combined statistical analysis (e.g., meta-analysis), including their case-control study with those of Cornel and Czeizel. They concluded that the three studies combined, although demonstrating an increased odds ratio, did not reach statistical significance.

But a later paper by Vollset[245] pointed out that their calculations had been in error, and that combining the three studies did indeed establish a highly significant increased risk (OR 2.94; 95% CI, 1.32-6.5; P = 0.004). The odds of these numbers occurring by chance were only 4 in 1,000. Vollset's comment: "I conclude that the three studies, when combined, do indicate that *the association between ovulation induction and NTD is real.*" [Emphasis added.] A reply by Cuckle and Wald to the correction is included in the same paper. "We agree with Vollset that the pooled results are formally statistically significant. This correction inclines us toward the view that *there is a real association between the use of clomiphene to induce ovulation and neural tube defects (NTD)* but we feel it would be prudent to reserve judgment." [Emphasis added.]

The paper by Milunsky et al. likewise established an increased risk. The study was conducted out of the Boston School of Medicine. The cohort of 438 women using clomiphene had two offspring (0.5%) with NTDs. Of the 22,317 women who did not report use of clomiphene, 47 of them (0.2%) had infants with NTDs. The odds ratio was 2.2, but not statistically significant (95% CI, 0.6-8.6). Yet although the numbers had not reached statistical significance, again the risk had more than doubled with use of clomiphene citrate.

The study by Karabacak and colleagues appeared on December 9, 1989. Using data from their clinic in Turkey, they reported on a case of spina bifida out of 128 ovulation-induced pregnancies. The researchers compared their rate with an NTD incidence for western Turkey, between 1980 and 1989, of 0.226% (174 cases of NTD out of 76,831 deliveries). "Thus in our clinic the prevalence of NTD was 0.78% in the induced pregnancy group, which represents a 3-4-fold increase over the rate at the Maternity Hospital (0.226%)." They also mentioned that two of the 174 NTD cases had been exposed to ovulation induction drugs, from which an *anencephalic girl had been part of a triplet delivery*. A female sibling had been born with hydrocephalus and a male with a hand deformity.

Reported in abstract (summary) form, the Goujard case-control study included data from a registry of congenital malformations in Paris for the period from 1986 to 1988. Although involving a 65% increase in NTD exposures, the numbers did not reach statistical significance (OR 1.65; 95% CI, 0.59-4.60).

In chronological succession I devoured each article, impatiently anticipating the next scientific nugget well before I finished the one I was reading. By the time I concluded, I had an unfamiliar pride for the medical profession. Maybe Merrell and the FDA had ignored their responsibilities, but medical science was now after an answer. In the span of less than five years there had been nine different studies (plus Lancaster's updates) that had demonstrated an increased odds ratio for neural tube defects following the maternal use of fertility drugs, including Clomid – five of them statistically significant. It had also been an international effort. Even though the studies had come from different parts of the globe, they were all coming up with similar results. Whether from Australia, Hungary, Netherlands, Turkey, France, England or the United States, or whether of a cohort or case-control design, the exposure to fertility drugs was resulting in an increased risk of delivering a child with a neural tube defect.

I also discovered a publication that seemed to put an official sanction on this series of papers. The Royal Commission on New Reproductive Technologies, a department of the Canadian Government, published in 1993 a complete analysis of all aspects of reproductive medicine, including Adverse Health Effects of Drugs Used for Ovulation Induction (Chapter 6). Like Vollset, they likewise did a meta-analysis of NTDs, and again came up *statistically significant* (odds ratio 1.86; 95% CI 1.2-2.9). Their calculations included the case-control studies of Cornel, Robert, Czeizel, Cuckle and Wald, and Mills, et al. (see below).

But were the drugs responsible or the underlying infertility condition, as had been suggested by some? Was it a combination of both? Did it really matter? If a fertility drug produces a defective egg because of the patient's underlying pathology, doesn't she still have a right to know about the increased risk? My bet was still on the drug.

At the time, I could only locate two NTD studies that failed to report an appreciable odds ratio above 1.0. One was by Mili and associates.[246] Mili, et al., were from the Centers for Disease Control (CDC). Their case-control study was first reported in April 1991. It was calculated from clomiphene-exposed cases and controls in Atlanta between 1968 and 1980. They reported no elevated risk for NTDs (OR 1.0; 95% CI, 0.23-4.50) and a slight increased risk for anencephaly of twenty percent (OR 1.20; 95% CI, 0.16-9.10). The numbers, however, were too small to place much meaning on the statistics. For example, the actual odds ratio for total NTDs could be as high as 4.50.

I would also question their number of exposed cases. Their data (through 1980) included only two Clomid exposures (1 with anencephaly and 1 with spina bifida) out of 345 purported infants with NTDs. When Dr. Godfrey Oakley (also from the CDC in Atlanta) presented his updated list for Merrell's use on March 11, 1976, it included 11 Clomid patients with congenital anomalies, *three of which were neural tube defects.* [See Chapter 7.] One had spina bifida, one had anencephaly with associated meningocele and one had meningomyelocele with hydrocephalus.[247] It appears that only the cases involving spina bifida and anencephaly were included in Mili's study. However, meningomyelocele is also a neural tube defect, which involves nonclosure of the spinal column with an exposed abnormal spinal cord. I would question not including all categories of NTDs, since they represent various forms and degrees of the same type of anomaly suffered by the embryo in early gestation. My suspicion is that Mili and her colleagues may have instead included the case of meningomyelocele in a separate category for "Central Nervous System Defects." If the meningomyeolocele case – and perhaps other similar NTDs – were incorporated into the CNS group, it may have obscured a possible significant increase in total NTDs. It is noted from available data that they found 9 Clomid exposures out of 694 (1.30%) cases with central nervous system defects compared to 20 exposures out of 2,979 (0.67%) controls – and the numbers were *statistically significant* (OR 1.93; 95% CI, 1.11-5.55).

The other paper was authored by James Mills, et al.[248] The study design included 571 cases with neural tube defects and two sets of controls; 546 infants with congenital anomalies other than NTDs and 573 offspring that were "apparently normal." Fertility

285

drug use was broken down between those who used ovulation induction to conceive the subject pregnancy and those who had used such drugs at any time in the past.

They reported that eight out of 571 cases (1.40%), six out of 546 abnormal controls (1.10%), and ten out of 573 normal controls (1.75%), had induced ovulation for the subject pregnancy. "The rate of maternal fertility drug use around the time of conception was not significantly higher for neural tube defects than for other abnormalities (odds ratio 1.3; 95% confidence interval 0.4, 4.5) or no abnormalities (odds ratio 0.8; 95% CI 0.3, 2.3). Fertility drug use at any time was not significantly more frequent for neural tube defects than for other abnormalities (odds ratio 1.3; 95% CI 0.7, 2.7) or no abnormalities (odds ratio 1.05; 95% CI 0.6, 2.0)." When one combined the two control groups, the odds ratio was essentially at one (e.g., no increase).

I had a major problem with the Mills study. My complaint relates to the use of an abnormal control group. This introduces a confounding factor because the controls may include abnormal infants *whose abnormalities were caused by fertility drugs*. This would occur if the drugs could cause other types of congenital anomalies, along with NTDs. For example, if fertility drugs could also cause limb reduction defects, and they were included as one of the subgroups in the controls, their inclusion could add exposures to the control group. The result could improperly skew the controls toward a one odds ratio (e.g., the null hypothesis), thus masking a real increased risk. This criticism is a legitimate concern when using abnormal controls to assess the possible risk of NTDs resulting from fertility drugs (see below).

Further, although the other half of Mills' study purportedly used *normal* controls, I learned that: (1) many infants were selected by prenatal ultrasound prior to delivery, rather than by a thorough physical examination at the time of birth; and (2) the "normal" controls included live-born infants without *major* malformations, defined as "anatomical defects that caused death, required surgical correction, or caused a serious functional handicap."[249]

Under this study design, a child with a minor malformation would be included within the "normal" control group, such as a child born without a finger or with a clubfoot, which did not cause death or require surgical correction, and was not a *serious* functional handicap. Further, prenatal ultrasound has been shown to be a highly ineffective means for detecting many types of congenital abnormalities. For example, in one study it was found that only 74.2% of spina bifida cases, 9.3% and 7.8% of ventricular septal defects and atrial septal defects (heart defects), respectively, could be detected by prenatal ultrasound.[250] There was thus a significant chance that infants with congenital heart defects could also have been included with the normal controls. This is perhaps why Mills and his colleagues described this group as "apparently" normal.

Abnormal Controls

Although I did not locate the following study until late in 1994, it would seem appropriate to include it at this point because of its relevancy to the topic of abnormal controls. It is, in fact, the classic example of why case-control studies involving such controls are unreliable – and can even be misleading, and sometimes outright deceptive. It was only through a fortuitous set of circumstances that I was to learn of a critically important part of the study, *undisclosed in the published paper*.

On August 13, 1994, a study by Martha Werler, et al., was published in *The Lancet*.[251] It was titled, "Ovulation Induction and Risk of Neural Tube Defects." As one might guess, I was hoping for yet another scientific article to strengthen the possible relationship between the use of fertility drugs and neural tube defects. But it proved to be of no help. They found that out of 1,032 cases with spina bifida, anencephaly or encephalocele, 31 (3.0%) had been exposed to fertility drugs at any time within 6 months of conception, whereas 113 out of 4,062 abnormal controls (2.8%) were similarly exposed (OR 1.1; 95% CI, 0.8-1.7). When they looked specifically at clomiphene, the statistics were even worse: 22 exposures in 1,032 cases (2.1%) and 96 exposures in 4,062 abnormal controls (2.4%), resulting in an odds ratio of 0.8 (CI, 0.5-1.3).

I tossed it in the pile with Mills – until a later discussion with my epidemiologist.

While preparing for my eighth and final Clomid case, I had retained a highly-qualified epidemiologist[252] to analyze all of the papers I had been collecting through my medical research. During one of our many telephone conversations, we had a chat about the recently-received Werler publication. I explained that it was unclear from the article what the exposure rates were among women who received treatment within one cycle prior to conception and/or during pregnancy; that in my view ovulatory stimulation two or more cycles prior to the inception of the subject pregnancies were meaningless exposures.

Unknown to me, my expert consultant did what most scientists do when confronted with a question about a published study: he called the lead author of the paper. During their talk, he solicited the data that the researchers had broken down on Clomid exposures for each of the cycles prior to conception. The information came to him in the form of a fax. [Exhibit 17] And as promised, it set out clomiphene exposures during cycles 4 through 6 prior to the last menstrual period (LMP); cycles 3, 2 and 1 pre-LMP; and for the first two months post-LMP. Werler even gave my epidemiologist the relative risks and 95% confidence intervals for each exposure group – and one additional unsolicited piece of information.

She also dropped a "smoking gun" in our two laps.

Werler explained in the fax how she and her colleagues arrived at the total number and types of abnormal controls. "As far as control subgroups go – we did our analyses of any use of a fertility drug among defect subgroups in the large pool of all subjects (i.e. *before a sample was selected* to reduce the control group to a more manageable size). *We were looking for either a doubling or halfing in rate of drug use compared to controls overall* – the larger pool gave us more power to do this. Those are the numbers and rates referred to in the article." [Emphasis added.]

In other words, rather than randomly selecting the non-NTD control subgroups (i.e. limb reduction defects, chromosomal defects, hypospadias, etc.) or matching *any* abnormal non-NTD control based only upon the selection factors (i.e. date, maternal age, location, etc.), they *pre-selected the controls with knowledge of their exposure rates.* They thus knew, while designing the study, which group of controls would have the highest exposure rates. With such knowledge, they were provided with the opportunity to stack the controls with those subgroups and dilute or offset the rate recorded for the NTD cases.

Did they do so? Read the balance of the fax and judge for yourself.

"The rates for chromosomal anoms (n = 1078) was 1.6%, for LRDs (n = 535) was 3.4%, and hyposp. (n = 740) was 5.1%. *Since the rate was high for hypospadias* I looked at clomiphene use among the sample control series – 11 exposed of 255 compared to 85 exposed of 3741 other controls. *Very interesting!"* [Emphasis added.]

Of course it was interesting. As reflected in the calculations added to the fax by my epidemiologist, when compared with the other abnormal controls, the frequency of clomiphene exposures for hypospadias was increased at a statistically significant level (OR 1.94; 95% CI, 1.02-3.68). Since they "were looking for...doubling...in rate of drug use compared to controls overall," and cite the 5.1% exposure rate in the paper (Exhibit 18), Werler was aware of this fact when they selected hypospadias as a control subgroup; she knowingly included a control subgroup (hypospadias) for which she had data supporting a causal association with clomiphene exposure. Her clomiphene sample of the hypospadias subgroup had 11 exposures out of 255 cases (4.3%) compared to 85 exposures out of 3,741 other controls (2.3%), yet she chose to dump them in with the rest of the controls.

Was she of the view that it would be improper to include an abnormal subgroup causally associated with the use of fertility drugs? It would seem so. After all, she excluded "defects of the central nervous system, eye, or bowel" because Mili et al. had found significant increases in the odds ratios for microcephaly (8.4), hydrocephaly (3.4), anophthalmia/microphthalmia (6.4) and atresia or stenosis of the colon, rectum and anus (4.6).[253] But she apparently overlooked the study by Macnab and Zouves,[254] published the same year as Mili's presentation. Although their numbers were small (two cases of hypospadias out of 53 pregnancies following IVF and GIFT procedures), they were statistically significant (P<0.01, with an expected incidence of 8.2 cases per 1,000). The induction of ovulation, of course, was through the use of fertility drugs. Lancaster also found a significant increase (P<0.01) in urinary tract anomalies in his 1990 paper on IVF and GIFT pregnancies. Perhaps she did not catch his study either.

But, then again, Werler already had her own data on hypospadias and clomiphene exposures. So why didn't she exclude hypospadias from the abnormal controls? Why didn't she mention her data on hypospadias in her article? After all, she found it "very interesting." Her justification for looking at the exposure rates of the control subgroups was "to assess consistency of exposure across diagnoses among (the potential controls)." As stated in her fax, they were "looking for either a doubling or halfing in rate of drug use compared to controls overall." Well, with hypospadias they found a doubling: 5.1% (38/740) exposure rate for all fertility drugs compared to a 2.3% (75/3,322) rate for the balance of the controls after excluding hypospadias. So much for consistency.

Oh, and one of the co-sponsors of the study was *Marion Merrell Dow*.

My opinion about the use of abnormal controls is not unique. In an article by Koury, James and Erickson[255] – all of the CDC – they demonstrated, by way of a study, the inherent problem in using abnormal or "affected" controls in case-control studies of birth defects. While studying the association between diabetes mellitus and birth defects, they found that by using affected controls they could change the odds ratio toward one with certain anomalies. "On the other hand, the use of affected controls to adjust for recall bias can introduce problems of its own, as discussed by Swan, et al. ('92) and by Drews, et al. ('93). In these instances, if an exposure is associated with more than one defect category, inclusion of other defect groups in the control group may make the controls unrepresentative of the exposure frequency in the population, and thus dilute the magnitude of the odds ratio toward the null (Swan, et al., '92)."

As I expressed earlier, there would not appear to be a *need* for the use of abnormal controls when studying fertility drugs. I cannot imagine a circumstance where a woman would not recall that her pregnancy – whether resulting in a normal or anomalous infant – had been produced by the induction of ovulation. Such drugs are only available by prescription, and in some instances are administered at a physician's office or clinic. Proof of exposure and timing of use can thus be documented by medical records. Although a case-control study using abnormal controls should not be discounted when demonstrating a *positive* association,[256] I would not give much value to such a study when the odds ratio was at or near zero.

The Infertility Factor

Are infertility patients predisposed to delivering infants with neural tube defects? For two decades I had been reading about concern that infertility patients were at a higher risk for NTDs; always with little or no proof. Did these claims have merit?

I would first want to know why the women had been unable to deliver a baby. Why were they considered infertile? If they were a habitual aborters, and the spontaneous abortions had been occurring in the first trimester, it may be that they were producing defective ova and they might well be at an increased risk for delivering a baby with an NTD.

But women who are infertile because they cannot ovulate (e.g., anovulatory), or suffer from some other ovulatory dysfunction, or have difficulty maintaining pregnancies beyond the second trimester, do not necessarily have defective eggs. As was demonstrated in Chapters 11 and 12, these types of "infertility" patients do not have a higher incidence of spontaneous abortions than those in the general population. The Boues also presented convincing proof back in 1973 that infertility patients using ovulation inducers two or more cycles prior to conception had the same incidence of abnormal chromosomes as those in the general population. Certainly one could view this data as at least presumptive evidence that, *absent the use of fertility drugs,* these women were producing the same number of normal eggs as women with normal fertility.

The ultimate test, however, is in comparing the NTD rate following unassisted pregnancies in such patients with the incidence of NTDs in conceptions among women without fertility problems. But by 1993 I could only locate three studies that had actually looked at this question.

One such study was the 1990 paper by Mills, et al.[257] Women who had been unable to conceive for a year or more were categorized as "infertile." Out of the 571 pregnancies resulting in NTDs, 103 (18.1%) fell into the infertility category; as did 84 of 546 infants with non-NTD abnormalities (15.4%); and 96 out of 573 normal controls (16.8%). They concluded that infertility did not play a role in the cause of NTDs. "Our data do not support the theory that infertile women or women whose pregnancies may have involved old gametes (unfertilized eggs) are at increased risk of conception of a child with a neural tube defect; there was no excess risk in women who had experienced difficulty in conception, rhythm method failure, or unplanned pregnancy." They also found that a prior history of spontaneous abortions was not causally associated with the occurrence of NTDs.

Presumably these numbers did not include infertility patients who had used ovulatory-stimulating drugs, in that the researchers were attempting to determine whether induction of ovulation *or* female infertility were risk factors in the cause of NTDs. I do, however, have a problem with Mills' use of abnormal controls, as mentioned earlier. If infertility could cause NTDS, along with "other abnormalities," their data would not be of much use. But although I viewed the results of their match with "normal controls" with caution (for reasons stated above), they are certainly supportive of the view that infertility does not predispose pregnancies to neural tube defects.

The study by Ghazi and colleagues in 1991[258] made a stronger case against a possible association between infertility and NTDs. The subjects of their study were 29,821 women, with a prior history of infertility of one or more years, who had delivered babies in Sweden between 1983 and 1986. Out of this population, only 10 pregnancies of 28 weeks or older resulted in neural tube defects (3 anencephaly, 5 spina bifida and 2 encephalocele), against an expected number of 16.8. They observed that "neural tube defects seem to be less common than expected among infants of women with infertility problems."

While assessing the risk of neural tube defects from the use of fertility drugs, Cuckle and Wald also took a look at the question of infertility. Did it contribute to the occurrence of NTDs? Was the underlying physiology that led to infertility a risk factor for these defects? They concluded that it wasn't. "A history of infertility was recorded in 13 patients (12%; 2 anencephaly, 11 spina bifida) and 24 controls (11%)." A similar ratio of mothers of NTD infants (13/107) had a history of infertility as women with normal infants (24/214). Difficulty conceiving did not present a risk for delivering an infant with an NTD.

A fourth study[259] added support for this premise. Although it did not address the specific concern about NTDs, the author conducted a large case-control study through the CDC in Atlanta involving 4,029 infants with all types of congenital anomalies and 3,029 control infants without defects. When he looked at the data for women who had sought "fertility advice," he found that there was not a significant difference between the cases and the controls (OR 1.04; 95% CI 0.9-1.2). Women who had sought advice for infertility problems were no more at risk for having an infant with a birth defect than women who had never consulted a physician for such problems.

I could not find one study suggesting that ovulatory dysfunction was a risk factor for neural tube defects.

Animal Studies

The clincher for me was the last paper I found on this very special day. It was an animal study published by Marie Dziadek out of Australia.[260] It was significant because it established that it was feasible to administer clomiphene citrate to an animal *prior to ovulation* and produce a neural tube defect. In fact, the study was specifically designed to address the question of whether it is "biologically plausible that a drug taken before conception could disrupt neural tube closure 24-27 days after conception (in humans)." In unequivocal fashion, Dziadek demonstrated not only that the drug was capable of producing neural tube defects when administered pre-conception, but also cause a reduction in the number of embryo implantations and retardation in fetal growth. Dziadek summarized the results of her study as follows.

"Preovulatory administration of clomiphene citrate caused decreased implantation rates and growth retardation of surviving fetuses, the degree of the effect being dependent on the dose and the time of drug injection relative to ovulation. The implantation rate was lowest, and the of fetal growth retardation highest, when clomiphene citrate was administered immediately before ovulation. An increased incidence of exencephaly was found in the fetuses of females injected with clomiphene citrate prior to ovulation. Transfer of blastocysts from treated mice to untreated fosters showed the effect of clomiphene citrate on implantation and fetal growth to be predominantly mediated through the female reproductive tract, rather than a direct effect on the embryo itself."

Exencephaly involves nonclosure of the cranial vault with the brain essentially intact. The author concluded from her study that clomiphene exerted its adverse effect *indirectly* by disturbing the hormonal support normally provided to the endometrium of the uterus. Although acknowledging that her findings could not be directly extrapolated to humans, she cautioned her readers. "Since there is concern about a possible association between ovulatory induction or subfertility and neural tube defects in humans, the outcome of this present study needs to be seriously considered as an explanation for this association, and further work in this area is indicated."

More on this important study later.

Clomiphene has also demonstrated a capability of producing neural tube defects in animals via a *direct* teratogenic action. Diener and Hsu had conducted a teratology study using rats and were able to produce exencephaly in the offspring;[261] Lopez-Escobar and Fridhandler were able to induce absence of the cranial vault in a rabbit fetus;[262] and Morris reported on rabbit fetuses with cranioschisis (incomplete formation of skull cap) following exposure to Clomid during organogenesis.[263]

Whether the product of chromosomal anomalies, such as trisomy 18, a prolonged half-life resulting in a direct teratogenic effect inhibiting closure of the neural tube, or an indirect action via hormonal influences on the uterus and other reproductive organs, or all of the above, strong epidemiological evidence existed implicating fertility drugs as a cause of neural tube defects.

I was now better-armed than I had ever been in any of my prior Clomid battles. At the end of that day I marched out of the UCLA Biomed Library, a briefcase brimming with copies of published papers, and a sense of accomplishment that only comes with success following persistent hard work at a seemingly-impossible task. It had taken years to get where I was at that day, but I had never felt so right in purpose and so rewarded for my resolve.

My weapons also included epidemiology studies establishing the existence of a significantly increased risk for a number of the congenital anomalies suffered by Brandon Gandy. These included *imperforate anus*: Lancaster (October 1991), Mili (October 1991); *hypospadias*: Czeizel (July 1989), Macnab (November 1991); *urinary tract malformations*: Lancaster (1990); *undescended testicles*: Czeizel (July 1989); and *multiple congenital anomalies*: Czeizel (July 1989), Lancaster (1990).

It was time to go to war.

* * * * *

CHAPTER 15

Back in the Saddle Again

The Gandy trial commenced on May 2, 1994.

My trial strategy was straight forward. With overwhelming evidence of culpability, the verdict would hinge on causation; whether I could convince a jury that Clomid was probably a "substantial factor" in causing Brandon Gandy's birth anomalies. This I would attempt to establish with a three-step approach.

My first goal would be to convince the jury that Clomid was a *human teratogen*, which I termed "general causation." My strongest evidence on this challenge would be the series of epidemiology studies on neural tube defects. But I would also need to counter the published suggestion by several experts that the connection between fertility drugs and neural tube defects was the underlying pathology causing the infertility, not the drugs ingested to address the problem. This I would do by demonstrating that subfertility patients have the same spontaneous abortion rate as women of normal fertility, and that two studies that had specifically looked at the question had concluded that women having difficulty conceiving had no greater incidence of NTDs than women in the general population. Given this data, if the statistical analyses established a *real* increased risk, as had been stated by Vollset and others, then the cause of the NTDs had to be the fertility drugs, not the underlying subfertility. Next, I would supplement the epidemiology studies with other supporting evidence, such as the timing/half-life factor, animal teratology studies – including Dziadek's paper – animal in-vitro and in-vivo studies, mutagenicity studies, and the similarity of the chemical structure of Clomid with another known teratogen.

The second part of my strategy would be to demonstrate that the *spectrum of anomalies* caused by Clomid and other fertility drugs *extended beyond NTDs* and included many of those suffered by Brandon Gandy. By 1994, several epidemiology studies had found a significantly increased incidence of other congenital abnormalities, including limb reduction defects, congenital heart defects, hypospadias and other urinary tract anomalies, undescended testicles, tracheo-esophageal fistula, esophageal atresia, atresia or stenosis of the colon, rectum and anus, including imperforate anus, exomphalos, prune belly syndrome, vertebral defects, anophthalmia/microphthalmia defects, and multiple congenital defects.

The third segment of my plan would be directed at *case-specific causation*, namely whether Clomid was specifically responsible for Brandon Gandy's multiple congenital anomalies. This would be accomplished by eliminating all other known causes of birth defects; by introducing evidence that Brandon's embryo had not been exposed to maternal illness, other drugs or chemicals, radiation, alcohol, smoking, trauma, extremes of temperature, or vitamin deficiency, and that his congenital malformations were not hereditary in origin. Linda Gandy had also delivered two other children *without the use of fertility drugs*, one before and one after Brandon, both of whom were born entirely normal.

Brandon's array of anomalies occurred between the 14th and 40th days post-conception as the result of some teratogenic insult. I would produce evidence that a drug capable of causing imperforate anus, hypospadias, undescended testicles, urinary tract abnormalities and multiple congenital defects, was circulating in Brandon's embryo during this window of time.

The trial, itself, was bifurcated – split into two parts. The first phase would be tried only on the issues of liability and causation. The jury would first determine whether the defendant had been negligent in conducting its studies or warning the users of its drug, as well as whether it had made fraudulent representations in its labeling or had acted in conscious disregard of the safety of the infants who were the product of their mothers' use of Clomid. Causation was also a necessary ingredient of liability. If the jury found that Brandon Gandy's congenital anomalies resulted from his mother's use of Clomid and the negligence of Merrell Dow, then we would proceed with phase two in order to determine the amount of compensatory damages. If they further found that Merrell had acted in conscious disregard of safety or made fraudulent statements, then any award of punitive damages would likewise be decided in the second part of the trial.

On the assigned date, the case was sent out to trial in front of the Honorable Macklin Wade. My old adversary, Robert Dickson, appeared as lead trial counsel on behalf of Merrell. He was to be assisted by Charles Messer. David Brown, an attorney in my office with whom I shared office space, was also present to assist me in the trial.

All pre-trial motions were decided and jury selection completed in the first two days. On May 4, 1994, both sides gave their opening statements, and by late morning that day I began calling my witnesses.

Linda Gandy, the physician who prescribed the Clomid and delivered Brandon, and my client's pediatrician, had all completed their testimony by the end of the day on Thursday, May 5th. Many of the essential facts were presented through these witnesses: Linda's inability to conceive and use of clomiphene; the assurances of safety about the drug; the pregnancies before and after Brandon; each of the pre-natal visits with the OB/GYN; the lack of exposure to other potential teratogens; a family history of both parents, including a lack of similar congenital malformations; all of the facts surrounding the delivery; and a description of all the anomalies.

On Friday, May 6, 1994, I called my pharmacologist/teratology expert, *Alan K. Done, M.D.* (pronounced as in "loan"). His testimony covered most of the issues involved in phase one, including violation of the standard of care in the industry regarding pre-market studies, lack of adequate warning on the labeling, Clomid half-life, and general and case-specific causation. By the time we concluded with his direct and cross-examination, Dr. Done had been on the witness stand two full days. My final witness was called Tuesday morning, May 9, 1994. *Dr. Leslie Ann Swygert*, a medical epidemiologist and former employee of the CDC, testified on general causation only. She concluded from the various epidemiology studies that Clomid was a human teratogen. After she was excused from the stand, the plaintiffs rested.

A motion for nonsuit was denied by the court.

Merrell's attorneys had scored some points during their cross-examination of my witnesses, yet nothing that was likely to derail my case. But now it was their their turn. Now was the opportunity to undermine the plaintiffs' contentions with their highly-credentialed physicians. This was to be accomplished through the testimony of five experts: a fertility specialist, a pharmacologist, a teratologist, an epidemiologist and the former Commissioner of the FDA, James Goddard, M.D. A judge had previously ruled that Merrell could only call one expert from each relevant specialty.

Merrell's first witness was *Daniel R. Mishell, Jr., M.D.*, a fertility specialist. Mishell had been one of the original clinical investigators in the Clomid pre-market clinical studies. He testified about his experience as a clinical investigator, about the use of various fertility drugs, including clomiphene citrate, and how they stimulated ovaries into expelling an egg. He discussed the side effects produced by fertility drugs, including ovarian hyperstimulation syndrome (OHSS). In his opinion, Linda Gandy had not experienced OHSS. He also expressed the view that the spontaneous abortion rate following Clomid was no different than in the general population. By the time we concluded my cross-examination, it was late morning on May 11, 1994. Mishell had done little to damage our case.

Ronald Okun, M.D. was the defendant's next witness. He was a pharmacologist and toxicologist and had been a professor on both subjects at UCLA. Okun's principal focus was on the subject of half-life. It was an issue that the defense team needed to defuse. They knew it would not go well to have the jury contemplating Clomid circulating throughout Brandon Gandy's body while his deformities were evolving. His conclusion was that Clomid had a half-life of only 4½ to 10 hours. Early on in my cross-examination I wanted to exploit his past association with Merrell and obvious bias for the company.

"At some point during the 1960s did you set up your own office?"

"No."

"Well, did you ever receive any financial assistance from the defendant in this case to set up your office?"

"No. I never did set up my office."

"Well, did they provide you with any kind of remuneration to assist you in the practice of medicine?"

"Not in the practice of medicine, no sir. The company then…I believe when I applied for monies from many companies and the National Institutes of Health to set up my laboratory at Cedars-Sinai and UCLA, many companies helped underwrite the cost of equipping the laboratory."

Because of Okun's equivocation, I decided to read from the deposition I had taken of him as recently as April 19, 1994, less than four weeks earlier. The following was read from the transcript verbatim.

"You have been a consultant for Richardson-Merrell for a period of time; is that correct?"

"Well, you will have to define what you mean by a consultant, but I had consulted for William S. Merrell, which is a division of Richardson-Merrell, in those days in the 1960s. I'm not sure that it extended into the '70s. I don't think it did, but I don't recall."

"With regard to the 1960s, what was the nature of your consulting which took place?"

"When I left my fellowship training, finished my fellowship training in clinical pharmacology in Baltimore and came back to Los Angeles, I applied to the National Institutes for funding of a laboratory, and some foundations and pharmaceutical companies, to attempt to get some funding to set up a laboratory. *Merrell was one of the people who responded positively and helped me financially set up a laboratory.* I agreed to do some consulting for them, and *they paid my expenses when I had expenses,* such as traveling to Cincinnati, in addition to moneys for the laboratory." [Emphasis added.]

I then reviewed with him, using company documents, a series of consulting fee payments, expense reimbursements and grant payments extending from the mid-1960s to the late-1970s, when he began receiving semi-annual retainers from Merrell. By the time I was ready to move on, his bias for Merrell – one of the hands that had fed him – had become quite conspicuous. The above testimony is highlighted to demonstrate by example how pharmaceutical companies can cultivate relationships and curry favors from physicians and scientists, not only for helpful testimony in litigation, but also by influencing papers that they might publish related to the company's products.

Okun had not based his opinion of Clomid's half-life on his own studies. Instead, he had relied upon his review of the package insert and 3 published papers which had reported on measuring the drug and/or its metabolites as they were being eliminated from the human body.

As to the package insert, on cross-examination he acknowledged that it reported a half-life of between 5 and 7 days. Further, markers of the drug had "appeared in the feces 6 weeks after administration." One of the 3 studies was in Hungarian, and although he read a translation, he admitted that it was difficult to interpret.

"And did they actually measure the half-life in that article?"

"No. As I mentioned earlier, they did not measure it, but there is a graph that enables you to *estimate* the half-life."

"Well, as a matter of fact, that's the only thing in the whole article that's of any guidance at all on the question of half-life; isn't that true?"

"I think so."

"And in terms of the graph, would you also agree it is very difficult to read it?"

"Well, the numbers are the same in Hungarian or English, but it is actually difficult to read, you're right, because they plot individual patients…and it is difficult to read, I guess is the best thing to say."

The second study was by Mikkelson, et al.,[264] in which they measured the isomers[265] of clomiphene citrate following a single dose of a 50 mg. tablet. Although Okun asserted that some level of clomiphene was already in the patients at the start of the study, I challenged this claim and had him acknowledge several statements made in the paper.

"And did they also find that when they looked at the drug accumulation, or the Z-isomer level after three months, that there was an accumulation of the drug?"

"Well, I believe that they said that. Again, I don't think that's correct, but I believe that they said that."

"In fact, at page 395 did they say, quote: 'Accumulation of the Z-isomer can be anticipated in patients who receive chronic CC (clomiphene citrate) therapy over a period of many months, and this may have important therapeutic implications.' That's what they said?"

"That's exactly what they said."

"And what would you interpret that to mean, 'important therapeutic implications'?"

"Pure conjecture."

"Oh, you believe that they're just conjecturing?"

"Yes."

"Would you agree that when one would take the drug, rather than one tablet a month, would take it five consecutive days and then wait a month and take it five consecutive days, and then a month, there would even be a greater accumulation of the Z-isomer? You would agree with that, wouldn't you?"

"No. I believe there's no accumulation of the Z-isomer."

"Well, that wouldn't be the interpretation of the authors of this article that you relied upon, though, is it?"

"Well, they didn't discuss what you just mentioned, but in all honesty I think they probably would agree with what you said, but their data does not show that."

"Let me refer you again to page 395. Is there the following statement, quote: 'For example, it is not uncommon for nonresponsive patients to receive escalating doses up to 250 milligrams a day of CC for five days a month, and then continue on therapy for many months. It can be anticipated that more extensive accumulation of the Z-isomer would occur in these patients.'? Is that what they said?"

"That's what they said."

"And you also disagree with that statement?"

"Yes, sir."

"Do they also state at the same page, 395, quote: 'After chronic treatment, accumulation of the Z-isomer probably also contributes to the ultimate pharmacologic effect exhibited over time.' End quote. Is that what they said?"

"That's exactly what they said."

Point made. The scientists that had conducted the study did not agree with Merrell's pharmacologist. Their view was that the most-active of the two Clomid isomers hung around for over a month and tended to accumulate with repeated treatments. It was time to move on.

For the third and final paper,[266] I took Okun through the whole procedure outlined in the paper, which entailed using the the uterus of a rat and extracting the estrogen receptor sites as part of the process of taking measurements of the level of Clomid. It struck me that the jury might question a study dependent upon ingredients of a rat organ for its accuracy. But in the end, Okun was still stuck with an uncomfortable conclusion by the lead author and his colleagues.

"Did Dr. Geier find *significant* plasma concentrations of the drug, still up until one month after treatment?"

"Well, I'm not sure that's correct. I understand that's what he said in the summary, but the reason I am not sure it is correct is that the technique that is used, which is the radioactive displacement from estrogen receptors, also picks up endogenous (internally produced) estrogen, as they describe in their paper; so that could easily be a measure of the endogenous estrogen."

"Well, Dr. Geier in his article did indicate there was *significant* amounts a month later; isn't that true?"

"He used the word 'significant.' I do not feel they are clinically significant because they are insufficient to have any clinical action. He must mean by 'significant,' the fact that he could detect it."

So there it was. Okun had based his opinion on the package insert and three published studies. But the package insert reported on markers of the drug found in the feces after 6 weeks; the authors of two of the studies had concluded that elements of the drug were present in *significant* amounts one month after ingestion; and the third paper was unintelligible. In my view, Merrell's witness had just crashed and burned.

We concluded with Dr. Okun at the end of the day.

On Thursday, May 12, 1994, Merrell called its third witness, *H. Eugene Hoyme, M.D.*, a teratologist. Hoyme expressed his opinion that Clomid was not a human teratogen and did not cause any of Brandon Gandy's congenital anomalies.

His opinions were based upon several factors. First, all of the best-designed prospective cohort studies had failed to demonstrate a statistically significant increase in a recognizable pattern of birth defects; second, the animal teratology studies all required a quantity several times the human dose, on a body weight basis, in order to produce the malformations; and third, it is not biologically plausible that a drug that produces high levels of estrogen would cause congenital abnormalities, because all pregnancies involve high levels of estrogen, including those without the use of fertility drugs. He described Brandon's array of anomalies as a "caudal regression sequence," since it was a problem of development in the lower half of the embryo very early in gestation. He suggested that there was a genetic component that contributed to the malformations because the mother, Linda, had been born with a hernia.

Since Hoyme had impressive qualifications in the field of teratology, it was important to establish that he was every bit as biased as Okun. This would be done through his desperate need for grants and other funds to continue his studies.

"Would you agree, Doctor, that over the years it's been quite difficult to get funding from the federal government?"

"Absolutely."

"It's been very frustrating, hasn't it?"

"Been frustrating, yes."

"They actually put very little money toward birth defects."

"Right."

"Not sexy enough."

"That's correct."

"Drug companies, however, do provide funds for grants for studies, don't they?"

"They do."

"Have you ever billed the defendant?"

"Oh, I have billed them within the last three weeks, yes."

"How much time have you put in on this case before testifying here today?"

"Probably 24 hours."

"And how much per hour are you billing them?"

"Two hundred and fifty dollars."

"Do you plan to use any of that money for research?"

"I plan to use some of it to fund travel to scientific meetings and things having to do with my professional work, yeah."

He acknowledged that he needed to see *conclusive* studies before he would consider a drug a human teratogen, and that he tended "to be very difficult to convince." Hoyme also had his limitations. He had never designed or participated in any type of an epidemiology study, had only contributed to one animal teratology study in 15 years, had never done an in-vitro study, and had never participated in a study involving Clomid or other ovulatory-stimulating drugs, or even sex hormones. He had also failed to review several important animal and in-vitro studies done with Clomid.

Hoyme agreed that although Brandon Gandy had a genetic predisposition to develop his congenital anomalies, they were *probably triggered by some environmental insult occurring between the 14th and 40th day post-conception.* By "environmental," he meant some embryonic exposure other than the normal and natural conditions produced by the mother.

"You do agree that (Brandon) had some genetic predisposition like all babies that have malformations, true?"

"Correct."

"And that there was some environmental factor that played a role, along with the genetic predisposition, in causing the birth defect?"

"Correct."

When asked whether he could find any evidence of exposure to other drugs, maternal illness, radiation, trauma, or other potential teratogens during this window of time, he agreed that he had found none.

The final attack was on the epidemiology studies he had relied upon in concluding that Clomid was not a human teratogen. These included the Clomid pre-market clinical investigations, a study by Ahlgren, et al.[267] and another by Kurachi, et al.[268] With the Clomid investigations, I ran through all of the deficiencies of the study, including lack of a control group, which he readily agreed bothered him to some degree. But the last point caught him by surprise.

"Doctor, would it bother you if these clinical investigators were relying upon getting birth announcements, and perhaps nothing more than birth certificates, to verify whether or not there were malformations? Would that bother you?"

"Well, I wasn't aware that that was the case."

"Well, just assume hypothetically it was. Would that bother you?"

"One would like the study designed where there was more scrupulous follow-up of the babies, yes."

The Ahlgren study also lacked a control group, which Hoyme had previously stated was an important component of a good epidemiology study. I also pointed to a statement from the paper that "(t)here was a probable increase in the number of infants born with major malformations." The authors also stated that this increase "might indicate a direct teratogenic effect" from the drug. Hoyme, however, passed this off for the reason that the numbers were not statistically significant, even though Ahlgren et al. observed that the "difference (did) not reach formal statistical significance but (was) *strongly suggestive*" of an association. [Emphasis added.] A total of 5.4% of his study group had major malformations compared to an expected rate of of 3.2%

I saved my cross on the Kurachi study for last, because I had a big surprise about its reliability. First I had Hoyme acknowledge that Clomid could cause multiple births and that the frequency could be as high as ten times what the rate is in the general population. I then ran him through the statistics cited in the paper, which reported on the incidence of malformations out of 1,034 Clomid pregnancies and 29,900 pregnancies that conceived without the use of fertility drugs. After deducting fetal wastage (spontaneous abortions, hydatidiform moles and ectopic pregnancies), the clomiphene group had 935 newborns from 881 delivered pregnancies and the controls 30,033 newborns from 25,744 delivered pregnancies. All of the data had been collected in Japan. By the time I had walked him through all of the steps, the final numbers indicated that 6.1% of the Clomid pregnancies resulted in multiple births and 16.7% of the control group had multiple births.[269] *Patients that had not used fertility drugs had almost three times the frequency of multiple births as the Clomid population.* Something was grossly wrong with these statistics and called into question how the authors had compiled their data.

On redirect, all Dickson could do was ask Hoyme whether the Kurachi study had been peer-reviewed, which of course it had. Other than that, he was stuck. The numbers were exactly as I had charted them. He could not even suggest that there was a higher incidence of multiple births among Japanese – for which he had no supporting data – because he would then be placed in the position of arguing that in Japan, unlike every other nation in the world, Clomid could actually cause a *reduction* in the rate of multiple births.

Merrell's fourth – and ultimately final – witness was *James Goddard, M.D.*, the former commissioner of the FDA. Goddard spent the remainder of the day explaining the procedures by which drugs are submitted to and approved by the FDA, the actual steps taken by Merrell to get Clomid on the market, including submission of its animal and clinical studies, not to mention personal conversations he had with Merrell personnel prior to the drug's approval.

As expected, he had concluded at the time that the drug had been properly tested and was safe and effective, and that the package insert and other labeling met all industry standards. He also testified about Dr. James Wilson's report and conclusion that Clomid was not teratogenic in humans. After identifying Dr. Edwin Ortiz' letter of June 4, 1969 (Exhibit 8), he assured the jury that it was nothing more than a recommendation and did not in any way mandate that Merrell pursue the requested studies, and that the company was in fact justified in failing to do the studies because of inherent difficulties in completing them. The recommendation of the Obstetrics and Gynecology Advisory Committee, communicated by Ortiz on August 15, 1975 (Exhibit 2), was another issue Goddard sought to minimize and reconcile. He again assured that Merrell's actions in response to the recommendations was appropriate and in compliance with industry standards.

Goddard returned to court the morning of Friday, May 13, 1994, to continue with his direct examination. It was my hope that it would turn out to be Dr. Goddard's unlucky day. He expressed his opinion that the package insert in use at the time Linda Gandy was prescribed Clomid provided reasonable and adequate warnings. It was also his view that there was "no causative evidence of a deleterious effect of Clomid therapy on the human fetus," and that this statement was true and correct.

My first goal on cross-examination was to expose his bias for the defendant and the drug industry. I covered in detail all of the facts set out in Chapter 9, including his favor for Merrell shortly before marketing Clomid, and the substantial compensation he had received from the defendant, and the rest of the industry, since becoming a consultant and expert witness. It had always been my strategy to bring out evidence of bias at the commencement of my cross-examination of a witness. This had two benefits. First, with many witnesses there is an effort to be a little more candid in their answers, in order to demonstrate that they have not been influenced by the facts of bias. Second, when they do challenge some of my questions, the jury may be less inclined to give the testimony any credibility.

Goddard agreed that when teratology studies demonstrated in 1962 that Clomid was teratogenic in the rat and the rabbit, a red flag was raised that there might be some risk to humans. I next showed him Dr. Pierce's letter of October 11, 1963 and Dr. Umberger's attached summary (Exhibit 6), neither of which had been previously provided to him by Merrell's counsel. He acknowledged that as early as 1963, the FDA was expressing concern that Clomid could carry over into early pregnancy and possibly interfere with the developing fetus. I next read the following testimony from Goddard's deposition.

"Doctor, would you agree that if Richardson-Merrell was engaging in the practice of reasonably prudent pharmaceutical companies between 1962 and 1967, that their pre-market clinical studies should have been designed to evaluate whether or not their drug product could cause an increased risk for birth defects?"

"Yes. I would say that."

I then pursued the same line of inquiry in open court.

"You would agree that if they did not design the study to evaluate whether or not there was an increased risk for birth defects, that they violated the standard of care? You would agree with that, wouldn't you?"

"Yes, in general."

"Now, I want you to assume that Dr. Bunde has testified under oath, in a deposition, that this particular study was never designed to evaluate whether or not there was an increased risk of birth defects with Clomid. Now, assuming that to be the case, wouldn't you agree that the company violated the standard of care?"

"If he did, I would think that was a lack of attention to the proper standard of care, yes."

The above testimony was followed by a series of questions pointing out the multiple defects in the design of the study, which by this time had been repeated on several occasions in front of the jury. I also led the witness through a number of records, establishing that Merrell had failed to report numerous pregnancy outcomes from at least 3 clinical investigators.

As to the June 4, 1969 letter, I produced communications from Merrell to the FDA in which it agreed that the requested studies were feasible, yet never pursued. The correspondence between the two entities clearly reflected that the FDA was still waiting for a "further report" from Merrell when the trail of letters ended in 1970.

After examining Goddard on a number of additional issues, we concluded with his testimony in the mid-afternoon. Since Merrell's final witness, *Darwin Labarthe, M.D.*, would not be available until Monday morning, we broke for the weekend. This was good news. It gave me two full days to refine my cross-examination of the defedant's epidemiologist. It was here that I expected to have my biggest impact on Merrell's defense; when I could make effective use of my major discoveries at the UCLA Biomed Library.

Two years earlier I had moved to Santa Barbara, and was quite anxious to get on the road for my 2½ hour drive up the coast. But before exiting the courthouse, I was approached by Bob Dickson. He wanted to talk money. Settlement discussions had been occurring throughout the course of the trial, but we had never been given a number that had stimulated any interest. Now, for the first time, they were coming close. But I needed time to speak with my clients. We exchanged numbers where we could be reached over the weekend, and I spent some time speaking to Linda and David Brown before what turned out to be a relaxing drive to my home. I could sense that the case was about to end. The next day we countered with a slightly higher number and reached an agreement. Linda and Curtis were both quite pleased with the result, as were both of their lawyers.

But Merrell insisted that we could never disclose the amount of the settlement.

On Monday morning, May 16, 1994, David appeared in court and put the settlement on the record with Dickson. I stayed home in Santa Barbara for a well-earned rest.

* * * * *

CHAPTER 16

Does Anyone Really Care?

Following the successful resolution of the Gandy case, I considered my long-ignored commitment to stay on top of the FDA, to exert what influence I could on bringing about some form of a public warning. In preparation for the trial, I had amassed, updated and organized a considerable amount of material. Beginning with the Lancaster study in 1987, and the series of published studies that followed, I now had some ammunition to fire at the FDA. I had also learned that none of the approved labeling, with its critical warnings, had ever been put into final print form and distributed with the drug. I decided to not only hit the FDA with another letter demanding action, but to actually lay out the substance of my case on Merrell's culpability and the FDA's indifference, as well as the evidence accumulated to date on the teratogenicity of fertility drugs.

On *October 11, 1994*, I sent the following letter to the Director, Division of Metabolic & Endocrine Drug Products of the FDA, with a complete set of supporting documents, making reference to CLOMID (clomiphene citrate):

"To Whom It May Concern:

"DOES ANYONE REALLY CARE?

"Clomid was approved for marketing on February 1, 1967, and has been available by prescription since May 1967, 'to induce ovulation in anovulatory women in appropriately selected cases.'

"Over the years, including the period of pre-market testing (1960-1967), one of the vital questions presented to FDA concerning the drug's *safety* has been the issue of whether or not Clomid could cause *congenital malformations* in humans. Yet since that time FDA has repeatedly and consistently failed to follow up and enforce its own suggestions, requests and requirements, all of which were intended (and presumably needed) to evaluate the drug's potential teratogenicity and warn physicians and their patients of the relative risks related to same. Consider the following:

> 1. *Recent Published Studies*. Epidemiology studies involving fertility drugs, including clomiphene citrate, beginning with Lancaster (1987) and followed by a series of additional case-control and cohort studies, have

demonstrated a *statistically significant increase* in the incidence of neural tube defects, cleft lip/palate, hypospadias, undescended testes, transposition of the great vessels (heart defect), tracheo-oesophageal fistula, vertebral abnormalities, multiple congenital malformations and chromosomal defects in the offspring of women using those drugs when compared to relevant control groups. Copies of these publications and/or their citations have been previously supplied to FDA. Yet to this date, *seven years later*, the current labeling contains absolutely no warning relative to these studies. Even more outrageous is the FDA approval of a current *misrepresentation* in the same labeling that 'no causative evidence of a deleterious effect of Clomid therapy on the human fetus has been seen.' If positive epidemiology studies are not 'causative evidence,' then what is?

2. *Reformatted Labeling.* A draft of Reformatted Labeling was prepared for approval by FDA in *August 1987*. This was to replace all existing labeling. It also contained, among other things, warnings that (a) Clomid and/or its metabolites might remain in the maternal body *during early pregnancy* in every woman who conceived during a cycle of treatment with Clomid; (b) among birth anomalies spontaneously reported since the marketing of Clomid, the proportion of *neural tube defects* has been high among pregnancies associated with ovulation induced by the drug; (c) population-based reports have been published on a possible elevated risk of *Down Syndrome* in ovulation induction cases; (d) population-based reports have been published on an increase in *trisomy defects* among *spontaneously aborted fetuses* from sub-fertile women receiving ovulation inducing drugs; and (e) that *patients* should be *counseled* by the prescribing physician with regard to these potential adverse reactions. Through this date, *seven years later*, the reformatted labeling has yet to be distributed to physicians and pharmacies. Nor have any of these warnings been included in any subsequent labeling.

3. *Earlier Draft Labeling.* An earlier draft of similar labeling was approved by FDA on *November 30, 1983*, with a request for final print copies. The draft labeling had been submitted by Merrell Dow over 2 ½ years earlier on *March 19, 1981*! This likewise was to replace all existing labeling. It also contained, among other things, warnings that (a) Clomid and/or its metabolites might remain in the maternal body *during early pregnancy* in every woman who conceived during a cycle of treatment with Clomid; (b) among birth anomalies spontaneously reported since the marketing of Clomid, the proportion of *neural tube defects* has been high among pregnancies associated with ovulation induced by the drug; (c) population-based reports have been published on a possible elevated risk of *Down Syndrome* in ovulation induction cases; and (d) population-based reports have been published on an increase in *trisomy defects* among spontaneously aborted fetuses from subfertile women receiving ovulation inducing drugs. To this date, *eleven years later*, the final print of this draft labeling has yet to be distributed to physicians and pharmacies. Nor have any of the previously approved warnings been included in any subsequent labeling.

4. *Requested Prospective and Retrospective Studies.* A hearing of the Obstetrics & Gynecology Advisory Committee was conducted by FDA on *July 18, 1975*. By invitation of FDA I personally made a presentation at that hearing which included copies of the literature forming the basis for the above-mentioned warnings (in the draft labeling and reformatted labeling), as well as a comprehensive criticism of the pre-market investigations (1960-1967) and why they were totally useless in evaluating the teratogenic risk of Clomid. Following that hearing, on *August 15, 1975*, FDA sent correspondence to Merrell Dow (then Merrell-National Laboratories) stating: 'The committee recommended that further prospective and retrospective data be collected by your firm regarding the occurrence of congenital anomalies, including Down Syndrome, in children of mothers treated with clomiphene citrate. We are requesting

that your firm initiate studies to collect such data.' To this date, *nineteen years later*, Merrell Dow has yet to conduct one retrospective or prospective study, nor even submit the protocol and study designs for FDA approval.

5. *Merrell Dow Summaries*. Subsequent to said hearing of July 18, 1975, Merrell Dow instead submitted to FDA *summaries* of pre-market investigations, Drug Experience Reports (DERs) and published scientific literature. The first summary (one volume) related to congenital anomalies in general, with additional emphasis on Down Syndrome, and is dated *January 16, 1976*. The second summary (nine volumes) related to neural tube defects (NTDs) and central nervous system (CNS) related anomalies, and is dated *November 14, 1980*. Both summaries were apparently submitted *in lieu* of conducting the prospective and retrospective studies previously referred to. Both summaries are based in part on the meaningless pre-market investigations (previously criticized to FDA), plus an obvious manipulation of statistics without scientific validity, and an outright misrepresentation of data (verifiable from FDA's own records). Both summaries were accepted *without challenge* and the prior request for original data studies *abandoned*.

6. *Follow-up and Autopsy Studies*. On *June 4, 1969* FDA requested Merrell Dow (then Richardson-Merrell) to perform *follow-up examinations* on all living infants, conceived in association with Clomid therapy, for a period of at least *two years*. In the same correspondence, FDA also requested *autopsies* to be performed on all abortions, stillborns and neonatal deaths resulting from the same group of pregnancies. Though it complained about the need for such studies, Merrell acknowledged the *feasibility* of performing them by using the pre-market clinical population. To this date, *twenty-five years later*, Merrell Dow has yet to conduct even one such study (neither reports on follow-up exams nor autopsy reports have been submitted to date).

"The above-described pattern of indifference has now extended for a period of 25 years. One might also argue that it even extends back to *November 1961*, when Drs. Lenz and McBride brought to the world's attention the tragedy of *thalidomide* and the reality that the maternal ingestion of drugs can reach the developing embryo and produce congenital malformations. The following year (1962) animal teratology studies with clomiphene citrate demonstrated said drug to be teratogenic in the Sprague-Dawley rat and Dutch Belted rabbit. [Thalidomide was likewise teratogenic in the Dutch Belted rabbit.] Although such studies could not be extrapolated directly to humans, they unquestionably were a *warning sign* of what could happen in man.

"The timing of ingestion of Clomid also offered no reassurance of safety. The drug was generally taken on days 5-9 of the menstrual cycle, with conception occurring on or about day 14 (only 5 days after last using the drug). With a half-life of 5 days (based on C_{14} studies) almost 50% of the drug and/or its metabolites thus remained in the maternal circulation at the time of conception. Theoretically, based on half-life principles, five days later one would still have a half of a half, then five days after that a half of a half of a half and so on. As stated in the Physician's Monograph of *January 11, 1965*, 'Excretion of C-14 label in 5 subjects who received Clomid C-14 orally averaged 51% of the administered dose after five days; * * * Excretion was principally in the feces; fecal levels exceeded urinary levels up to 6 weeks after administration, suggesting that the remaining drug/metabolites were being slowly excreted from a sequestered enterohepatic recirculation pool.' This potential carry-over effect was well recognized by FDA as early as October 1963. On *October 11, 1963*, Dr. Grace Pierce of FDA forwarded to Merrell a pharmacologic evaluation by a Dr. Umberger (also of FDA). That summary stated in part:

> 'Teratogenicity has been demonstrated in animals. Human pregnancy cases are quite limited and therefore inconclusive. Animal fertility studies are suggestive of prolonged action of the drug, perhaps due to deposition and sustained release from fat deposits. The drug could therefore be effective longer than the duration of its administration. It may carry over from the phase of induced ovulation *into early pregnancy to interfere with the zygote and fetus.*' [See Exhibit 'A' attached hereto, emphasis added.]

FDA was thus fully cognizant, well before Clomid was approved for marketing, that at the critical period of organogenesis (about day 14 post-conception) a substantial portion of the drug and/or its metabolites would still remain. At this point it was also inescapable that an evaluation of the teratogenic risk of Clomid to humans could only be determined with a properly structured *epidemiological study*, using a *control population* with similar study designs. *This was never done.* In fact, not only did FDA allow Merrell to obtain approval of its NDA without a properly designed epidemiological study (see below), FDA has also continued to allow Merrell to cite that study as proof of its safety for Clomid offspring, even after the deficiencies of the study were pointed out to the FDA on July 18, 1975 and before.

"For all of the above-stated reasons, and as supported by the evidence identified hereafter and exhibits attached hereto, it is strongly urged that FDA, with as much dispatch as it is capable of bringing about, order Merrell Dow Pharmaceuticals to (1) prepare *final print* reformatted labeling with language already approved, within *thirty days* after FDA's receipt of this correspondence; (2) distribute the final print reformatted labeling, with a recall of all existing labeling, within thirty days after completion of final print labeling; (3) prepare draft labeling, with updated warnings consistent with the current scientific literature identified herein, and submit same for approval by FDA within 60 days of FDA's receipt of this correspondence; (4) give strong consideration to contraindicating the use of Clomid during a conception cycle and possibly one cycle before conception; and (5) to the extent that a hearing is required to bring about any of the requests set forth herein, to schedule same at the most expeditious date allowed under current regulations and statutes.

"*1. Recent Published Studies.*

"In 1987 Lancaster reported on the outcome of a cohort study on pregnancies from in-vitro fertilization (IVF) and gamete intrafallopian transfer (GIFT) in Australia and New Zealand. When compared to national data he found a *statistically significant increase* in *spina bifida* (P=.0015) and *transposition of the great vessels* (P=.0034). Three of the 6 cases of SB and 2 of the 4 cases of TGV were from *multiple births*. One of the SB infants also had *trisomy 18* with an absent left auditory canal, renal dysplasia, absent urethra, and imperforate anus. Another SB infant had a twin with *trisomy 18*.

This was the first in a series of epidemiology studies related to *neural tube defects*. [Lancet, Vol. II, No.8572, p.1392, December 12, 1987; Exhibit 'B'.] Clomiphene was one of the drugs used in this study [see Exhibit 'C']. Then in 1989, Cornel, et al. reported on a case-control study from the Netherlands with *neural tube defects*, and likewise found a *statistically significant increase* (95% confidence interval 1.03 – 15.2). They stated 'the specificity of the anomalies reported here (mainly NTD) suggests a genuine increase in risk.' [Lancet, p.1386, June 17, 1989; Exhibit 'D'.] Czeizel then reported on still another case-control study, this one from Hungary. Several congenital malformations were studied, including *neural tube defects*. Again, a *statistically significant increase* was reported (odds ratio 5.75, 95% CI 1.62-20.4). [Lancet, p.167, July 15, 1989; Exhibit 'E'.] From Oxford, England, Cuckle and Wald then reported on still another case-control study involving *neural tube defects*. Although the data did not reach statistical significance, there again was an increased relative risk (1.62). [Lancet, p.1281, November 25, 1989; Exhibit 'F'.] More importantly, when the Cuckle study was combined with those by Cornel and Czeizel by Vollset, they demonstrated a *highly significant increased risk* (OR 2.94, 95% CI 1.32-6.50). Vollset concluded 'that the three studies, when combined, do indicate that the association between ovulation induction and NTD is real (Mantel-Haenszel test, p=0.004).' [Lancet, Vol.335, p.178, January 20, 1990; Exhibit 'G'.] On December 9, 1989, Karabacak, et al. reported on another study involving *neural tube defects*. In a study conducted in Turkey, they also found a *statistically significant increase* in the incidence of NTDs (95% CI, 1.09-7.05). 'Thus, in our clinic the prevalence of NTD was 0.78% in the induced pregnancy group, which represents a three-four-fold increase over the rate at the maternity hospital (0.226%).' [Lancet, Vol.II, p.1391, December 9, 1989; Exhibit 'H'.]

"Then in December 1989, Cornel, et al., reported on a compilation of data from five international IVF centers (including the U.S.) again with regard to NTDs, and again found a *statistically significant* association (2.7 per thousand, 95% CI 1.6-4.8 per thousand, with a base line rate of 1.3-1.4 per thousand). [Lancet, p.1530, Dec. 23/30, 1989; Exhibit 'I'.] Milunsky, et al. reported on yet another case-control study involving *neural tube defects*. Although too small to reach statistical significance, this study again found an increased relative risk (RR 2.2, CI 0.6-8.6). [Teratology, 42: 467, 1990; Exhibit

'J'.] Finally, Robert, et al., reported on still another case-control study involving *neural tube defects*. And one more time a *statistically significant* increased risk occurred [OR 2.36, 95% CI 1.25-4.46; P=0.013; Exhibit 'K'.] Concerning *biological plausibility* for a drug taken before conception to disrupt the neural tube closure during early pregnancy, the recent animal study by Dziadek takes on considerable importance in view of the above-mentioned human epidemiology studies. Dziadek found that by administering clomiphene citrate to mice prior to ovulation, she was able to produce *neural tube defects* (i.e., exencephaly). [Teratology, 47: 263-273, 1993; Exhibit 'L'.]

"In addition to the TGV anomalies referred to by Lancaster (1987), epidemiology studies have also shown an increased risk for other types of congenital malformations. Supplemental to neural tube defects, Czeizel (1989) also found a *statistically significant increase* for *cleft lip/palate* (OR 7.1, 95% CI 2.0-25.3; P=.0004), *hypospadias* (OR 3.4, 95% CI .9-12.0; P=.045), *undescended testes* (OR 5.1, 95% CI 1.4-18.1; P=.005), and *multiple anomalies* (OR 7.7, 95% CI 2.5-23.4; P=.0001). [Exhibit 'E'.] In an update of his IVF studies from Australia and New Zealand, Lancaster in 1990 also reported on a *statistically significant increase* in the incidence of *tracheo-oesophageal fistula, urinary tract malformations* and *vertebral abnormalities* (P less than 0.01). 'Multiple malformations were also more frequent than expected.' [Teratology, 42: 325, September, 1990, Exhibit 'C'.] An increased incidence of *hypospadias* (in offspring of mothers using various fertility drugs, including clomiphene citrate), has also been reported by Macnab & Zouves (P = less than 0.01). [Fert. & Ster. Vol. 56, No.5, November 1991; Exhibit 'M'.] Finally, a study collecting data from the Registry of Congenital Malformations in Paris has reported on a *statistically significant increase* in the incidence of infants with *chromosomal abnormalities* (OR 1.92, 95% CI 1.02-3.59). [Goujard, et al., Teratology, 45: 326, March 1992; Exhibit 'N'.]

"On or about *November 29, 1989* and *March 30, 1990*, Merrell Dow provided to FDA citations for the Cornel article [Exhibit 'D'] and Czeizel article [Exhibit 'E'], Nos. 034139 and 034140, respectively. The Cornel article refers to and cites the 1987 article by Lancaster [Exhibit 'B']. On or about *April 1, 1991*, Merrell Dow provided *copies* of the published epidemiology studies by Cuckle [Exhibit 'F'], Vollset [Exhibit 'G'], Karabacak [Exhibit 'H'], Cornel [Exhibit 'I'] and Milunsky [Exhibit 'J'], Nos. 034836,

034760, 034759, 034812 and 035908, respectively. A publication authored by Franz Rosa of FDA, published in Lancet in 1990 [Lancet, 336: 1327], reflects that FDA was well aware of all the relevant literature of neural tube defects, at least through the date of the publication [see Merrell SL No. 035981]. During the same year, Cornel sent a letter to the editor of Teratology [42: 201-203, 1990], pointing out the inadequacy of the studies and data prior to 1987 to determine whether or not ovulation induction could cause neural tube defects. [See Merrell SL No. 035624.] Dr. Cornel then went on to point out several studies suggesting an association between the two.

"How many positive epidemiology studies must FDA see before it considers the need for a warning? How much evidence is needed before patients using fertility drugs, and their prescribing physicians, are entitled to be put on notice of the risks? Does FDA suggest that causation must be proven *conclusively* before a warning of the risk is justified? If not, why has there been such a protracted delay in getting this information to the public and to the prescribing physicians?

"The *current* labeling presently carries a statement that 'no causative evidence of a deleterious effect of Clomid therapy on the human fetus has been seen.' This is set forth under Contraindications-Pregnancy. See current package insert attached hereto. [Exhibit 'O'.] Why does FDA continue to allow this representation to remain in the current labeling? How can such a statement be justified in the face of a number of positive epidemiology studies, even if they are not conclusive on the issue? The statement represents that there is '*no* causative evidence.' What 'causative evidence' must FDA see before it will require Merrell Dow to delete this statement?

"2. *Reformatted Labeling.*

"In *August 1987*, a revision draft of Reformatted Labeling was prepared by Merrell Dow, and thereafter submitted to FDA for approval. [See attached Exhibit 'P'.] Among other things, the labeling includes the following statements:

> 'Some Clomid and/or its metabolites (here measured only as $14C$) may, therefore, remain in the body during early pregnancy in every woman who conceives in the menstrual cycle of Clomid treatment.' [Page 3]

* * *

317

'Information for Patients. The purpose and risks of Clomid therapy should be presented to the patient before starting treatment. Advise and counsel the patient that the goal of Clomid therapy is ovulation for subsequent pregnancy. * * *' [Page 9]

'Patient counseling. The physician should counsel the patient with special regard to the following potential adverse reactions that may be encountered. [Page 10] .... 4. Pregnancy Wastage and Birth Anomalies .... Among the birth anomalies spontaneously reported as individual cases since commercial availability of Clomid, the proportion of neural tube defects has been high among pregnancies associated with ovulation induced by Clomid, but this has not been supported by data from population-based studies.' [Page 12; of course this has *now* been supported by data from population-based studies.]

* * *

'Population-based reports have been published on possible elevation of risk of Down Syndrome in ovulation induction cases and of increase in trisomy defects among spontaneously aborted fetuses from subfertile women receiving ovulation inducing drugs (no women with Clomid alone and without additional inducing drug). However, as yet, the reported observations are too few to confirm or not confirm the presence of an increased risk...' [Page 13]

* * *

'Nevertheless, the studies in humans cannot rule out the possibility of harm. The studies done in pregnant women are limited because drug administration is not indicated once pregnancy has been achieved. (See WARNINGS and CONTRAINDICATIONS.) There are no adequate and well-controlled studies in pregnant women.' [Page 14]

Further, noticeable in its absence, is the statement that 'no causative evidence of a deleterious effect of Clomid therapy has been seen.' It has been completely deleted from the entire Reformatted Labeling draft. If this statement was inappropriate in August 1987, why does it continue to exist in the present labeling? In fact, the presence of this

318

misrepresentation in the current labeling is even more astonishing when one considers the above-mentioned epidemiology studies that were published *after* August 1987. Of greater importance, however, is the question of why the Reformatted Labeling has not been printed and distributed for a period in excess of 7 years. If patients were justified in receiving the warnings, set forth above, in August 1987, why haven't they been given the benefit of those warnings for the past 7 years? If prior to August 1987, 'the studies in humans (could not) rule out the possibility of harm' to the fetus, why aren't women who are pondering the possible use of this drug entitled to know what the risks are going in? Given the state of the literature that existed prior to August 1987, I personally feel that these warnings are somewhat *watered down*; however, they at least provide the patient with *some* indication that there may be a legitimate risk for congenital malformations in the event that she might conceive during a treatment cycle with Clomid.

3. *Earlier Draft Labeling.*

"On *March 19, 1981*, Merrell Dow submitted to FDA a draft of revised labeling for Clomid. The cover letter states, 'This revised labeling has been discussed on several occasions with Dr. Ridgley Bennett and all suggested modifications have been incorporated into the text.' [Exhibit 'Q'.] Apparently, Dr. Bennett of FDA had been working on this draft for some time. It bears a date of August 12, 1980, with revisions of February 6, 1981. [Note that underlines on attached draft and cover letter are my own.]

"Thereafter, for some unknown reason, it took over *2½ years* for this draft labeling to be approved! On *November 30, 1983*, Solomon Sobel, M.D., of FDA, referencing this submission of March 19, 1981, forwarded correspondence to Merrell Dow with the following statement:

> 'We have completed the review of this supplemental application as submitted with draft labeling. However, before the supplement may be approved, it will be necessary for you to submit final print labeling. The labeling should be identical in content to the draft copy except that a HOW SUPPLIED section should be added and inclusion of the prescription caution statement is also recommended.' [Exhibit 'R'.]

Merrell then found a way to further delay distribution of this labeling. On February 1, 1984, it forwarded a letter explaining that it was updating its Clomid labeling to include product information through October 1983. [Exhibit 'S'.] Reformatted Labeling also now was required by 21 CFR 201.57. It is interesting, however, that in *10 years* Clomid has yet to be distributed with Reformatted Labeling. In the meantime, Merrell has continued to distribute Clomid with its previously outdated labeling, other than updating the product information from time to time. Then, moving along at its typical snail's pace, on November 3, 1986, Dr. Sobel responded to this submission of February 1, 1984. [Exhibit 'T'.] Again a request was made for 'final print labeling.' This presumably would have been with the Reformatted Labeling required by 21 CFR 201.57. Reference was also made to the requirement that pregnancy category X be used since the drug is contraindicated in pregnant women. Merrell responded to this request on December 11, 1986, complaining that 'Pregnancy Category X,' would be confusing. [Exhibit 'U'.] Dr. Sobel responded to this concern on March 5, 1987 [Exhibit 'V'] and made a suggested revision. Finally, on July 31, 1987, Merrell Dow submitted its draft for Reformatted Labeling to FDA. [See Cover Letter, Exhibit 'W'.] This apparently follows the history of the draft labeling from August 12, 1980 through August 1987.

"A review of this earlier draft labeling reflects that as early as August 12, 1980, FDA was of the opinion that the following similar statements were appropriate to properly warn patients:

> 'Some Clomid and/or its metabolites (here measured only as 14C) may, therefore, remain in the body during early pregnancy in every woman who conceives in the menstrual cycle of Clomid treatment.' [Page 3]
>
> * * *
>
> 'Patient Counseling. The purpose and risk of Clomid therapy should be presented to the patient before starting treatment. Advise the patient that the goal of Clomid therapy is ovulation for subsequent pregnancy. * * * The physician should counsel the patient with special regard to the following potential adverse reactions that may be encountered.' [Page 8]
>
> * * *
>
> '4. Pregnancy Wastage and Birth Anomalies. ... Among the birth anomalies spontaneously reported as individual cases since commercial availability of Clomid, the proportion of neural tube defects has been high

320

among pregnancies associated with ovulation induced by Clomid, but this has not been supported by data from population-based studies.' [Page 10; again, this has *now* been supported by data from population-based studies.]

* * *

'Population-based reports have been published on possible elevation of risk of Down Syndrome in ovulation induction cases and of increase in trisomy defects among spontaneously aborted fetuses from subfertile women receiving ovulation inducing drugs (no women with Clomid alone and with additional inducing drug). However, as yet, the reported observations are too few to confirm or not confirm the presence of an increased risk...' [Page 11]

Even as early as August 12, 1980, FDA also determined that the aforementioned *misrepresentation* was inappropriate and *deleted* 'no causative evidence of a deleterious effect of Clomid therapy on the human fetus has been seen.' Yet *14 years later* it has survived the scrutiny of FDA and still finds life in FDA's indifference and/or procrastination.

"4. *Requested Prospective and Retrospective Studies.*

"A hearing of the Obstetrics & Gynecology Advisory Committee was conducted by FDA on <u>July 18, 1975</u>. This followed a jury verdict I obtained on behalf of a deformed child, which was rendered in Los Angeles County on April 15, 1974. The mother had ingested Clomid. This also followed a series of letters from myself to FDA, dated January 13, 1975, March 21, 1975, May 9, 1975, June 13, 1975, June 17, 1975 and July 2, 1975, with enclosures relative to my analysis of the literature and data [attached hereto as a group and marked Exhibit 'X']. These materials, along with my oral presentation, presented evidence which I believed supported a case for causation between the maternal ingestion of Clomid and the development of Down Syndrome and neural tube defects in the offspring. I also outlined a number of flaws in the pre-market investigations which rendered them meaningless for assessing the drug's teratogenicity. Following the hearing, based upon the recommendations of the Advisory Committee, FDA communicated to Merrell:

'The committee recommended that further prospective and retrospective data be collected by your firm regarding the occurrence of congenital anomalies, including Down Syndrome, in children of mothers treated with clomiphene citrate. We are requesting that your firm initiate studies to collect such data.' [Exhibit 'Y'.]

The date was *August 15, 1975*. Since that request, no study designs were ever submitted to FDA for approval and no *studies* 'to collect such data,' were ever initiated, let alone completed and reported on. Instead, Merrell sent two sets of *summaries* which collected Clomid case histories from the pre-market investigations, DERs and scientific literature and compared them to reference populations for incidences of congenital malformations. These summaries were dated *January 16, 1976* and *November 14, 1980*. In reality Merrell simply took information FDA already had, distorted and manipulated the statistics to suit its needs, then sat and hoped. As usual, it worked. No further measures were ever taken by FDA (to this day) to see to it that Merrell collected the data requested with properly designed *studies*.

"What should have been demanded from Merrell, and nothing less, were properly designed *epidemiology studies*, focusing on congenital malformations in general and *Down Syndrome* and *neural tube defects* in particular; studies similar to those performed by Lancaster (1987), Cornel (1989), Czeizel (1989), Cuckle (1989), Karabacak (1989), Milunsky (1990) and Robert (1991) for neural tube defects and Goujard (1992) for chromosomal abnormalities [unfortunately, a well-designed epidemiology study specifically for Down Syndrome has yet to be performed]. The problem is that *Merrell* should have conducted these studies and they should have been performed *eleven to sixteen years earlier!* Because of FDA's procrastination and indifference there has been a delay of well over a decade in realizing these studies. Worst of all, there may be a generation of *thousands of deformed children* that might otherwise have been avoided had FDA enforced its own mandate.

"*Pre-market Investigations*. That FDA would rely, even in part, on Merrell's pre-market investigations is indeed shocking. As was explained back in 1975, *that study was never designed to evaluate the risk of birth defects*. Consider again all of the following:

1. This was not an epidemiology study. There was *no control group* with similar histories and study designs, including use of the same definition of congenital malformation, same methods of examination of infants, same geographical population group, and examinations over the same period of time following birth. Nor were the protocols and guidelines for the study patterned after another study designed to determine the incidence of congenital malformations in either an infertility population or the general population. [Admissions of Fact (under oath) No.24, Manzo vs. Richardson-Merrell, Inc.; Exhibit 'Z'.]

2. None of the clinical investigators were given a standard or uniform *definition* for 'congenital malformations' or 'birth defects;' nor were they given a *list* of abnormalities to be included when reporting 'congenital malformations' or 'birth defects.' [Admission of Fact Nos.19 and 20]

> (a) Carl A. Bunde, M.D. was Director of Medical Research of Richardson-Merrell during the pre-market clinical investigations with Clomid, and was the head of the Department of Medical Research which conducted said studies. Dr. Bunde testified in a deposition (on March 3, 1979) his agreement that to arrive at an accurate statistic in evaluating whether or not there was a greater incidence of birth defects with Clomid patients, as compared to another population not taking Clomid, it was necessary that both groups used the *same definition* of birth defect. [Bunde depos., pp.39-40, 42; Exhibit 'AA'.]

3. None of the clinical investigators were requested or required to do routine *follow-up examinations* of *each* child born of a pregnancy resulting from, or in association with, maternal ingestion of Clomid. [Admission of Fact No.21.]

> (a) Dr. Bunde also acknowledged that to make an accurate comparison between birth defects from Clomid patients and those from another population without Clomid, the period of observation

should be approximately the same in both groups. [Bunde depos., p.40.]

4. None of said clinical investigators were specifically requested to include both *major* and *minor* congenital abnormalities in their reports. [Admission No.23.]

5. None of the clinical investigators were requested to *routinely* do *any* of the following procedures to *each* patient or child where birth defects occurred following maternal ingestion of Clomid: (a) document all *medicine* taken by the mother during pregnancy; (b) document all *trauma* occurring to the mother during pregnancy; (c) document all *x-rays* received by the mother during pregnancy; (d) document all *illnesses* suffered by the mother during pregnancy; (e) have chromosomal studies performed on each deformed child; or (f) examine the family background of both parents to determine whether or not any *hereditary traits* might be responsible for the birth defects. [Admission No.22.]

6. None of the clinical investigators were required or requested to routinely perform *autopsies* on *stillbirths* or *neonatal deaths* of infants following maternal ingestion of Clomid.

(a) Out of 27 stillbirths, one autopsy was performed and reported. [Answers to Interrogatories (under oath), Manzo vs. Richardson-Merrell, Inc., No.1(c)-(f), Fourth Set; Exhibit 'BB'.]

(b) Out of 59 neonatal deaths, five autopsies were performed and reported. [Answer to Interrogatory No.1(g)-(j), Fourth Set.]

7. Dr. Bunde also testified under oath that at no time prior to the marketing of Clomid was there any protocol specifically designed or set up to evaluate whether or not Clomid could cause birth defects. [Bunde depos., p.32, pp.84-85.]

8. The most egregious deficiency of the study, however, was the fact that perhaps the majority of all pregnancies were *not delivered by the investigator or his staff nor did they examine the infants*. Most, if not all, investigators were fertility specialists who received a large proportion of

their patients by outside referrals from OB/GYNs. After they achieved a pregnancy with Clomid, the patient would be *sent back* to the referring physician for delivery. Thus, the delivering physicians and later examining pediatricians were not part of the study and had no obligation to report the results of any examinations of the infants. Edward T. Tyler, M.D., was one of the principal clinical investigators on Clomid, and also testified on behalf of the defendant in the trial of Breimhorst vs. Richardson-Merrell (on April 2, 1974). Dr. Tyler's testimony shed considerable light on the situation. He testified that he did not deliver any of the babies nor did he maintain records on all of the physicians that delivered them. He said they would 'get letters and birth announcements from (their) patients,' and that 'some doctors were nice enough to send (them) the delivery room report.' However, this was not done as a matter of custom. He felt confident that the delivering physicians would 'like to let (them) know what happened.' [Tyler trial testimony, pp.28-29; Exhibit 'CC'.]

9. Aside from the above glaring deficiencies, there is also evidence that Merrell Dow *withheld records* on Clomid pregnancies. Each investigator was aasigned a number [see Exhibit 'DD']. Dr. G. Bettendorf was assigned No.157. Dr. David G. Becker was assigned No.271. And Dr. Sheldon A. Payne was assigned No.066. All of the Clomid pregnancies from the pre-market investigations (2,635 pregnancies out of which outcome known in 2,369) were stored in a computer, and a readout of a summary of all these pregnancies is set forth in a multi-paged document entitled 'Clomid Pregnancy Data as of January 1970.' From this document, it can be determined that Merrell reported on *two cases* from Dr. Bettendorf, *eleven cases* from Dr. Decker and *136 cases* from Dr. Payne. [See Exhibit 'EE'.] From a company document, however, it is clear that Dr. Bettendorf treated *forty* Clomid pregnancies, twelve of which resulted in spontaneous abortions [Exhibit 'FF']. And from published articles by Decker [Exhibit 'GG'] and Payne [Exhibit 'HH'], reporting on the pre-market investigations, it can be determined that Dr. Decker had

fifteen Clomid pregnancies and Dr. Payne treated *180 pregnancies* out of which the outcome was known in 140. This type of cross-checking has only been done with a few investigators, and the above examples may represent only the 'tip of the iceberg.' Needless to say, FDA has not been given the full story on the Clomid pre-market investigations.

"Given all of the above-mentioned problems with the pre-market clinical studies, one would ask why FDA continues to allow Merrell to cite that study, and all of its statistics, in its current labeling, such to suggest that it represents a valid and scientific study suggestive of the safety for the offspring of women using Clomid to conceive. To sanction the continued display of this study in the labeling on the drug only compounds the problems created by not enforcing the prior request for retrospective and prospective studies.

"5. *Merrell Dow Summaries.*

"In response to the request for prospective and retrospective studies, issued by FDA on August 15, 1975, Merrell submitted two reports, each containing summaries of the investigational population, Drug Experience Reports (DERs) and published scientific literature. On *March 30, 1976*, Merrell submitted to FDA a *one volume* report entitled, 'Pregnancy Outcome of Humans Following Clomid (clomiphene citrate USP) with Summary of Detail of Reported Information on Birth Anomalies of Offspring,' dated January 16, 1976. This report summarized the investigational population (2,369 cases), DERs to date (57 cases) and the published scientific literature (848 cases). It compared the Clomid summaries with four specific sources of birth defect incidence rates [Myrianthopoulos and Chung; CDC; McIntosh; and Shapiro and Abramowicz]. Although comparisons are made with regard to overall incidences of congenital malformations, special comment is made with regard to Down syndrome, which was specifically addressed at the hearing of *July 18, 1975*. The second report is dated *November 14, 1980*, contains *nine volumes* and is entitled 'Pregnancy Outcome of Humans Following Clomid – Neural Tube Defects & CNS Related Anomalies.' This latter report similarly compares the same Clomid populations, with updated literature references, to the same standard incidence sources. However, it focuses specifically on neural tube defects and central nervous system congenital anomalies. As will be demonstrated below, these two sets of summaries go to considerable lengths to compare 'apples with oranges,' and in fact have made a science of it.

"(a) Investigational Population.

"The deficiencies of the pre-market investigations conducted by Merrell are outlined above. They obviously are meaningless for comparing with *any* other source for birth defect incidence rates. However, Merrell went even further to distort the statistics and induce a favorable review by FDA.

"FIRST, to give a *lower* incidence rate of congenital malformations it divided the 'reported' number of birth defects (58) into the total number of *pregnancies* (2,369), rather than into the total number of *deliveries*, after excluding abortions, ectopic pregnancies and hydatidiform moles (1,887). [See p.28 in submission of March 30, 1976.] Thus, rather than a rate of *3.1%*, Merrell reported a rate of *2.4%*. It is proper to exclude abortions, ectopic pregnancies and moles because they are severely *deformed*, especially first trimester spontaneous abortions. Of those that are not observably abnormal, many might deliver abnormal if they are allowed to go to term. If one is truly going to give an incidence figure of congenital anomalies out of total *pregnancies*, then the numerator should include abnormal abortuses and hydatidiform moles (and where appropriate ectopic pregnancies). This is why most studies look only at the rate of anomalies in immature, premature and term births.

"SECOND, if one is going to compare an incidence rate calculated from total *pregnancies*, then the study compared to should also use total pregnancies as the denominator. *Merrell has instead chosen four reference populations that calculated rates from total deliveries.* Myrianthopoulos & Chung calculated their incidence rate from 53,257 single *deliveries*; McIntosh et al. calculated their rate from 5,739 single and multiple *deliveries*; and Shapiro & Abramowicz calculated their rate from 9,851 single *deliveries*. The surveillance data given by CDC is from *live births*. [See Vol. 9 of November 14, 1980 submission.] By the very design of its presentation, Merrell was assured that the Clomid populations would have a lower incidence of birth defects than the reference populations compared with. The deception is exemplified by the following statement from the March 30, 1976 submission (at p.7):

327

'In general, the overall incidence of reported birth anomalies from pregnancies associated with maternal Clomid ingestion was within the range of that reported in published references for the general population (see Table 4). The overall incidence was below the percentage of that quoted by the Collaborative Perinatal Project (15.56%), even if adjustment by calculation is made of the 2.4% reported among single births to 6.4% (calculated per reference in footnote a of Table 5) with the assumption that the reported anomalies were detected and reported only at birth and that the literature reference data include information to one year of life.'

Merrell deceptively compared its Clomid incidence rate based on *pregnancies* (2.4%) to a reference source based on *deliveries* (6.1%). Merrell's 'apples' were compared with Myrianthopoulos' 'oranges.'

"THIRD, when one examines a population of infants at one to two years following birth, he will generally find *2 to 3 times the frequency* of anomalies than were found shortly after birth. It is therefore important to compare populations who are *examined at the same time* subsequent to delivery. As indicated above, the Clomid investigational population was at best examined only *at birth*. None of the 363 investigators were requested to routinely perform follow-up exams of delivered infants [Exhibit 'Z']. The reference populations compared with, however, involved follow-up exams at *one year* [Myrianthopoulos], *one year* [McIntosh] and *two years* [Shapiro]. Myrianthopoulos found only *one-third* of total malformations at birth and McIntosh calculated an incidence rate at birth at *3.2%* compared to *7.5%* at one year. Shapiro did not break out anomaly rates for time of delivery. Again Merrell twisted the statistics to achieve an incidence rate lower or on parity with malformation rates in the general population. Again, apples were compared with oranges. [NOTE: Merrell had the same rate at birth (3.1%) as did McIntosh (3.2%), despite the reporting deficiencies referred to above, and the failure to provide a standard definition of congenital malformations and lack of autopsies on neonatal deaths and stillbirths (see below).] Finally, the importance of timing of examination and ascertainment techniques were best expressed by Myrianthopoulos & Chung as follows:

'This is undoubtedly, *one of the highest rates of malformations ever reported.* This high frequency is, of course, easily explained on the basis of *period of time* through which the malformations were observed and the conditions which made *almost complete ascertainment* possible. As Stuart et al. [10] succinctly pointed out, the incidence of malformations depends largely on the method of data collection; relatively high rates are obtained in studies involving direct examination by trained observers and even higher rates when infants are observed over a period of time.' [Emphasis added; pp.4-5.]

"FOURTH, it is also critically important to use the *same definition* of 'congenital malformation' in both populations being compared. Many will consider some conditions found at birth as congenital anomalies whereas others will not. One of the reasons why Myrianthopoulos & Chung had such a high incidence rate is because they included such things as tumors, anomalies of dentition, supernumerary nipples, strawberry/port wine hemangiomas, cystic kidneys, cataracts, preauricular skin tags, delayed teeth eruption, hairy pigmented nevus, café au lait spots, and other abnormalities that many do not describe as congenital malformations. McIntosh and Shapiro also both used very specific definitions of congenital malformations, although neither was quite as inclusive as Myrianthopoulos. Conversely, the Clomid investigational population did not use *any* definition of congenital malformation, nor did it specify a list of anomalies to be included or specify that the malformations should be divided up between major and minor anomalies. [See Exhibit 'Z'.] Without a working definition, the investigators in the pre-market Clomid study would be *less inclined to include an anomaly* than the referenced population investigators who were given specific directives. Again the summaries were slanted for low ascertainment for the investigational population compared to the reference population.

"FIFTH, Myrianthopoulos performed *autopsies* on *92%* of the stillborns and neonatal deaths and McIntosh *86.5%* of stillbirths and *85.2%* of neonatal deaths. Shapiro and CDC only reported on live births. Conversely, Merrell performed autopsies on *3.7%* of stillbirths and *8.5%* of neonatal deaths. The importance of this difference is quite significant. Myrianthopoulos found *8.2% of all stillbirths* and *29.0% of all neonatal deaths* with *congenital malformations* and further stated:

'It is well known that the incidence of congenital malformations is higher when based on autopsy findings than when based on clinical diagnosis only [3, 4], and the fetal and neonatal deaths would tend to inflate the incidence of malformations usually observed in a population of newborns.' [p.2]

McIntosh found *6.2% of all stillbirths* and *29.6% of all neonatal deaths* likewise with *congenital malformations* and stated:

'The high percentage of autopsies performed on stillbirths and neonatal deaths does not permit comparison of malformation rates in even these groups with rates found in other studies in which information was taken from death certificates or from hospital records.' [p.519]

It is thus quite clear that because of the high frequency of performing autopsies, Myrianthopoulos and McIntosh should *not* be used for comparison against a study with such low rates of autopsies. This was again another effort by Merrell to utilize inappropriate reference populations for comparison with the investigational population.

"Thus, summarizing and comparing the pre-market investigations on Clomid was absolutely inappropriate and lacked scientific validity. This also should have been readily apparent to FDA. The two sets of summaries should have been suspect when they compared the investigational population to one study that had 'one of the highest rates of malformations ever reported,' and two others which were likewise at the higher end of those reported in the scientific literature. Many publications report 3% or less. If Merrell wanted to give a thorough and objective presentation on the issue, why did it select only reference populations which had the higher incidences of congenital malformations ever reported?

"(b) Down Syndrome.

"In the summary of March 30, 1976, Merrell made the following statement under a heading entitled '*Comment on Down Syndrome*':

'Among the 2,082 live born and stillborn infants (single and multiple births) of Clomid associated pregnancies during the investigational studies, 1960-1970, there were 5 reports of offspring with Down syndrome. This calculates to an incidence of 2.40 per 1,000. The mean incidence figure for 1968-1973 for the metropolitan Atlanta population was 1.00 per 1,000 (Table 9). Of the mothers of these offspring, one (069-014) discontinued Clomid on 9/12/63 and had an estimated date of conception 2/1/64; *one patient* (100-176) *discontinued Clomid on 10/21/65 with a record of LMP of 12/30/65*; one patient (208-033) had no Clomid in the cycle of conception with ovulation induction attributed to prednisone; and one patient (066-233) received Donnatal, Stelazine, Librium, and prednisone at or near the estimated date of conception of 9/22/65 and later that month. If for reasons presented above, 1 to 3 patients are excluded, then the incidence for 4 is 1.92 per 1,000, for 3 is 1.44, and for 2 is 0.96.' [Emphasis added; pp.21-22.]

The reference (emphasized) above is an outright *misrepresentation* of the facts and records already submitted to FDA. Case no. 100-176 involved a woman who did *not* discontinue Clomid on 10/21/65, but was last treated *January 3, 1966 through January 7, 1966* (with LMP of 12/30/65). This case unquestionably involved conception during the treatment cycle. [See Exhibit 'II'.] Additionally, although case no. 208-033 did not involve a conception within a treatment cycle with Clomid, conception occurred only *one cycle* after last ingesting Clomid (treatment 8/27/65-8/31/65, with LMP of 9/10/65 and conception date of 10/6/65). Based upon the Boue study, demonstrating a similar incidence of trisomy chromosomal abnormalities in abortuses following conceptions during a treatment cycle and one cycle after treatment, this case was likewise in the *high risk group*. In other words, four of the five reported cases occurred either in a treatment cycle or one cycle after last treatment. Further, the one case that did not fall into this critical timing category (069-014) had the *oldest* maternal age of the five cases (37). Again, Merrell has distorted the statistics and even made an outright misrepresentation with regard to key records pertaining to this issue; a matter which was a focus of the hearing of July 18, 1975.

"(c) Drug Experience Reports.

"The DERs referred to in both of the aforementioned summaries have little scientific value with regard to the issue of whether or not Clomid can cause congenital malformations, and particularly whether or not it can cause Down syndrome or neural tube defects. This is because there is no known denominator. They are only case reports. However, because of the high number of DERs involving *neural tube defects*, a *red flag* was waved calling out for epidemiology studies designed to evaluate the risk of NTDs when using Clomid.

"(d) Scientific Literature.

"Another gross misstatement of statistics involves Merrell's recitation of data from the scientific literature. This problem existed for both summaries (1976 and 1980).

"The submission of March 30, 1976, refers to reports on birth anomalies in the scientific literature (at p.20) and cites '13 published papers having original information without duplication of population, having a sufficient number of patients, and in which there was mention of one or more anomalies of offspring of Clomid associated pregnancies.' From this literature, Merrell cites an incidence of birth defects of 4.1%. This literature was identified in Table 16. However, when one looks at the 13 published papers identified in Table 16, it becomes apparent that the aforementioned representation is *not true*. Goldfarb (no.2919), Greenblatt (no.2216) and Karow (no.2963) are all from the investigational population, and all three of the papers do not contain 'original information without duplication of population.' [We, of course, know about the deficiencies in the investigational population.] When the total number of pregnancies are deleted from these three, the remaining pregnancies total 406 (not 848). After deduction for abortions (64), the delivered pregnancies equal 342, from which there were 19 congenital malformations (5.6%, not 4.1%). These calculations use Merrell's own statistics. [See Exhibit 'JJ'.] Few of the cited publications give insight into the methods of ascertainment, timing of examinations or definitions of malformation (if any) that were used. Several of the remaining ten authors were also clinical investigators. In fact, one (Murray) refers to data, some of which clearly comes from the investigational population (see paper no.5516).

"The submission of November 14, 1980, also contains a major distortion of the statistics derived from the scientific literature. In an effort to demonstrate that the incidence of Down syndrome and neural tube defects following Clomid use was the same as existed in the general population, Merrell again resorts to the questionable use of *pregnancies* as its denominator, rather than *deliveries*. In its paper, it again identifies the

2,369 pregnancies from the investigational population and 'a cumulative 2,880 pregnacies/infants in a total of 27 population-based scientific literature publications which presented original data on 25 or more pregnancies and had mention of one or more identified birth anomalies.' [p.2, Vol.1] The 27 cited publications, and their statistics, are attached hereto. [Exhibit 'KK'.] When one separates deliveries (after spontaneous abortions) from pregnancies/infants, the numbers break out as follows:

1. Goldfarb (2919):	160/160	(investigational population)
2. Karow (2963):	183/113	(investigational population)
3. Pildes (3222):	49/36	(investigational population)
4. Ibuki (4559):	32/20	
5. Greenblatt (4815):	156/71	(investigational population)
6. Bret (4865):	26/21	
7. Shearman (5925):	42/38	
8. Kullander (6063):	25/23	
9. Hagenfelt (6426):	48/31	
10. Env.-Santos (6777):	36/35	
11. Rust (8080):	25/24	
12. Henry-Suckett (8238):	31/28	
13. Harlap (11604):	225/196	Down syndrome (1)
14. Fayez (11649):	46/40	Down syndrome (1)
15. Baron (13456):	92/79	Rachischisis (1)
16. Ahlgren (13583):	159/141	Meningocele (1); Down syndrome (1)
17. Guistini (14085):	91/61	Meningocele (1)
18. Gorlitsky (15234):	45/41	
19. Bettendorf (15264):	64/52	
20. Tadashi (15297):	233/211	
21. R. Velasco (15433):	103/86	
22. Scheunpflug (15689):	128/92	
23. Sas (16152):	349/206*	Anencephaly (1); Spina Bifida (2)
24. Maunilova (17217):	43/24	
25. Adashi (18181):	86/63	

26. Hack (18267):   344/294

27. Barrat (20341):   59/41

                         2,880/1,847   (after deletion of investigational population)

* Approximation

Six NTDs out of 1,847 deliveries (1/308). Three Down syndrome out of 1,847 deliveries (1/602; unadjusted for maternal age).

"Further note that Merrell did not identify one case of neural tube defect (rachischisis) from the Baron paper, even though it was specified at page 5 (Table 3). Rachischisis is unquestionably a neural tube defect, involving a congenital fissure of the spinal column. In other words, Merrell presented to FDA a neural tube defect rate of 1 in 576 (2,880 divided by 5) rather than an incidence of 1 in 308 deliveries (1,847 divided by 6).

"Of the cited general sources, only Myrianthopoulos is useful. CDC and Shapiro only looked at live births, and McIntosh did not break out statistics for NTDs per delivery, but by malformation (one infant might have 2 or more malformations). Combining anencephaly, meningomyelocele/meningocele and rachischisis, Myrianthopoulos calculated an NTD incidence rate of *1.54 per thousand (1/649)*, suggesting that the combined literature revealed *twice the expected frequency* of NTDs following use of Clomid (1/649 vs. 1/308). Comparing apples with apples can make a difference. When Cornel, et al. looked at several different populations, including several identified by Merrell in its summaries, they made the following statement: 'We conclude that, apart from the case reports, there are three lines of inclusive evidence on an association between disturbed fertility and NTD, *all three suggestive of a relative risk of at least 2.*' [Emphasis added; Exhibit 'I'.] When Vollset combined the case-control studies by Cornel, Czeizel and Cuckle & Wald, he found an odds ratio of 2.94 [Exhibit 'G']. Milunsky, et al. [Exhibit 'J'] found a relative risk of 2.2 and Robert, et al. [Exhibit 'K'] found an odds ratio of 2.36. Is it just a coincidence that all of these studies show an increased risk for neural tube defects at approximately *twice the expected frequency*?

"What is truly astounding is that FDA bought this package with open arms, apparently without analyzing, questioning or cross-checking the data. In fact, so manipulated by this presentation was FDA that in 1990 *Franz Rosa* of FDA actually *duplicated* it in the Lancet. [See Exhibit 'LL'.] If one compares the figures from Merrell's table [Exhibit 'KK'] with the Rosa publication [Exhibit 'LL'], one will see the *identical* set of figures for each identified publication. Dr. Rosa used the identical criteria for inclusion from the scientific literature (excluding 'cohorts without mention of birth defects, or those with less than 25 outcomes'). He even failed to pick up the case of rachischisis set forth in the Baron paper. The sample of 448 cases he refers to in Lancet ('12 additional cohorts with 25-49 outcomes') also come from Merrell's list (those not 'listed by Cornel, et al. 1989'). It would seem that Dr. Rosa should have acknowledged, at the very least, the true source of his data.

"For all of the above-stated reasons, the two sets of summaries identified above should have been disregarded by FDA, and the prior request for prospective and retrospective studies enforced.

"6. *Follow-up and Autopsy Studies.*

"On *June 4, 1969*, FDA requested Merrell Dow (then Richardson-Merrell, Inc.) to perform *follow-up examinations* on all living infants, conceived in association with Clomid therapy, for a period of at least *two years*. In the same correspondence, FDA also requested *autopsies* to be performed on all abortions, stillborns and neonatal deaths resulting from the same group of pregnancies. [See Exhibit 'MM'.] Thus, as early as 1969, FDA recognized at least two of the major deficiencies of the pre-market clinical studies, to wit: (1) Failure to conduct follow-up examinations of infants born following maternal ingestion of Clomid; and (2) An extremely low number of autopsies performed on stillborns and neonatal deaths. When Dr. Ortiz sent that letter, he knew that the data FDA was receiving from Merrell was not telling the full story in terms of potential risk to the fetus. On June 19, 1969, Merrell acknowledged the *feasibility* of doing the study, though complaining about the need [Exhibit 'NN'].

"Enclosed herewith find an Interdepartment Memo, dated July 14, 1969, related to a meeting between FDA and Merrell which took place on July 9, 1969 [Exhibit 'OO']. Of particular note is the reference with regard to recommendation number 2. Note the following:

'Be that as it may, Dr. Dill has an impression that we should want to be able to show that Clomid does not increase the abortion rate. His thought is that

335

chromosomal studies would clarify this point. It is well known, of course, that chromosomal aberrations are common in aborted human fetal material (XO aneuploidy, triploidy, tetraploidy, trisomics of Groups A, B, C, D, E, F and G, etc.). Dr. Dill thought that if Clomid-related abortuses proved to have a 10% higher rate of chromosomal aberrations than non-Clomid ones, this would be significant.'

These comments take on considerable significance when one considers the Boue paper published in Lancet in 1973 (four years later). In that study, there was a *40% higher rate* of chromosomal aberrations in patients using ovulatory stimulating drugs compared to non-users and users who conceived two or more cycles after last treatment. This study was also *statistically significant*. [Exhibit 'C' to correspondence of March 25, 1975 (Exhibit 'X').] In other words, at least in Dr. Dill's way of thinking, when the Boue study was presented to FDA prior to the hearing of July 18, 1975, this should have been considered *significant*. It is thus all the more mystifying why the FDA never would have pursued the recommended studies requested by Dr. Ortiz on June 4, 1969. In reality, Merrell never performed these recommended studies and, again, FDA dropped the ball. To date, 25 years later, these studies have yet to be performed.

"In conclusion, I would again ask: DOES ANYONE REALLY CARE? If so, given all of the above, it is urged that FDA finally do something to protect the public, and in particular the babies who are being delivered following their mother's use of fertility drugs. This is the FDA's obligation by law, and it is urged that this obligation be met as expeditiously as possible." [All emphasis in the original.]

Did anyone at the FDA really care? Perhaps, but I never received a response back from the FDA. This time there was no invitation to return to Rockville, Maryland – not even an acknowledgement of the submission. This time there would be no hearing, and no one at the FDA wanted to hear any more from Terry Mix.

Several years later I would learn that forces had already been set in motion to mold the labeling for Clomid and its generic, clomiphene citrate. Four and a half months before I had sent my letter, the FDA had requested Merrell to submit new labeling, incorporating a number of changes desired by the agency. The drug company's draft of the package insert was sent off on August 23, 1994, and thereafter approved on September 30, 1994.[270] Two weeks after Dr. Solomon Sobel sanctioned Merrell's proposed language, he received my package of accusations, criticisms and evidence (he no doubt already knew about). Although it would have been nice to envision Sobel running out of his office door with his hand elevated, screaming, "Hold the press! I wanna see what our friend in California has to say," the reality is that the language had already been chiseled in stone.

Not knowing what was going on behind the scenes, I could have made myself a pest again. But the evidence was so overwhelming and my presentation so inclusive that it did not seem warranted.

This assumption was a mistake I would later regret.

* * * * *

CHAPTER 17

The Federal Court of Science

Not only must a plaintiff prove that the ingested drug was capable of causing birth defects, it must also be proven that the drug caused *this* plaintiff's congenital anomalies. The difficulty is that any side effect that can be caused by a drug, including birth defects, can also be caused by other factors as well.

For example, there is now a concensus that Vioxx can cause heart attacks and strokes. But we also know that there are other risk factors for cardiovascular disease. Assume that a 58-year-old man suffered a fatal heart attack after using Vioxx, at high doses, for over a year and a half. But we also learn that he was overweight, a heavy smoker, did not exercize, and had a total cholesterol count of 285 a month before he died. Obviously, an autopsy might shed some light on the question. But what if it disclosed that he had a moderate degree of arteriosclerosis or that an autopsy had not even been performed? Even if a pathologist could examine the clot or clots that killed him, they would not contain markers unique to Vioxx. How would we know that it was the drug that took his life rather than his pre-existing health and lifestyle?

What if it was all of the above? What if it was a combination of his pre-existing physical condition and the use of the Vioxx? In some states they use the "but for" rule; but for the use of Vioxx, the man would not have suffered a fatal heart attack. In California, a plaintiff can prove his case if he can establish by a preponderance of the evidence that the use of the drug was a "substantial factor" in causing the injury or death.

With birth defects, there is usually an aspect of *genetic predisposition* that plays a role in whether a drug will produce a given anomaly in the embryo. Even with thalidomide, not every embryo that was exposed to the drug, during the critical window of gestation, developed phocomelia or some other congenital malformation. In other words, the hereditary composition of our genes can make us more *vulnerable* to an environmental insult while we are developing in the uterus. This is why one person will develop lung cancer after smoking a pack of cigarettes a day for ten years, while his next-door neighbor smoked three packs a day over 30 years without a similar consequence.

When a defense attorney would argue that my client had a family history of a similar (but not the same) or related birth defect, I would welcome the contention. It only meant that the plaintiff was *predisposed* to develop the congenital anomaly with the help of the defendant's drug. In my view, it was easier to convince the jury that the drug was a substantial factor in producing the anomaly. In California we say that "you take the plaintiff the way you find him." Being an "eggshell" plaintiff does not hurt the case, it helps it. If a victim of an auto accident bleeds to death because she was a hemophiliac, it is still a legitimate claim for wrongful death, even if the average person would have survived with a few sutures.

The issue of causation is thus a complex web of surrounding facts and factors. And when it comes to birth defects, there are a multitude of circumstances that need to be considered when assessing whether or not a drug was a substantial factor in producing the anomaly.

Another challenge, especially in federal court, is convincing the trial judge that the plaintiff's experts used the proper method of analysis in arriving at his or her conclusion. If the plaintiff cannot meet this preliminary test, the expert will be excluded and he will be unable to present sufficient evidence to have the case decided by a jury. This gives a judge tremendous power over the cases in front of him or her.

These issues contributed to the disaster of my eighth and final Clomid case.

On March 30, 1988, Alexander Lust had been born with right hemifacial microsomia, involving a complete absence of the right ear and auditory canal and an underdeveloped right mandible (lower jaw bone). His mother had ingested 100 mg. of Clomid on days 5 through 9 for six consecutive cycles prior to conception. Thus, due to the half-life factor, there would have been a substantial buildup of Clomid over the months. Conception had also occurred during a treatment cycle and she likely experienced OHSS at the time. An additional enticement was the fact that Alex's mother had delivered two other children – without the benefit of fertility drugs – and neither was born with congenital malformations. On the surface, the case was attractive.

On November 11, 1992, I sent off a retainer agreement to Alex's parents for signature and return. After three months of reviewing medical records and consulting with my experts, we filed a lawsuit in the Los Angeles Superior Court on February 2, 1993. Service immediately went out to Merrell. As I had in the Gandy case, I sought out another lawyer in my office to assist in prosecuting the lawsuit. This time it was Charles Sneathern, an attorney with whom I had shared office space for over ten years.

A Trip to Federal Court

On the morning of May 5, 1993, Charlie presented himself at the doorway to my office. I could see that he wasn't happy. "Bad news," he said, holding up the paperwork in his hand. "Merrell removed to federal court."

"They what!" I was absolutely shocked. Not only had Merrell never removed an eligible Clomid filing before, to my recollection Bob Dickson's firm had never removed a state court lawsuit to federal court on any other drug case that I had prosecuted against his firm. I had always presumed that they equally shared my disdain for the federal court system.

"You heard me right," said Charlie, as he entered and dropped into one of my client chairs.

"Shit! Never before, Charlie, never before."

"Well, they did it this time. And there's nothing we can do about it. They've got diversity and we've got a case stuck in federal court."

What Charlie was referring to was the fact that the plaintiffs were California residents and Merrell Dow Pharmaceuticals was an out-of-state corporation, thus creating "diversity." If we had named another defendant who was also a California resident, or local business entity, we could not have been removed from state to federal court. But we could not justify a malpractice action against the prescribing physician.

I pondered a moment, then nodded, "It's Bendectin, Charlie. Merrell's been kicking butt in federal court. Every time you hear of a plaintiff's verdict, the district court or circuit court of appeals takes it away."

"Doesn't sound good for us, does it?"

"Well, it may be a bit more of a challenge, but we have a good case. This is not Bendectin. We have published epidemiology studies in support. Who did we get?"

"Edward Rafeedie. He's a Reagan appointee. Conservative. Used to sit in state court in Santa Monica until he caught Reagan's eye. Don't know a plaintiff's lawyer that's been happy with him, but who knows."

340

I had never been in front of Rafeedie, but had also heard of his reputation for being conservative and pro-defense, at least while he was sitting with the Los Angeles Superior Court. Yet I had appeared before many conservative judges over the years, and they had not been all bad experiences. More critical in my mind was how much deference Rafeedie gave to jury verdicts. All I wanted was to get our case to a jury and to keep a good result. Many federal court judges seem to take delight in setting up an obstacle course to achieving that goal. Motions for summary judgment before trial, motions for nonsuit during trial, and post-trial motions for judgment notwithstanding the verdict were commonplace in front of federal district court judges only because of their high rate of success.

Throughout my entire career I had fought to stay out of federal court. Appointed for life,[271] the only way to remove a federal judge is through impeachment – and we all know what a difficult challenge that can be. Perhaps as a consequence, many have a reputation for being somewhat arrogant, impersonal, and at times outright dictatorial. The bench is their throne, and they generally leave little doubt who rules their little kingdom. They also run a much tighter ship than their counterparts in state courts. The federal court rules are not only different, but also more demanding, dictating extra work and a constant eye on the calendar to avoid missing a critical deadline. Federal civil trials are also in front of six-person juries and require a unanimous verdict. But the most onerous facet of appearing in the federal court system is that most district court judges seem to go out of their way to deny plaintiffs the right to have their cases decided by a jury.

By the summer of 1994 we were looking at a fall trial date. All interrogatories had been answered and depositions of the plaintiffs and treating doctors taken. By early fall, we had also taken the depositions of our expert witnesses and were putting the final touches on our trial preparation.

As previously mentioned, the biggest challenge of our case would be establishing that Clomid was the probable cause of Alex's specific anomaly. A jury might be convinced that Clomid was a human teratogen, but this would be of little value if they were not equally persuaded that it could likewise produce hemifacial microsomia. The burden of this challenge would fall squarely on the ample shoulders of Alan Kimball Done.

But would Alan Done be up to that task? This was the weakest link in our case. Through late 1994, *not one epidemiologic study had looked at Alexander Lust's specific anomaly*. Without studies demonstrating a statistically significant increase in this type of malformation, how does a teratologist establish a link between the ingestion of Clomid and a baby delivered with hemifacial microsomia? Done had his ideas on this issue, and was satisfied that they were valid and would be convincing to a jury. However, standing in his way would be an aggressive motion to exclude his testimony by Merrell and a very conservative district court judge ruling on the motion. Though unsuccessful, they had moved to exclude Done in Gandy, so there was every reason to believe it would be tried again. After all, this was federal court.

Alan K. Done, M.D.

Using Alan Done as our primary causation expert had its drawbacks. Between 1975 and 1983 he had been a professor of pediatrics and a professor of pharmacology at Wayne State University School of Medicine in Detroit, Michigan. During the same period, he was also an attending pediatrician at Children's Hospital of Michigan. But in late 1983, at the age of 57, he decided to move to Salt Lake City, Utah – where he had been born, raised and educated – and become a full-time consultant. There his consulting clients ranged from pharmaceutical companies to government offices to attorneys for litigation. But now, rather than seeing patients, he was seeing clients; rather than educating medical students and interns, he was educating juries; and rather than publishing papers in medical and scientific journals, he was writing medical-legal reports. Because of his effectiveness in front of juries, he was increasingly being used to testify in court. In short, whether by design or circumstance, he was becoming a professional witness.

From a lawyer's perspective, this was a mixed bag. It was comforting to know that your expert could handle himself on a witness stand. And being a forensic expert, in the minds of most jurors, is a reflection of his or her level of expertise. An expert witness is used frequently in court because of the quality of that expert's education, training and experience, and the ability to educate. Conversely, opposing attorneys and many judges see them simply as "hired guns," selling their opinions for excessive fees. For juries, such accusations can generally be overcome by establishing the quality of their credentials, the reasonableness of their billings, consistency in their opinions, and that they offer their services to both sides. Many judges, however, see them as nothing more than a witness with an opinion for sale. Although I was quite comfortable with selling a jury on Done's candor and objectivity, I was uncertain how Rafeedie would be affected by his status as a professional witness.

I would not have to wait much longer to find out.

As I had anticipated, Merrell filed a motion seeking to knock out Done as our principal witness on causation. The challenge of his qualifications as a teratology expert was of little concern, since he had overcome such attacks in over 40 earlier trials, including Gandy. The more serious contention would be on the issue of whether his scientific methodology (analytical method to arrive at his conclusions) met the legal standards set out by the United States Supreme Court in *Daubert vs. Merrell Dow Pharmaceuticals, Inc.* in 1993.[272] The hearing eventually took place on December 5, 1994.

On the scheduled date, Charlie and I appeared on behalf of the plaintiff, along with Alan Done. Consistent with my aversion to federal court, I had always seen the old building as a mausoleum – a burial ground for plaintiff's lawsuits – and the anxiety churning inside was a product of my concern that Rafeedie was going to add yet another headstone to that growing list. The fall trial date had been vacated, pending his ruling on the defendant's motion. Jefferey Carlson and Charles Messer appeared for Merrell, both from the firm of Dickson, Carlson & Campillo.

Rafeedie was quick to remind all present about the purpose of the hearing. The court would determine whether Done's reasoning and methodology on causation was scientifically valid, using the standards set forth by the Supreme Court in Daubert.

I then put Dr. Done on the stand and for the next couple of hours reviewed his education, training and experience covering the fields of teratology, endocrinology, pharmacology, toxicology and pediatrics; followed next by a recitation of his scientific methods for verifying that Clomid was a human teratogen. Included within his analysis were case reports, timing of dosage, epidemiological studies, animal teratology studies, animal in-vitro and in-vivo studies, mutagenicity studies, and an assessment of biological feasibility.[273]

Our next challenge was case-specific causation. If one lacks epidemiology studies that have looked at a rare birth defect, how does one arrive at a conclusion that it was probably caused by a given drug? There were a number of factors, assured Done.

First, he had found at least three case reports of hemifacial microsomia, reported in the literature, associated with the maternal use of Clomid. He thus knew that it was among the defects that *might* be caused by the drug. Second, because epidemiology studies had shown an increased risk in a wide variety of congenital anomalies, this would increase the likelihood that the spectrum could also include hemifacial microsomia, depending upon the timing of exposure of the drug. Third, when a drug is mutagenic, it is more likely to cause a wide spectrum of anomalies, which further increases the possibility that it would encompass the malformation suffered by Alexander Lust. Fourth, based upon an extensive review of the relevant medical records and the depositions of his parents, Done had been able to exclude all other known causes of birth defects as being responsible for Alex's anomalies. Fifth, at the time Alex was developing hemifacial microsomia, Clomid – a human teratogen – was present in the embryonic circulation. And sixth, since Alex's anomalies involved the first and second branchial arches, and his father had a minor joint anomaly involving the same branchial arches, this would suggest that Alex had a genetic predisposition toward developing the malformation upon exposure to a human teratogen. Based upon all of these factors, Done was of the opinion that it was probable that Clomid was the principal cause of the plaintff's malformations.

All attorneys and Dr. Done returned the following morning, at which time Jeff Carlson cross-examined the witness. He then called Eugene Hoyme, M.D., to challenge some of the testimony expressed by Dr. Done. After my cross-examination, the hearing concluded. The parties had until December 12, 1994 to submit post-hearing briefs, after which the matter would be submitted for decision.

Rafeedie's Decision

My secretary, Debbie Nawa, would routinely open my mail every day and then place it on my desk by mid-morning. On February 16, 1995, she entered my office with an unusual pout on her face and announced, "You're not going to like this." She handed me the stack of mail with Rafeedie's order prominently on top. "Looks like he granted their motion to exclude Dr. Done."

I picked the order off the top of the stack and angrily exploded to no one in particular, "Damn it! That goddamn Rafeedie. Federal court, I hate it!"

Debbie quietly closed my door while I read the opinion, dissecting each statement, which in my view ran contrary to the facts and the law. Numerous misstatements about the testimony were made throughout the decision. Finally I snapped and flung the opinion across the room. But for the fact that Debbie had stapled the nine pages of the order together, they would have decorated my office couch like large pieces of confetti. For a good five minutes I just stared at the packet, which was sitting upside down and propped up against a decorative throw-pillow. There it sat – taunting – reminding me how my own professional world had likewise been set on its ear.

Five days later, I was standing in front of Rafeedie at the mausoleum. He had called the attorneys in to decide on the next step. When I was invited to speak, I used the opportunity to raise a critical issue. The judge's decision had made numerous references to a recent decision by the Ninth Circuit Court of Appeals, filed on January 5, 1995.[274] That decision had been rendered *after* our hearing and the post-trial briefs. I wanted an opportunity to address the issues raised in the new decision and to offer additional testimony from Dr. Done. With the concurrence of counsel, Rafeedie decided that the most effective approach would be for Merrell to pursue a motion for summary judgment (which it had recently filed). He then directed his comments straight at me.

"Now, in your response to the motion, and in your opposition, you can have your witness supplement his testimony. That business that you didn't know about this case, and therefore, the witness can now change his testimony to conform to the case is hardly inspiring. The case of Daubert is a 1993 case. And the testimony that your witness gave was in light of Daubert. In fact, it was a hearing mandated by Daubert in order to determine his qualifications to testify. The Daubert case sets forth what is required. The Supreme Court has said what is required. All this Ninth Circuit did was further apply the Supreme Court case in a particular fact situation."

These were curious comments coming from the district court judge, given that every citation and reference to Daubert in his order related to the 1995 Ninth Circuit opinion, not the Supreme Court's. The Ninth Circuit may have been applying the 1993 standards to qualify an expert witness, but its decision *included specific criteria not mentioned by the Supreme Court.* My initial inclination was to bring out these points to Rafeedie, but he had already extended the opportunity to supplement Done's testimony (through a declaration under oath). I was also convinced they would fall on deaf ears and a closed mind.

Our only hope with Rafeedie was to not only supplement what Done had previously testified to, but present a scientific work of art.

The Motion for Summary Judgment

On March 20, 1995, I was back again in the mausoleum and appeared in front of our district court judge to argue the motion for summary judgment. Charlie remained at the office, as I saw no purpose for his presence at the hearing. The court called our case and we announced our appearances. Jeff Carlson and Charles Messer again answered on behalf of Merrell. In addition to our legal points and authorities, I had filed and served an extensive declaration from Dr. Done, setting out his scientific methodology and analysis, consistent with the refinements mandated by the Ninth Circuit.

Eager to administer the coup de gras, Rafeedie wasted little time in announcing his intentions. "This is a renewal of the defendant's motion for summary judgment. And the basis of it, of course, is that the court in its 104 hearing determined that the plaintiff's expert witness was not qualified under Daubert to testify on the issue of causation. The issue of causation is a required element in each of the claims made by the plaintiff in this case. The plaintiff, therefore, has an element missing on which there is no triable issue of fact. It would, therefore, appear...and the Court is not prone to reconsider its decision as has been suggested here by the plaintiffs regarding the Court's ruling on Dr. Done's qualifications and the admissibility of his testimony. Therefore, it would seem to me that the defendants are entitled to summary judgment because you have no proof of causation."

There it was. Rafeedie was refusing to reconsider his original decision, even though he had invited me to supplement Done's testimony. But I was not about to throw in the towel. "Your honor, I would agree. If your honor is going to exclude the opinion testimony of Dr. Done on the basis that he did not..."

"I already ruled that his testimony would be excluded," interrupted the judge. "It does not meet the requirements of the Daubert case."

"Your honor also indicated on February twenty-second that the plaintiff would be allowed to submit further declaration testimony from Dr. Done, which your honor would look at, I presumed in the context of reconsideration of the evidence. We have submitted a forty-page declaration from Dr. Done..."

"That does not change the Court's ruling," Rafeedie again interrupted.

"Is your honor inclined to hear any argument from me on this point?"

"Not really, Counsel. I think we've heard a lot of argument already. We've had a hearing that lasted a couple days. We have had extensive briefing. I don't know what more there is to be said."

Here I was again, hammering my head against the wall. Yet I was not about to give in. "Well, as I have indicated before, your honor, the order that you issued on February 14, 1995, cited extensively the Ninth Circuit opinion of Daubert filed by the Court on January 5, 1995. That opinion came out approximately a month *after* the hearing."

"Counsel, that's not a very good argument," responded Rafeedie. "You made that in your papers. First of all, it didn't do anything except apply the Supreme Court's Daubert decision. I don't know what it is that you would do. This didn't change the law. It simply applied the Supreme Court's decision."

"Well, first of all, the Daubert decision, as I understand, is not final. There has been a petition for rehearing filed."

"The Supreme Court's decision is final," countered the judge.

"The Ninth Circuit," I again reminded.

"We are relying on the *Supreme Court's* decision in the case. My ruling was made, I think, with that in mind, the Supreme Court decision, not the Ninth Circuit decision – that just happened to come out during the time period."

Not only was I pounding my head against the wall, I was apparently talking to it as well. Nothing seemed to be penetrating. Whereas the Supreme Court laid out some general guidelines, the Ninth Circuit set out several requirements that had never been mentioned by the Supremes in 1993. "Your honor has cited the Ninth Circuit opinion extensively in your order," I asserted.

"Because it simply supported the view that we took of the Supreme Court's decision. What is your point?"

"My point is, your honor…"

"You didn't have a chance to discuss the case?"

"That is correct, your honor. I did not have a chance to argue…"

"What would you argue that would make a difference, because that case certainly does not help you in the slightest?"

"I would have pointed out, your honor, as I attempted to do in my opposition papers, that the facts in that case were very distinguishable when compared to the case presently before the bench. That with Bendectin, for example, there were no epidemiology studies. In the situation involving Clomid, there are extensive epidemiology studies published in peer-reviewed publications indicating that there is a significant increased risk, statistically, using all the methodology used by teratologists, which support Dr. Done's opinion. We have also…"

"I haven't said so, but frankly, I think Dr. Done and his testimony is the very type of evidence that the Supreme Court was intending to keep out of these courts. It is the view of the Court, that his evidence and his testimony are designed for this case. *It conforms to the prevalent view in California that harm or injury plus expert witness equals liability.* It is the type of thing that the Supreme Court was trying to keep out of the courts, and it simply is not reliable scientific evidence. We've stated the reasons for it. And I don't think that anything would change the Court's view on that."

Evidently not. There it was, the Court's bias laid wide open. The "prevalent view in California" was that all a plaintiff needed to establish liability was harm or injury and an expert witness. Got an injury? Hey, come with me to the expert shopping mall and I'll make your case. Forget the merits. As long as I have a big enough checking account, I'll sell your case and we'll make millions. Welcome to Edward Rafeedie's view of the world. Done is a professional witness, isn't he? So out he goes. Sure he had his reasons, but so does every con man. Don't want to be sucked in with his scientific double talk? Simple. Just don't listen to him – or his attorney.

"Your honor," I pleaded, "as Dr. Done's declaration pointed out, he formulated his opinion as to whether or not Clomid was a human teratogen long before he had any connection with me or any other lawyer on Clomid. He published his opinion in that regard. In fact, I have a copy of his article here published in 1983, years before he was ever contacted by any lawyer to render an opinion on Clomid. So Dr. Done did formulate his opinion…"

"You are simply repeating what you have already said in your papers, and I have considered that." Rafeedie was now as resolute as a rock.

"All right," I weakly uttered.

"So the Court grants summary judgment."

It was now evident that Rafeedie had never read the declaration. He was so intent on dumping Alan Done, he apparently saw no point in reviewing and analyzing his forty-page declaration. Because if he had, he would have been faced with the monumental task of discrediting what amounted to a scientific treatise. The easy way out was to refer to the testimony at the 104(a) hearing and ignore the declaration of March 2, 1995 – a declaration that had been prepared to address the expanded standards set forth in the Ninth Circuit Daubert decision of January 5, 1995 that *did not exist at the time of the earlier hearing.* At this point our only hope was an appeal.

But would we have any better luck with the Ninth Circuit?

When the U.S. Supreme Court rendered the Daubert decision on June 28, 1993, it *overturned* an earlier Ninth Circuit decision on the same case which had upheld the granting of a summary judgment against the plaintiff by the trial court. The trial judge and the Ninth Circuit Court of Appeals had both applied an old and restrictive standard on the admissibility of scientific opinions and disallowed all of plaintiffs' expert testimony. The Supreme Court, however, said that they were both wrong. It invalidated the source of their rulings[275] which had held that scientific evidence was only admissible if it was based on a scientific technique *generally accepted* as reliable within the scientific community. The court held that this old standard had been replaced by the more recent Federal Rules of Evidence,[276] and that general acceptance among the scientific community was no longer necessary.

Justice Blackmun delivered the majority opinion for the higher court. Although indicating that the list was not definitive, the standards he set out for qualifying expert scientific opinions were (1) whether the reasoning or scientific methodology could be and had been tested; (2) whether the reasoning or methodology had been subjected to peer review and publication;[277] (3) whether there were standards controlling a known or potential rate of error; and (4) although not required, whether there had been general acceptance by a relevant scientific community.

The upper court remanded (returned) the case "for further proceedings consistent with (the) opinion." Since the Supreme Court had apparently *liberalized* the standards for qualifying an expert for testimony,[278] it was assumed by many that the case would be returned to the federal trial judge for "further proceedings" and the plaintiffs given an opportunity to qualify their experts under these new standards. But the Ninth Circuit was not about to let this one get away. Rather than forwarding the lawsuit on to the trial judge, it *kept* the Daubert case and rendered still another opinion, giving its own spin on the new Supreme Court decision. It was not about to let the Supremes interfere with its desired ruling in the case.

On January 5, 1995, the U.S. Ninth Circuit Court of Appeals entered the scientific field of teratology and published its standards on how to determine whether a drug is a human teratogen. Ignoring the protestations of plaintiffs' counsel, and to the great delight of Merrell – and the rest of the pharmaceutical industry – the appellate court set out the "scientific method" by which it can be determined whether a drug was the cause of the birth defects in a specific case (case-specific causation).

The two minor plaintiffs contended that their limb reduction defects were caused by their mothers' ingestion of Bendectin. The plaintiffs had previously submitted in-vivo and in-vitro animal studies, analysis of the chemical structure and a reanalysis of earlier published epidemiology studies in support of their claim that Bendectin was the cause of the congenital anomalies. The Ninth Circuit *again* affirmed (approved) the trial court's order excluding the expert opinions and granting the motion for summary judgment.

Proudly proclaiming that federal judges had been assigned the role of "gatekeeper" by the Supreme Court, Justice Kozinski proceeded to set up the Ninth Circuit's obstacle course for any plaintiff seeking to qualify an expert to render a scientific opinion.[279]

Obstacle Number One. The Ninth Circuit instructed that the trial courts should consider "whether the experts are proposing to testify about matters growing naturally and directly out of research they have conducted independent of the litigation, or whether they have developed their opinions expressly for the purpose of testifying." The court's concern was that an expert's scientific methods to arrive at a conclusion would be influenced by his or her *possible bias* due to the compensation to be received for the research and testifying.[280] The apparent goal of this requirement was to avoid a party "buying" a desired conclusion from a retained expert witness.

The criticisms of this criterion are many. It reflects not only the Ninth Circuit's naivete of what goes on in the pharmaceutical industry, but the court's own bias against plaintiffs seeking compensation from members of that industry. It presupposes that research independent of litigation is essentially free of bias, when in fact it is frequently burdened by the very problem the court is purporting to solve. Scientific research of pharmaceutical products is either dependent upon funding from the manufacturers of those products or grants from institutions (i.e., National Institutes of Health, universities, etc.). Few scientists fund studies out of their own pockets, and the source of funding can provide an enticement of its own to reach a desired result.

The Clomid clinical investigations were conducted independent of litigation, but even under the purported oversight of the FDA it provided little of the "scientific method" the court was arguably after. The design of such studies are not only first approved or established by the drug company, but compiled, analyzed and reported on by an entity with a financial motive far stronger than any plaintiff's expert in a lawsuit. Prior to marketing, Merrell had spent close to a decade and tens of millions of dollars in research to produce a fertility drug which could only justify that investment with FDA approval. Recall that employees of Merrell were criminally prosecuted for falsifying records related to its drug, Triparanol. Can there be any question that it might be a little biased in favor of a study giving its drug a clean bill of health? Should not an expert opinion based upon a study sponsored by the drug company likewise be subject to possible exclusion?

Following marketing, it is common practice among pharmaceutical companies to supply grants for studies on its drug products. In order to successfully apply for such a grant, a study design must be approved by the company. Then before the study is published, drafts of the paper are submitted to the manufacturer for feedback, including any criticisms.[281] Even when the company only supplies the drug for the study, it is understood that it will get a "first look" before publication. Such input can potentially influence the final conclusions of the study. If a study by such a grantee were to trash a drug because of its severe side effects, it is not likely that the researcher would be seeing much grant money for any future studies – at least from the drug's manufacturer.[282] Indeed, it is not unusual to find such a researcher on occasion acting also as a "consultant" for the company. Travel expenses and other perks are frequently picked up by the drug company for researchers to speak on the benefits of a drug at a seminar or symposium. Should opinions based upon studies involving drugs conducted pursuant to grants from their manufacturers be subject to possible exclusion as well?

Even when a drug is being studied under a grant from a public or private institution, there still exists the potential for bias. Many times the researcher has a vested interest in the outcome of a study. For example, the vast majority of clinical investigators in the Clomid pre-market study were fertility specialists. The principal objective of their specialty was to get women pregnant, and Clomid offered them another tool of their profession to bring in patients – if it could in fact make women ovulate and conceive. Thus, although studying the efficacy of the drug was of vital concern, anything that might impede possible approval of the drug or deter potential users, such as a capability for producing birth defects, might be quite undesirable. This is why Edward Tyler was willing to accept birth announcements and letters from his patients to verify that they had delivered normal infants.[283] But it was not because Tyler and the other physicians were indifferent to whether Clomid might cause birth defects. It was because of their inherent bias that predisposed them to believing that such a possibility was so remote as to not be a concern. It is for this very reason that *double blind* epidemiology studies were designed; studies in which neither the investigator nor the subject patients are aware of whether he or she is using the studied drug or the placebo until conclusion of the study.

Since only double blind studies are insulated against such bias, should all others be considered off limits and subject opinions based upon them to exclusion simply because they may be influenced by bias? Of course not. Historically and traditionally – at least in the state courts – the issue of bias has never been grounds for excluding an expert's conclusion, nor for that matter any other testimony a witness might be prepared to give. That has always been dealt with by cross-examination and the presentation of contrary evidence.[284] The issue of bias has always gone to the *weight* to be given to such evidence, not to its *admissibility*. Just because an expert *might* be influenced by bias, does not mean that he or she has actually succumbed to it. A further criticism is that this criterion does not even assess the actual methodology used. Even if an expert used a methodology generally accepted in the scientific community, he would still be branded as biased if he originated his work for purposes of litigation. Yet notwithstanding all of the above, the Ninth Circuit will call "strike one" should a study be conducted for the purpose of testimony.

Obstacle Number Two. "If the proffered expert testimony is not based on independent research, the party proffering it must come forward with other objective, verifiable evidence that the testimony is based on 'scientifically valid principles.' One means of showing this is by proof that the research and analysis supporting the proffered conclusions have been subjected to normal scientific scrutiny through peer review and publication." In other words, if the expert's research and analysis was specifically for the purpose of testifying, then he or she must next show that the work was submitted for publication and subjected to the peer review process.

The problem is that the methodology for assessing whether a drug is a human teratogen encompasses more than one field of study. Epidemiology, although important, is by no means the only discipline used to make that assessment. Animal teratology, animal in-vitro and in-vivo studies, chemical analysis, half-life studies, and mutagenicity studies all enter into the mix – along with epidemiology studies – to arrive at a conclusion about human teratogenicity. Those assessing the risk of birth defects rarely rely exclusively on their own study to arrive at a conclusion; they invariably refer as well to other published studies conducted in their own field, not to mention those in other scientific specialties. Inevitably *all* experts must rely upon published studies conducted by others to conclude whether a drug is a teratogen. So if an expert is conducting research to testify in litigation, how is he or she to qualify under the second criterion, even if the results of his or her study are published? The result of that single study cannot stand on its own – it will rarely be a sufficient basis by itself to render a conclusion that a drug causes birth defects in humans. Even an epidemiologist would not conclude, on the basis of one study showing a statistically significant association between a drug and birth defects, that a drug is a human teratogen. A "strike two" would be inescapable.

Obstacle Number Three. "Establishing that an expert's proffered testimony grows out of pre-litigation research or that the expert's research has been subjected to peer review are the two principal ways the proponent of expert testimony can show that the evidence satisfies the first prong of Rule 702. Where such evidence is *unavailable*, the proponent of expert scientific testimony may attempt to satisfy its burden through the testimony of its own experts. For such a showing to be sufficient, the experts must *explain precisely how they went about reaching their conclusions and point to some objective source* – a learned treatise, the policy statement of a professional association, a published article in a reputable scientific journal or the like – *to show that they followed the scientific method, as it is practiced by (at least) a recognized minority of scientists in their field.*" [Emphasis added.]

Failing this criterion it is "strike three" and the expert is gone. But given the Supreme Court decision on *Daubert*, this would seem to be a reasonable expectation to qualify an expert witness. In fact, it should be the *only* condition needed to be met to solicit a conclusion from an expert witness in a federal civil case. Just because an expert conducted his study and analysis independent of litigation, does not mean he or she followed the "scientific method." And having published a study in a peer-reviewed journal would rarely provide a sufficient basis to arrive at an opinion on human teratogenicity. But very few plaintiffs' counsel would complain about the imposition of the above standard – if it applied equally to defendants and *the Ninth Circuit would only abide by it.*

The opinion readily agrees that if the only issue was whether or not Bendectin was a human teratogen, then justice would dictate that the case be remanded back to the trial court to provide plaintiffs with the opportunity to meet the conditions set out by the Supreme Court and the Ninth Circuit Court of Appeals.[285] But when it came down to the question of *case-specific causation*, the three jurists were of a different mindset. The reason? Because according to that appellate court the *only* way the plaintiffs could prove that Bendectin was the cause of plaintiffs' specific limb reduction birth defects was through epidemiological studies demonstrating a statistically significant increase of those specific anomalies by more than 100% (that exposure to Bendectin during pregnancy was associated with a relative risk or odds ratio of more than 2.0). "In terms of statistical proof, this means that plaintiffs must establish not just that their mothers' ingestion of Bendectin increased somewhat the likelihood of birth defects, but that it more than doubled it – *only then can it be said that Bendectin is more likely than not the source of their injury*. Because the background rate of limb reduction defects is one per thousand births, plaintiffs *must show* that among children of mothers who took Bendectin the incidence of such defects was more than two per thousand."[286] [Emphasis added.]

Since the incidence of limb reduction defects among mothers ingesting Bendectin, as previously testified to by plaintiffs' experts, was less than two per thousand, the Ninth Circuit deemed that the plaintiffs could never meet their burden of proof that Bendectin was the *probable* cause of their defects, and that it would serve no purpose to remand the case back to the trial court to allow plaintiffs the opportunity to meet the new Daubert standards for "scientific methodology." Although the court recognized that there could be factors contributing to proof of causation other than relative risk in an epidemiology study, it still blindly assumed that it must come down to a statistical number.[287]

Aside from the question of statistics, there can be many facts unique to the case that can lead an expert to conclude that a given drug is the *probable* cause of the congenital anomalies. Once an expert concludes (from epidemiology studies, animal teratology studies, and all other factors enumerated above) that a drug is a human teratogen, he or she then takes a critical look at those facts. *Timing of exposure* can not only be a factor in disqualifying a drug as the cause, it can also be a highly persuasive element in convincing one of a causal association. Many epidemiology studies only look at drug exposures during pregnancy, or during the first trimester, but rarely report on exposures during the narrow window of time needed to produce the specific anomalies under study (i.e., limb reduction defects). If one concludes that a human teratogen – based upon animal teratology, in-vitro and in-vivo studies, and perhaps epidemiology studies – can only produce the anomaly if exposure occurred during a 5 day period (i.e., days 23 through 27), it might be very convincing if the drug exposure occurred during that period of time. When one can also *eliminate all other known causes* of the congenital anomaly, such as heredity, radiation, other drugs, maternal illness, trauma, and other known causes of birth defects, such individual factors can potentially convince an expert that the drug is more likely than not the cause of the malformation, even though the epidemiology studies demonstrated, for example, a statistically significant increase of 60% (a relative risk of only 1.60). It is reminded that thalidomide was determined to be a human teratogen, *not by epidemiology studies*, but my case reports. When Lenz (in Germany) and McBride (in Australia) saw a flood of cases of a rare congenital anomaly (phocomelia), their independent investigations found thalidomide to be the common denominator. The point is that there are other ways used to arrive at a conclusion of whether or not a drug, or other environmental event, is a human teratogen.

The Ninth Circuit refused, however, to give little deference to an expert's trained ability to assess the level of risk posed by a drug capable of deforming a human embryo. By insisting that the only way an expert could reach such a conclusion was through an epidemiology study with a relative risk above 2.0, it not only imposed its lay view into a field of science, it at the same time rejected a standard set out in its own decision. Rather than sending the case back down to the trial court with instructions to allow the plaintiffs an opportunity to: (1) explain precisely how they could conclude that Bendectin was a probable cause of the plaintiffs' limb reduction defects, and (2) point to an objective source supporting their scientific method, the appellate court chose to end the case and effectively deny the minor plaintiffs' right to a jury trial.

No, I was not optimistic that I would fair any better than the Daubert plaintiffs.

Unless I could alter the Lust decision on appeal, the impact would be felt by every other Clomid victim that could not avoid federal court. It is true that an appellate decision upholding the district court rulings would carry more weight. But even if we did not take the case up to the Ninth Circuit, Merrell's attorneys would be reminding every federal trial judge throughout the United States of the Lust rulings, seeking to have them follow suit. Mix put on his entire case through his expert and still couldn't meet the minimum standards to get an opinion on causation. They no doubt would even parade Done's forty-page declaration in front of each judge, arguing that it was ruled inadequate to establish the proper "scientific method," notwithstanding my view that Rafeedie failed to give it the slightest consideration.

Another factor of dubious value, but inherent in the ultimate decision to appeal, related to a character trait of yours truly. Bulldog Mix was never quick to cave in on *any* case. While this had its distinct advantages at times, this never-say-die attitude was frequently not tempered with reason – and rightly described by those close to me as nothing more than utter stubbornness. Always a fighter to the end, the destiny of the case to end up on appeal was no doubt determined the very moment Rafeedie announced, "So the Court grants summary judgment."

Within 30 days of Rafeedie's ruling we had filed our Notice of Appeal, and by August 1, 1995, all appellate briefs had been filed by both sides. Oral argument before the three justices to decide the case was not heard until June 3, 1996.

Out of an abundance of caution, I had determined that it would be preferable to have an experienced appellate attorney argue the case. Since I had only prosecuted an occasional appeal over the years, I was somewhat out of my comfort zone when standing in front of an appellate court arguing the esoteric spin on a particular rule of law. Whereas I could warm up to just about any jury, the sterile and formal atmosphere of an appellate courtroom precipitated enough anxiety to bring into question my sanity for not long ago passing this off to others more experienced in the forum. An added consideration was that this was a *federal* appellate court. Only once before had I appeared in front of the Ninth Circuit, and that had been over ten years earlier. Besides, our briefs had been thorough and hit every point we wanted to make.

After placing a few phone calls around town, I had secured a seasoned appellate attorney to argue the case. On the appointed date, Coleen Gillespie appeared before the Ninth Circuit and gave it our best shot. The report back was that with only ten minutes of argument per side, the court was a difficult read. Sometimes the questions posed by a justice can give insight into his or her view about the case. But there were very few questions and none of them turned on any lights. We would simply have to wait for the decision.

The Ninth Circuit Decision

July 11, 1996, was a very dark day in the history of Mix verses Merrell. On that date the Ninth Circuit Court of Appeals affirmed (upheld) Rafeedie's exclusion of Done as a witness and his subsequent granting of Merrell's summary judgment motion.

Though somewhat expected, I was crushed. What was especially devastating was the Ninth Circuit's disregard and misinterpretation of the evidence presented to it on the issue of Done's scientific analysis. As with Rafeedie, all of my efforts to communicate the true state of the record had apparently fallen on deaf ears and blind eyes. Upon completion of my review of the appellate opinion written by Justice Jerome Ferris, it was quite evident that the Ninth Circuit had done nothing more than hastily rubber stamp Rafeedie's rulings. I was in a state of utter frustration, and my only outlet – until now – was to fire off a petition for rehearing to the same appellate tribunal. I had little hope that it would have any impact, but it certainly helped to vent my displeasure and the reasons for it. The full text[288] of that petition follows.

"In addition to the *testimony* presented by Dr. Done at the FRE 104(a) hearing, plaintiff also submitted for the District Court's consideration a *40-page declaration* from said expert witness. This written testimony was allowed by the Trial Court, and it was considered by it before reaching its final decision. After a careful analysis of the Circuit Court's opinion of July 11, 1996, it would appear that this Court has made significant and material misinterpretations of Dr. Done's testimony, and may have overlooked his declaration entirely.

"Professional Witness.

"In the decision of <u>Daubert vs. Merrell Dow Pharmaceuticals, Inc.</u>, this Court held that '(e)stablishing that an expert's proffered testimony grows out of pre-litigation research *or* that the expert's research has been subjected to peer review are the *two* principal ways the proponent of expert testimony can show that the evidence satisfies the first prong of Rule 702.' [Emphasis added.] In other words, the proponent of the expert testimony can establish that such evidence reflects 'scientific knowledge,' that the findings of the expert were 'derived by the scientific method,' and that his work product amounts to 'good science,' if *either* his opinions grew out of 'pre-litigation research' or that the research was subjected to peer review. Further, only when such evidence is 'unavailable' must the proponent then 'explain precisely how (he) went about reaching (his) conclusions and point to some objective source…to show that (he has) followed the scientific method, as it is practiced by (at least) a recognized minority of scientists in (his) field.'

"Although plaintiff conceded that Dr. Done's research was not subjected to peer review, *it is strongly contended that he developed his opinions on Clomid by way of pre-litigation research.* It is on this issue that the Court made its first material misinterpretation of the evidence offered by Dr. Done. This is reflected by the following:

'We begin our inquiry by determining whether Dr. Done's research satisfied the applicable guarantees of reliability. Lust does not contend that Done subjected any of his research to peer review, but he does contend that Done developed his opinions on Clomid outside the litigation context. We reject the argument. Although Done published the 1984[289] article prior to this litigation, he was at that time *already a professional plaintiff's witness.* It is not unreasonable to *presume* that Done's opinion on Clomid was *influenced by a litigation driven financial incentive.*' [Emphasis added.]

This interpretation of the evidentiary record is *totally and materially in error*, and is not supported by any evidence before this Court. Dr. Done was not a 'professional plaintiff's witness,' either when he conducted his initial research on Clomid or when he published his articles listing it as a human teratogen. When asked about the date of publication at the 104(a) hearing, he expressed *uncertainty*, stating 'I believe it was 1984, but I'm not sure.' He also acknowledged that there were two separate publications. In his declaration he clarified that the dates were 'approximately 1981 and again in 1983.' From *1975 to 1983*, Dr. Done was a *full professor of pediatrics and pharmacology* at Wayne State University in Detroit, Michigan. In fact, he was the *founder and Director of the Division of Clinical Pharmacology and Toxicology at Children's Hospital*, and remained in this position until 1983. During this same period of time he taught medical students, interns and even graduate physicians about birth defects and their causes, and attended pediatric patients in said hospital, including those with birth defects. Dr. Done did not leave academia and become a full time consultant until 1983.[290]

"This entire issue was addressed by Dr. Done in his declaration of March 2, 1995, to wit:

'I also understand that the Court is of the opinion that I developed my conclusions concerning the teratogenicity of CLOMID specifically for the purpose of testifying in court. If this is the Court's understanding, it is in error. I initially became concerned about possible risks for birth defects associated with the use of CLOMID when I was conducting research at FDA in the late 1970s with regard to Bendectin. At the time, I was reviewing all of the Drug Experience Reports on congenital malformations in association with all drugs, and observed that CLOMID, by a 25% margin, was the drug most commonly associated with reported birth defects. Although I had been retained by counsel to do research concerning Bendectin, I had never been retained or even contacted by counsel with regard to CLOMID. In fact, it was not until approximately five years later that I was ever asked by an attorney to render an opinion concerning CLOMID. Because my review of DERs prompted me to suspect that CLOMID might be a human teratogen, I thereafter reviewed the existing medical literature concerning animal and human epidemiologic studies on the drug existing at the time. My analysis of that material followed the same methodology and analysis set forth below. On the basis of this review of the literature, I came to the conclusion that CLOMID was a probable human teratogen. *This literature search and analysis had absolutely nothing to do with litigation or attorneys; it was done as part of my educational process as a pediatrician and pharmacologist.* At the time, I was a professor of pediatrics and pharmacology at Wayne State University in Detroit, Michigan, and was a clinician as well. *Since I was an educator that taught principles of teratology to physicians*, I determined that it would be important to educate myself concerning the teratogenic potential of this drug. In approximately 1981, and again in 1983, I published a list of drugs which were in my opinion human teratogens, and included Clomiphene Citrate in that list. The publication was 'Emergency Medicine,' and it was *read by the medical community*, and to the best of my knowledge was *never distributed to attorneys.* Although my article was not peer-reviewed, *my intent on publishing the list was to educate physicians and not to derive business from attorneys.* In summary, following the reasoning and methodology outlined below, I came to the conclusion that CLOMID was a human teratogen long before an attorney ever asked me to express such an opinion in a courtroom.' [Emphasis added.]

There is nothing within the testimony given at the 104(a) hearing that in any way contradicts the above statement from Dr. Done's declaration. Although one might want to term Dr. Done as a 'professional witness' *after* leaving Wayne State in *1983*, to brand him with such a designation at the time of his research and later publications is *grossly unfair*, both to Dr. Done and to the plaintiff herein. Researching another drug (Bendectin), for attorneys representing some plaintiffs, did not make him any more of a 'professional witness' than Dr. Hoyme, when he agreed to be an expert for defendant in this case.

"The uncontradicted evidence before this Court is that Dr. Done's proferred testimony grew 'out of pre-litigation research,' and plaintiff thus was not required to explain precisely how Dr. Done went about reaching his conclusions nor to point to some objective source showing that he followed the scientific method recognized by a minority of scientists in the field.

"Chief Premise.

"This Court also concluded that Dr. Done failed to explain precisely how he went about reaching his conclusions and to point to an 'objective source demonstrating that his method and premises were generally accepted by or espoused by a recognized minority of teratologists.' Justice Farris explained the Court's finding as follows:

'Despite his claim that he relied on a generally accepted method, Done's *chief premise* was that if there is evidence of a positive association between an agent and a wide variety of birth defects in human epidemiological and animal studies, then the agent *substantially increases the probability* of *all* types of birth defects. Merrell Dow's expert testified to the effect that this premise is not espoused by a relevant minority of teratologists, and the articles Done submitted do not suggest otherwise.' [Emphasis added.]

This reference apparently comes from an earlier statement in the same opinion that 'Done responded by *pointing to some articles* that, he argued, supported his *premise* that a positive association between an agent and a wide variety of birth defects establishes that the agent substantially increases the probability of all types of birth defects.' [Emphasis added.]

"Dr. Done never stated that the above quote was the *chief premise* upon which he concluded that Clomid was the probable cause of plaintiff's birth defects. His only comment in the entire record, even touching this question, was his statement that 'a' basis of his opinion in this case was that several studies had shown a 'statistically significant increase in a number of other types of malformations in addition to neural tube defects.' He then added, 'since it is my opinion that Clomid is the known specific drug capable of causing *all kinds* of birth defects, depending upon the timing, *it should be able* to include this specific defect.' [Emphasis added.] Significantly, he did not state that this was the *chief premise* or basis or the principal or predominant one – only 'a' basis for his opinion. In fact, he provided *a substantial number of other reasons* to support his opinion that Clomid was a probable cause of the plaintiff's birth defects. These additional bases included (1) elimination of other possible causes for the anomalies, including other drugs, x-rays, maternal illness, alcohol, tobacco and heredity; (2) whether or not it was biologically feasible; (3) the timing of the exposure; (4) whether or not there was genetic susceptibility to this specific defect; and (5) an assessment of the individual case reports reported in the literature.

"Since this hearing preceded the <u>Daubert</u> Ninth Circuit opinion (decided January 5, 1995), plaintiff did not attempt to cite authorities for these approaches or methodologies. However, these methodologies were *explained in detail* and *cited extensively* in Dr. Done's declaration of March 2, 1995, after the District Court allowed plaintiff's expert to 'supplement his testimony.'

"With direction from the Ninth Circuit that, under certain specified circumstances, the expert was required to 'precisely' explain his methodologies and cite 'a published article in a reputable journal' to demonstrate that the methodologies were practiced by 'a recognized minority of scientists in the field,' the declaration of March 2, 1995 was prepared and submitted.

"Dr. Done explained that his approach was to *first determine whether or not Clomid was a human teratogen* (general causation) and then assess whether or not it was a cause of plaintiff's congenital anomalies (case specific causation). Although the declaration substantially expands on – and even supplements – the bases given in oral testimony, *there is nothing in the declaration that conflicts with or contradicts his 104(a) testimony.*

"Concerning *general causation*, Dr. Done identified the following factors used in his methodology:

'(1) Whether or not the *timing* of the exposure is appropriate to have caused the congenital anomaly or anomalies under consideration; (2) the results of *animal teratology studies*; (3) the results of *animal in-vivo and in-vitro studies*; (4) whether the *chemical structure* is similar to another drug generally accepted as a known human teratogen; (5) whether the drug under consideration is *mutagenic*; (6) the results of *human epidemiology studies*; and (7) whether or not it is *biologically plausible* for the drug to be causing the congenital anomaly or anomalies under consideration.

He then went on to not only detail 'how he went about reaching his conclusions' for each identified criterion, he also cited the *authority* for using each such basis, as well as each *Clomid study* that supported his conclusions. The authority for the methodologies included papers by Shepard and Jelovsek, et al.; where appropriate, rule numbers and page numbers were also cited, and relevant quotes given. In all, Dr. Done's declaration covers *23 pages* explaining how he arrived at the conclusion that Clomid was a HUMAN TERATOGEN (capable of causing birth defects in humans).

"Dr. Done then outlined his approach to assessing *case specific causation.*

"He first explained that plaintiff suffers from a condition known as *hemifacial microsomia*, and that no epidemiology studies had been done on that specific anomaly to date. He stated that when such studies are lacking, there are other methodologies that are followed by recognized experts to assess the *full spectrum* of birth defects. This involves looking at *anecdotal (case) reports*, including timing of exposure, animal studies, existing human epidemiological data, and possible mechanism of action. [See Rules 112 and 113;[291] and article by Hoyme, et al.[292]]

"Following the approach outlined by Hoyme et al., Dr. Done evaluated the full *history* involving the plaintiff, including the timing of exposure, the absence of exposure to other known environmental teratogens, heredity, genetic predisposition toward this type of congenital anomaly (the first and second branchial arch), as well as the fact that animal teratology studies had demonstrated a biological plausibility to cause anomalies of the first and second branchial arch (hemifacial microsomia is an anomaly of the first and second branchial arch of the developing fetus).

"To summarize, the only time Dr. Done made reference to the *wide variety of birth defects* was at the 104(a) hearing, when he stated that it was 'a' basis of his opinion, and when it was not understood that there was any necessity to cite a specific source of authority. In his declaration, the only related reference was to animal studies, and then to only demonstrate biological plausibility. When used in the declaration, it was supported by appropriate published articles in reputable scientific journals. At no time was such an approach cited by Dr. Done as the *chief premise* for his conclusion." [Emphasis in the original.]

The Petition for Rehearing was denied without comment within a week. The only surprise was how quickly the decision had been made. Had it even been read? If it had, I doubted that it had been reviewed with an open mind. To grant a rehearing and reverse its earlier decision would require an acknowledgement that the appellate court had made an error the first time around. No way was that going to happen. A careful reading of its July 11, 1996 opinion reflected a court intent on upholding Rafeedie's ruling to knock out another plaintiff's expert, just as it had done with plaintiffs' experts in the Daubert Bendectin case on January 5, 1995.

After all, Dr. Done was "already a professional plaintiff's witness." Not a professional witness; a professional *plaintiff's* witness. The "P" word. This was why it was "not unreasonable to presume that Done's opinion on Clomid was influenced by a litigation-driven financial incentive." The apparent mindset of the Ninth Circuit was that most, if not all, professional *plaintiff's* witnesses are biased in their analysis because they are compensated for their time related to preparing for and testifying in court.

But from what evidence did the court conclude that Dr. Done was a "professional *plaintiff's* witness"? It was no secret that Done had been a professional witness and consultant since the beginning of 1984. He in fact acknowledged that about 70% of his income was derived from "medical-legal matters." But nowhere in his testimony or declaration did he state that he exclusively testified for plaintiffs. This was something else the court "presumed" because he had testified several times against Merrell Dow.

More critical, however, was the Ninth Circuit's assumption that Done's 1983 article, that included Clomid on a list of probable human teratogens, "was based on research conducted in preparation for expert testimony in a different case concerning a different drug manufactured by Merrell Dow." Although Done became *suspicious* about Clomid while conducting research at the FDA concerning Bendectin litigation, the actual research about clomiphene citrate was conducted later and independent of any litigation. At no time did Done state during the 104(a) hearing that his research on Clomid was based upon work related to Bendectin, and this was made quite clear in his declaration of March 2, 1995 (see above). But this made little difference to the appellate court.

In the end, it was a painful irony that with all of the positive epidemiology and animal studies, and an exhaustive and detailed analysis of the scientific data on Clomid, I could not even qualify my expert witness to express his conclusions to a jury. Yet in Breimhorst, without a single supporting epidemiology study and a minimal amount of scientific evidence, I was able to present all of my expert testimony and achieve a satisfactory verdict. The difference? Although 21 years had passed between the two cases, there can be little question that the federal court system, with its conservative judiciary and restrictive laws, was the sole and exclusive reason that Alexander Lust was denied his day in court. After all, less than a year earlier, a similar challenge was made in state court against the same expert witness, but with an entirely different result.

* * * * *

CHAPTER 18

I Rest my Case

My review of the literature through 1994 was sufficient to motivate me to write this book; that and my experiences and discoveries through Clomid litigation over 24 years. Still, it would not have been justified if subsequent published studies had exonerated the family of fertility drugs. I thus did a comprehensive investigation into the relevant post-1994 literature before putting pen to pad - actually, fingers to laptop. My recent research, in fact, even extended as far back as 1980, recognizing that I may have overlooked papers during my earlier efforts. This chapter contains the end-product of my early and recent labors, not to mention those of my retained experts and, at times, a medical researcher.

Every relevant epidemiology study has been included, even those containing negative findings. If I have missed any, it was through inadvertence, not out of design. I have no difficulty with presenting papers that do not support my views. Indeed, it is the very purpose of this book to give the reader *all* of the evidence; something that has not existed before this publication.

It must be recognized that criticism can be found with almost any epidemiology study. It is a rare event when one is published without flaws, including many that might have materially affected the outcome. This is the reason that most experts in the field of teratology will not rely on the findings and conclusions of one study, even one that has very high statistical significance. They want to see duplication. When an increased risk has been duplicated in repeat studies, especially if they are consistent following differently-designed studies, such experts begin to accept the hypothesis of a causal relationship. For the same reason, the existence of studies that have failed to demonstrate an increased risk does not establish that a drug is a non-teratogen.

What has impressed me most about the risk of birth defects from fertility drugs are the studies related to neural tube defects – and to a lesser extent the closure defects involving the alimentary (digestive) tract and heart defects. In my view, there have been too many studies demonstrating an increased risk of NTDs (whether statistically significant or not) to pass them off as chance occurrences. Although one will occasionally see a negative study, those demonstrating a positive association overwhelm those that do not. [See Table 1] Further, a current look at whether subfertility patients are at a greater risk of delivering an infant with an NTD reveals that this is not the case; patients requiring use of ovulatory-stimulating drugs are no more likely to deliver an infant with an NTD than women of normal fertility.

Another clincher – at least for this observer – is the now well-establshed association between multiple births and neural tube defects. Put simply, NTDs – especially anencephaly – occur much more frequently with multiple conceptions than with singleton pregnancies. Up to ten percent of Clomid (clomiphene) pregnancies and up to twenty percent of Pergonal (hMG) pregnancies result in multiple births. Fertility drugs induce ovaries to expel multiple ova, which result in multiple pregnancies, which in turn create an increased risk of neural tube defects. This statistic, standing alone, establishes at the very least an inference of a relationship between the two events.

The strongest piece of evidence, however – and a very integral part of this complex puzzle – is a discovery I made while updating my research for this book. It relates to the question of a *mechanism of action*, primarily for neural tube defects, although it is applicable to several other anomalies as well. Over the past decade, science has made great strides in discovering how environmental insults can adversely influence the development of an evolving embryo. This recently opened a door for me that I never knew existed. It will be discussed at length in Chapter 19.

This chapter lays out the entire case against fertility drugs; all of the proof establishing them as human teratogens. Nothing has been withheld. The scientific method of analysis is also presented for all to consider and judge, including the criteria used to determine whether a drug is a human teratogen. I then document the proof from medical and scientific studies involving the issues of: timing of exposure; human epidemiology; mutagenicity; animal teratology; animal in-vitro and in-vivo findings; similarities with the chemical structure of another known teratogen; and, finally, biological feasibility. All are presented in logical and understandable language. This chapter brings together all of the fragmented evidence previously reviewed by the reader and presents the complete picture.

Based upon all that follows, in my opinion it is *virtually certain* that clomiphene citrate is a human teratogen and a *high probability* that other fertility drugs – those that share the common side effects of multiple ovulation, elevated estrogen levels and OHSS – are also human teratogens. However, notwithstanding my thirty-plus years of research on the subject, I am still a layman with neither a degree in science nor medicine. I am also biased and an advocate. I would thus urge that you give very little weight to my personal view on the subject. Instead, consider all of the recited evidence and discuss it with a physician whose opinion you trust and value – after he or she has read this and the next chapter and, perhaps, some of the cited papers.

In the end, it is not important that I have convinced you to share my opinion about fertility drugs. The primary purpose of this text has been to give those who are considering or using fertility drugs an opportunity to make up their own minds based upon *all* of the evidence; to make a truly informed decision. Up to the date of this publication, that opportunity has been denied to all.

Not anymore.

General Reasoning and Methodologies

In reviewing, interpreting and analyzing the research identified below, I have followed the reasoning and methodology generally accepted by teratologists, dysmorphologists, geneticists, neonatalogists, pediatricians, obstetricians, pathologists, epidemiologists and other specialists who have studied the question of human teratology. This generally includes an evaluation of: (1) whether or not the *timing* of the exposure is appropriate to have caused the congenital anomaly or anomalies under consideration; (2) the results of *human epidemiology studies*; (3) whether the drug under consideration is *mutagenic*; (4) the results of *animal teratology studies*; (5) the results of *animal in-vivo* and *in-vitro studies*; (6) whether the *chemical structure* is similar to another drug generally accepted as a known human teratogen; and (7) whether or not it is *biologically plausible* for the drug to be causing the congenital anomaly or anomalies under consideration.

In a survey of national teratology experts by Jelovsek, et al.,[293] a *consensus* of rules used to evaluate human teratogenicity were listed, which included all of the above-mentioned methodologies. Each of the rules is reflective of the *weight* to be given to the study or studies under consideration. All of these methodologies were used by me in my evaluation of clomiphene and fertility drugs as a group. Citations to rules below refer to this publication. These principles have been supplemented and refined by further issue-specific articles set out in the subcategories below.

Shepard's *Catalog of Teratogenic Agents* (1992) sets out his criteria for concluding that a drug, chemical or other environmental event is a human teratogen. They are listed as follows (p.xxii):

"1. Proven exposure to agent at critical time(s) in prenatal development (prescriptions, physician's records, dates).

2. Consistent findings by two or more epidemiologic studies of high quality:

    a. Control of confounding factors;

    b. Sufficient numbers;

    c. Exclusion of positive and negative bias factors;

    d. Prospective studies, *if possible*; and

    e. Relative risk of six or more *(?)*.

3. Careful delineation of the clinical cases. A specific defect or syndrome, *if present, is very helpful*.

4. Rare environmental exposure asscociated with a rare defect. Probably three or more cases (examples: oral anticoagulants, methimazole and scalp defects (?), and heart block and maternal rheumatism).

5. Teratogenicity in experimental animals important *but not essential* (i.e., oral anticoagulants as exception).

6. The association should make biologic sense.

7. Proof in an experimental system that the agent acts in an unaltered state. Important information for prevention.

Note: Items 1, 2, and 3 or 1, 3 and 4 are essential criteria. Items 5, 6, and 7 are *helpful but not essential*." [Emphasis added.]

In Shepard's view, the critical and essential criteria are that the timing of exposure be appropriate for the specific anomalies being evaluated, that there be two or more epidemiology studies of high quality with significant and consistent findings of an elevated risk, and that the clinical cases be carefully reviewed and described; *or* items 1 and 3 with a rare environmental exposure to three or more cases with a rare defect. This last criterion is no doubt an acknowledgment that a human teratogen can be discovered from case reports, exclusive of epidemiologic studies, when the anomaly and environmental agent are rare and found in association on at least three occasions.

Timing of Exposure

Timing of exposure relates to the question of whether or not the drug had the *opportunity* to cause the congenital anomaly; whether it was present in the maternal and/or embryonic circulation when the malformed organ was susceptible to damage. A drug administered too late during gestation cannot be causally related to a birth defect that was formed in the absence of the drug. The same argument could be made when the drug is ingested too early. Clomid is generally administered *prior* to conception (days 5-9 of the menstrual period), usually about five days before fertilization. Other fertility drugs are also administered prior to conception. It is thus even more important to make a careful study of this criterion.

Carbon 14 (C_{14}) studies performed by Merrell Dow, and reported in its package insert, demonstrate that Clomid has a *half-life of five days* – some even say seven days. In other words, 5 days after ingesting a single 50 mg. tablet, 50% of the drug and/or its metabolites still remain in the body. Thereafter, in theory, fifty percent of the remaining half of the drug continues to be eliminated over the next 5 days, then another fifty percent of the residual drug components over the next five days and so on. During Merrell's studies, the C_{14} markers of the drug were found in the feces as late as *six weeks* after the drug was last ingested.

With a half-life of 5 days, if one assumed that: (1) a patient took two 50 mg. tablets (100 mg.) per day on days five through nine of the menstrual cycle; (2) she ovulated and conceived on day 14; and (3) the above theoretical rate of elimination applied for each 5-day period, then: 200 mg. of the drug and/or its metabolites would be circulating on the date of conception; 50 mg. (one tablet equivalent) would still remain on post-conception day 11, when the period of teratogenic susceptibility commences;[294] and 19 mg. would still remain on day 18 when organogenesis starts and the neural plate begins to form into the neural groove. [Exhibit 18] This would also assume that there had not been a buildup of clomiphene because of earlier treatment cycles.

Recall also the testimony and writings of James G. Wilson, when he acknowledged that "chemically differentiated cells may be subject to teratogenesis several hours or possibly days before their ultimate role in development is indicated by morphological differentiation."[295] Interpretation: an embryonic organ can be subject to a teratogenic insult hours, possibly days, before it actually starts to form.

Clomiphene citrate is composed of two isomers; the zuclomiphene (Z) isomer and the enclomiphene (E) isomer. Isomers are molecules within a drug that share the same formula, but in which the atoms are arranged differently, resulting in different properties or effects. In a later study by Mikkelson, et al.,[296] they measured the rate of elimination of the Clomid isomers. Twenty-four women were given a single 50 mg. tablet, after which blood samples were taken at regular intervals and assayed. Readings were taken of both isomers and their metabolites. They found that the more active Z isomer could be found in *significant* plasma concentrations up to one month after treatment, and longer.

The authors also measured the plasma concentration of the Z isomer over three consecutive months and found that it *accumulated.* "Because of the unexpected long half-life of the CC (clomiphene citrate) Z isomer, subjects in this study, despite receiving only one 50 mg. tablet monthly, nevertheless displayed some accumulation of this isomer throughout the three phases of the study." They added, "(A)ccumulation of the Z isomer can be anticipated in patients who receive chronic CC therapy over a period of many months, and this may have important therapeutic implications. For example, it is not uncommon for non-responding patients to receive escalating doses of up to 250 mg./day of CC for five days/month and then continue on therapy for many months. It can be anticipated that more extensive accumulation of the Z isomer would occur in these patients." Because of the accumulation phenomenon, *the subjects had over twice the concentration of the Z isomer after 70 days than they did after 28 days.*

One additional study by Geier and colleagues[297] warrants a discussion. Their effort did not measure clomiphene or its isomers or metabolites, but instead its ability to bind with (attach to) estrogen receptors. Various female reproductive organs, such as the uterus, have receptors in target cells that estrogenic compounds are drawn to and bind with. Since clomiphene has estrogenic and antiestrogenic activity, they considered such a study as a means of measuring its biological activity. However, since it was preferable to measure the binding activity from blood serum rather than actual female organs, they used estrogen receptors from pulverized rat uteri. After administering Clomid to the patients, they would take their blood plasma containing the drug's molecules at regular intervals and mix them in a laboratory with a preparation containing the rat receptors. The binding activity would then be measured until the levels reached the pre-treatment baseline numbers. They found that one woman ingesting the drug for 5 consecutive days reached a peak of the measured component (7,300 pg/ml) 12 hours after the last tablet, then reached 1,300 pg/ml on day 14 of the cycle, 700 pg/ml on day 22 of the cycle and 500 pg/ml on day 35. A second patient had a similar rate of elimination and others were shorter.

Guess what else they found? One patient did not reach pretreatment levels until *54 days after cessation of clomiphene therapy.*[298] If she had conceived five days after her last tablet, this would equate to day 49 post-conception, just one week short of completion of organogenesis. And this would be when the drug's *biological activity* would cease, not necessarily the presence of its molecules.

Clomid would thus be present in significant concentrations in the maternal and embryonic circulation at the time most congenital anomalies are occurring. This, of course, is only important when considering whether clomiphene citrate has a direct teratogenic effect on certain target organs. To the extent that it possesses the capacity to produce birth defects by inducing chromosomal errors or via indirect action through the female hormonal system, it would not be essential to establish that the drug remains circulating into the period of organogenesis.

"Compounds that are metabolized and/or excreted slowly result in increased duration of exposure and have more potential for adverse effects." [Rule 81]

Epidemiology Studies

There can be little question that (human) epidemiology studies are the most important, and are given the greatest weight, when it comes to assessing the teratogenic risk of a drug. *"In general, given equivalent qualities of studies, human data would be weighted more heavily than animal data in extrapolation to the human."* [Rule 136]

Although individual case reports have value and are considered by most teratologists, the greatest weight is given to more than two epidemiologic studies with statistical quality. *"There is a relative ranking in the positive weight that case reports and studies contribute to extrapolation of an effect in humans; that rank order in a positive fashion would be: 1.0 More than two epidemiologic studies; 0.8 Two epidemiologic studies; 0.7 Multiple reports of multiple cases; 0.7 An epidemiologic study, prospective or cohort; 0.5 Multiple reports of single cases; 0.4 An epidemiological study, retrospective; 0.3 Two to five cases in one report; 0.1 A single case report."* [Rule 115] For example, two or more reports of two or more NTD cases, in association with clomiphene use, would be given equal value to a positive association seen in a single prospective/cohort study; and either of them would have 70% of the value of more than two epidemiologic studies demonstrating a statistically significant increased risk.

    "In evaluating epidemiologic studies of developmental toxic effects in humans, it is important that there is control of confounding factors, sufficient numbers, exclusion of bias factors, both positively and negatively (i.e., statistical quality of a study is used as a weight factor)." [Rule 118] "Control of confounding factors" refers to either eliminating or equalizing other factors that might contribute to an increase in the birth defect rate, such as maternal age, prior pregnancy history, quality of examinations, ethnicity, uniformity of the description of anomaly or anomalies, etc. The ideal design of a study is to have similarity between the controls and the treated group, except for the studied drug (cohort study) or similarity between the controls and the cases, except for the studied abnormality (case-control study). "Bias" could exist, not only because the researcher or researchers have their own agenda, but also because of *recall bias*, when the subjects are more motivated to recall certain events, or *selection bias*, when the researchers might unwittingly select a control group that is at a higher or lower risk for exposures (in a case-control study) or a control group that is at a higher or lower risk of delivering infants with anomalies (in a cohort study).

    When assessing epidemiologic studies, one is initially looking for an increased rate or incidence that is *statistically significant*; the possibility of the increased numbers occurring by chance alone is 5% or less (P=0.05 or less). The study should have some control group or reference population. *Case-control* studies involve a case population with the congenital anomaly or anomalies under study, a control population without the anomaly or anomalies, and measure the relative exposures of the drug to each group. *Cohort* studies involve a population exposed to the drug under study, a control group without exposure to the drug, and measure the relative difference in outcomes (i.e., birth defects) between the two populations.

As mentioned in earlier chapters, over the years many researchers have looked at the question of whether there has been an increase in the rate of *total (combined) birth defects* following exposure to fertility drugs. With the introduction of in vitro fertilization (IVF) in the 1980s – and its subsequent proliferation throughout the world – this opportunity has broadened considerably. Virtually all assisted reproductive technology (ART) procedures utilize fertility drugs to produce the eggs being inseminated, including intracytoplasmic sperm injection (ICSI). ICSI involves a direct injection of a single sperm into the ovum. But similar to other IVF procedures, fertility drugs are used to stimulate the patient's ovaries to produce multiple ova, which are extracted through the use of a thin needle and then inseminated outside the body. Upon confirmation that conception has occurred and the cells have begun dividing (usually 2-4 days), the impregnated ovum (zygote) is inserted into the uterus. To insure that at least one zygote will "take," normally two or more are placed in the womb at the same time. Because of this practice, approximately 25% of pregnancies following ICSI and other IVF procedures are multiple births.

As recent as February 9, 2007, it was reported in the lay press that "Fertilty Treatments Increase Birth Defects, Study Finds."[299] The article reported on a Canadian cohort study presented at a medical conference of the Society for Maternal-Fetal Medicine. The study revealed that there was a 58% increased risk of delivering a baby with a congenital malformation following IVF and other ART procedures. "Nearly 3 percent of (fertility treatment) babies had a birth defect versus just under 2 percent for babies conceived naturally." This, by itself, should raise some eyebrows. It was also not the first such report.

An earlier study by Hansen, et al. (2002) was published in the prestigious New England Journal of Medicine.[300] They likewise evaluated the potential risk of major congenital anomalies associated with the use of ART procedures, including ICSI and IVF. Their data demonstrated a 114% increased risk (9.0% vs. 4.2%; P< 0.001) when looking at all infants (including multiple births) following IVF and 105% increased risk (8.6% vs. 4.2%; P< 0.001) when using ICSI. Merlob and colleagues (2005)[301] found similar statistics in their IVF study involving major congenital malformations: a 2.3-fold increase (9.35% vs. 4.05%; P< 0.0001) during the period of 1986-1994 and a 1.75-fold increase during the period of 1995-2002 (9.00% vs. 5.18%). Later the same year, Olson and others (2005)[302] published their study and likewise found that women undergoing IVF were at an increased risk of having babies with major birth defects – this time a 41% increase (6.2% vs. 4.4%; P= 0.004).

This is not to suggest that there is an absence of studies failing to find an increased risk of congenital anomalies following ART. Indeed, there are such studies. And it was for this very reason that Hansen and fellow researchers (2005)[303] set out to do a *meta-analysis* of the higher quality studies available in the literature. After compiling a list of 25 papers published between 1989 and 2003, they selected *seven* individual studies that met their demanding criteria. Upon combining the data from the selected papers, they found a 40% increased risk (OR 1.40, 95% CI 1.28-1.53). Even when they pooled all 25 studies, they still found a significant risk (OR 1.29, 95% CI, 1.21-1.37); namely, about a 29% risk of developing congenital anomalies.

An *odds ratio* (OR) is the ratio of the odds of an event (i.e., birth defects) occurring in one group to the odds of the same event occurring in a compared group. An odds ratio of 1.00 indicates that the event has an equal likelihood of occurring in both groups. An odds ratio greater than 1.00 implies that the event is more likely in the first group. This is not to be confused with a *relative risk* (aka *risk ratio*) – which in my view is a more accurate assessment of the risk factor – and is simply the ratio of the percentages in both groups, and calculated by dividing the percentage of occurrence in one group into the percentage of the other. Just as with odds ratios, relative risks of 1.00 indicate that the risk in both groups is the same. Generally, although the odds ratio and relative risk numbers are calculated differently and are not the same, with birth defect rates their respective calculations are usually quite similar.

Now that I have you totally confused, I will throw another important epidemiologic term at you, namely *confidence interval* (CI). The 95% CI calculated from a study addresses the issue of statistical significance. Since both compared groups are random samples from the general population, it indicates with 95% certainty that the actual incidence falls within the range of the lower and higher confidence limits. In order to be statistically significant, the lower limit of the confidence interval must be above 1.00. The narrower the range of the confidence limits, the greater the certainty that the numbers accurately represent the true level of risk.

Although the above studies are of significant value when exploring the potential risk of fertility drugs, it is when epidemiologists and other experts sharpen their pencils and narrow the focus onto *individual* congenital anomalies that the real picture is brought to light. Assume for the moment that fertility drugs can only cause one type of anomaly (i.e., neural tube defects) and that their use doubled that risk. With a hypothetical NTD rate in the general population of one in a 1,000 deliveries, one out of every 500 pregnancies resulting from fertility drugs would produce a baby with spina bifida or anencephaly (or variations thereof). Such an increase in risk, however, would only have a small impact on the rate of *total* birth defects. If one assumed a rate of 2.0% of major defects in the general population (e.g., ten out of every 500 deliveries), then exposure to fertility drugs would move the rate of all birth defects to 2.1%, or an *increased risk of ten percent*. More importantly, to detect such a small increase in a cohort study – at a statistically significant level – would require a very large population in the treated and control groups. Smaller study groups would never pick up the increase. This is why the true risk of fertility drugs was never fully appreciated until researchers began taking a serious look at individual congenital anomalies.

Neural Tube Defects

The association between neural tube defects (NTDs) and Clomid, individually, or with other fertility drugs as a group, have been the most widely studied congenital anomalies to date. These include anencephaly, encephalocele, exencephaly, iniencephaly, craniorachischisis, spina bifida occulta, and spina bifida cystica, including meningocele, meningomyelocele and myelomeningocele. All have been previously described and involve non-closure of the neural tube (skull and/or spinal column) very early in the period of organogenesis. Study designs have involved both case-control and cohort groups.

Most of the studies that predate 1995 have been discussed in detail in Chapter 14. In 1995, two additional NTD studies emerged. Both were of a case-control design; one involving normal controls (Shaw, et al.),[304] the other, abnormal controls (Lammer).[305]

Shaw drew from infant deliveries in California between 1989 and 1991. Lammer selected his infant population from Atlanta for the period between 1970 and 1979. Although the numbers did not reach statistical significance, Shaw et al. found a fifty percent increase in the number of Clomid exposures to cases over the controls (OR 1.50; 95% CI, 0.43-6.10). When the data were expanded to include exposures to all fertility drugs, the calculations represented an 80% increase (9/538 cases compared to 5/539 controls). The authors acknowledged that their small numbers were a handicap in measuring the true risk for NTDs. "This study, as did others, had too few preconceptional clomiphene users to estimate NTD risk precisely."

Lammer's study was afflicted with even more problems. His NTD cases were limited to only anencephaly and spina bifida aperta (including meningocele and meningomyelocele). Mothers of "all of the other malformed case infants" were used as the control group. As a consequence of this selection bias, limb reduction defects, trisomy 21 (Down syndrome), hypospadias and intestinal or anal atresia – all anomalies which had been implicated with the use of fertility drugs – were included as controls. By design, the inclusion of these anomalies increased the likelihood of securing exposures in the control group, the consequence of which would be to bias the study toward an odds ratio of one. Lammer's data was thus not surprising: 3/289 cases – 6/504 controls (OR 0.87; 95% CI, 0.14-4.11). Once again, a case-control study using abnormal controls produced a negative association.

Later the same year, Greenland and Ackerman took a critical look at all of the epidemiology studies published through 1995.[306] A number of their observations were right on the mark.

On the use of abnormal controls: "Because in some studies CC (clomiphene citrate) has been found to be associated with several defects besides NTDs, we recommend that future case-control studies of CC include an unaffected control group. (T)here currently are no controlled studies indicating a potential for recall bias in fertility drug cases, and there have been strong arguments against use of malformed controls because of the potential for selection bias. To avoid the potential for recall bias, we recommend that medical records be used to ascertain CC use."

On excluding multiple pregnancies: "We caution, however, that over-control should be avoided. For example, CC may induce multiple births and multiple birth is associated with an elevated risk of perinatal morbidity and birth defects; multiple births thus would be an intermediate factor rather than a confounder, and control for them would produce severe bias toward no association."

On the (1983) Kurachi study: "The *un*exposed cohort in the Japanese study had an NTD prevalence of 2.7 per 1,000, far in excess (P < 0.0001) of the 1.2 per 1,000 reported for Japan by the World Health Organization and thus suggestive of some sort of bias." The Kurachi article reported the occurrence of two NTDs out of 935 infants from clomiphene pregnancies, a rate of 2.14 per 1,000. If the authors had used the WHO prevalence rate for Japan, they would have come up with an *80% increased risk*. Their control group was 29,900 women who conceived following spontaneous (unassisted) ovulation and delivered 30,033 infants at nine university hospitals throughout Japan. From this population, they purportedly documented 84 NTDs, for a prevalence of 2.8 per 1,000.[307] Their *control* population had 2.3 times the expected incidence of NTDs. Greenland and Ackerman thus concluded that there was some form of bias in the study. That conclusion would have been strongly reinforced had they known of my discovery that the same control group also had nearly three times the incidence of multiple births as the pregnancies induced by clomiphene (16.7% vs. 6.1%; see Chapter 15 and cross-examination of Hoyme).

On the Werler (1994) study: "Werler et al. included controls with hypospadias, which has also been associated with CC use (citing papers by Czeizel[308] and Macnab and Zouves[309])." See my discussion on Werler's use of hypospadias controls in Chapter 14.

My recent research uncovered a number of additional studies which explored the potential risk of NTDs following the use of fertility drugs, including many papers examining the risk of birth defects among infants produced through ART. Unfortunately, most ART studies have one or both of two major flaws in their design which bias them against an association.

First, most used protocols which were structured to calculate the incidence (percentage) of congenital anomalies in the treated (ART) group from total *offspring* rather than total *deliveries*. Approximately 25% of ART deliveries are multiple births.[310]

Because of the nature of the ART procedures, the resulting multiple pregnancies are predominantly dizygotic, namely involving two or more ova. As a consequence, up to 99% of the twins, triplets and other multiple conceptions following ART are non-identical.[311] The problem arises due to the fact that NTDs occur more frequently in multiple births – especially anencephalics;[312] and when it occurs, usually one of the siblings is spared.[313] An example will illustrate the problem.

Assume that out of a group of 1,000 *singleton* pregnancies, fifty (5%) of them were born with congenital abnormalities. A second group of 1,000 *twin* pregnancies resulted in one hundred infants born with defects, but only one from each set of twins (10%). Although the second group had twice as many pregnancies resulting in congenital malformations, when one compares the respective incidence figures using the total number of delivered infants, there would not have been an increased rate (e.g., 50/1,000 vs. 100/2,000). The rate for each group would be five percent.

When the controls come from the general population, whether as a selected group or national incidence figures, the problem is exacerbated by the fact that 99% of the controls consist of singleton pregnancies.[314] In one such study, 44.3% of the ART infants were from multiple births, compared to 2.3% in the control population.[315] Using total delivered infants in both groups to calculate the incidence of NTDs thus dilutes the ART group and biases the study against an association. Some studies attempt to compensate for this selection bias by adjusting for multiplicity; others do not. *Such studies should be designed to look at NTD incidence figures from total deliveries, not total infants.*

Second, it is an unquestioned fact that a large majority of NTDs occurring following ART are detected prenatally, frequently by the middle of the second trimester. By ultrasound and/or by detection of alpha-fetoprotein (AFP) in the amniotic fluid, many NTDs are discovered prior to completion of the second trimester. AFP leaks from the fetus into the amniotic fluid through exposed capillaries of the NTD, and can be discovered as early as 12-14 weeks after conception. When such a discovery is made, the pregnancy is often terminated by a therapeutic abortion. This is especially true with anencephaly, an abnormality incompatible with life. The second problem arises when a study limits its population to completion of pregnancies occurring either after or late in the second trimester. When this occurs, NTDs terminated by an earlier therapeutic abortion might be missed. Such selection bias can, again, dilute the exposed group of ART pregnancies and predispose it to no association. In order to make an accurate assessment of an increased risk for NTDs, the epidemiology study *should be designed to pick up all early terminations due to anomalies.*

Yet, notwithstanding these major design flaws in some papers, *every relevant[316] cohort study involving ART pregnancies that I could locate demonstrated an increased risk of 50% or greater for NTDs.* Some were statistically significant and others were not (because of insufficient numbers), but all consistently reflected an increased risk for patients using IVF and related procedures.

Table 1 includes all relevant epidemiology studies I could locate which examined the risk of NTDs in association with the use of fertility drugs. I limited my final search to only three criteria: (1) the study was designed to assess the risk of NTDs following fertility drug exposure, including IVF and related procedures; (2) the studied anomalies specifically included neural tube defects, either individually or as a group; and (3) the study group included a large enough population to demonstrate an increased risk. With these requirements, the vast majority of studies included an increased risk (IR) of 50% and higher.

Table 1
_____

EPIDEMIOLOGY STUDIES: NEURAL TUBE DEFECTS

1. CASE-CONTROL STUDIES (Increased Risk of 50% or Higher):

Study	Cases – Controls: Exposures	IR	Significance
Cornel (1989)[317]	NTD: 3/94 – 8/970 **	**287%**	**(95% CI, 1.03-15.2)**
Czeizel (1989)[318]	NTD: 3/825 – 12/18,904 *	**473%**	**(95% CI, 1.62-20.4)**
Cuckle (1989)[319]	NTD: 4/107 – 5/214 *	**60%**	(95% CI, 0.43-6.20)
Robert (1991)[320]	NTD: 11/180 – 114/4,247 **	**128%**	**(95% CI, 1.25-4.46)**
Goujard (1992)[321]	NTD: Not Given **	**65%**	(95% CI, 0.59-4.60)
Shaw (1995)[322]	NTD: 6/538 – 4/539 *	**50%**	(95% CI, 0.43-6.10)
	NTD: 9/538 – 5/539 **	**80%**	Not Given
Medveczky (2004)[323]	NTD: 7/1202 – 96/38,151 *	**131%**	(95% CI, 1.0-4.5)
	NTD: 19/1202 – 202/38,151 **	**189%**	Not Given
Wu (2006)[324]	SB: 3/18 – 32/1,608*	**738%**	**(95% CI, 2.0-44.8)**
	SB: 4/18 – 48/1,608**	**644%**	**(95% CI, 2.5-36.7)**

2. COHORT STUDIES (Increased Risk of 50% or higher):

Study	Exposed – Unexposed Controls	IR	Significance
Lancaster (1987)[325]	SB: 6/1,697 – 1.2/1,697 (Expect) **	**400%**	**(P = 0. 0015)**
Karabacak (1989)[326]	NTD: 1/128 – 174/76,831 **	**245%**	Not Given
Cornel (1989)[327]	NTD: 12/4385 – 1.35/1000 (Expect) **	**103%**	**(95% CI, 1.6-4.8/1000)**
Milunsky (1990)[328]	NTD: 2/438 – 47/22,317 *	**117%**	(95% CI, 0.6-8.6)
Beral (1990)[329]	NTD: 7/1,581 – 2.9/1,581 (Expect) **	**141%**	Not Given
Rizk (1991)[330]	NTD: 5/961 – 2.8/961 (Expect) **	**79%**	Not Given
Rufat (1994)[331]	NTD: 3/1,263 – 0.62/1,263 (Expect) **	**384%**	Not Given
FIVNAT (1995)[332]	NTD: 8/6,879 – 2.75/6,879 (Expect) **	**191%**	**(P < 0. 01)**
Westergaard (1999)[333]	NTD: 4/2,245 – 2/2,245 **	**100%**	Not Given
Bergh (1999)[334]	AN: 4/5,856 – 0.31/5,856 (Expect) **	**1,191%**	**(95% CI, 3.5-33.0)**
	SB: 6/5,856 – 2.55/5,856 (Expect) **	**135%**	(95% CI, 0.9-5.1)
Wennerholm (2000)[335]	NTD: 2/1,143 – 0.63/1,143 (Expect) **	**217%**	Not Given
Lancaster (2000)[336]	NTD: 9/4,260 – 5.15/4,260 (Expect) **	**75%**	Not Given
Ericson (2001)[337]	NTD: 12/9,175 – 4.1/9,175 (Expect) **	**193%**	**(95% CI, 1.5-5.1)**
Kallen (2005)[338]	NTD: 25/16,280 – 7.4/16,280 (Expect) **	**238%**	**(95% CI, 3.3-6.9)**

3. CASE-CONTROL STUDIES (Increased Risk Below 50%):

Study	Cases – Controls: Exposures	IR	Significance
Mills (1990)[339]	NTD: 8/571 – 6/546 Abn **	27%	(95% CI, 0.4-4.5)
	NTD: 8/571 – 10/573 Norm **	----	(95% CI, 0.3-2.3)
Mili (1991)[340]	NTD: 2/345 – 16/2,829 Norm*	2%	(95% CI, 0.23-4.5)
Werler (1994)[341]	NTD: 31/1,032 – 113/4,062 Abn **	7%	(95% CI, 0.8-1.7)
	NTD: 22/1,032 – 96/4,062 Abn*	----	(95% CI, 0.5-1.3)
Lammer (1995)[342]	NTD: 3/289 – 6/504 Abn *	----	(95% CI, 0.14-4.11)
Whiteman (2000)[343]	NTD: 13/655 – 13/616 Norm/Abn *	----	(95% CI, 0.4-2.3)
	NTD: 14/655 – 15/616 Norm/Abn **	----	(95% CI, 0.4-2.0)

4. COHORT STUDIES (Increased Risk Below 50%):

Study	Exposed – Unexposed Controls	IR	Significance
Kurachi (1983)[344]	NTD: 2/935 – 80/30,033 *	----	(95% CI, 0.01-3.02)
Kallen (2002)[345]	NTD: 0/4,029 – 1.83/4,029 (Expect) **	----	Not Given

NTD: Neural Tube Defect; AN: Anencephaly; SB: Spina Bifida.

* Clomiphene Citrate; ** Fertility Drugs (including clomiphene citrate).

Fraternal Twinning

From my review of the current literature, it appears that most writers in the field agree that NTDs occur more frequently in the presence of multiple births, especially anencephaly. However, when one attempts to nail down the possible association between NTDs and dizygotic (fraternal) twinning, the supporting data is a little vague. The difficulty originates from the fact that very few epidemiology studies provide accurate statistics on the zygosity of the multiple births. Usually, all that is available from their data sources is the sex of each twin; rarely do birth defect registers provide information on whether the twins were conceived from two diffent zygotes (fertilized ova) or from a single – monzygotic (MZ) – ovum. Male/female twins, of course, are all dizygotic (DZ). But with this limitation, the researchers make *estimates* on zygosity for male/male and female/female twins (e.g., like-sex twins) based upon an epidemiologic formula.

The literature, nevertheless, still supports the conclusion that NTDs occur more frequently with fraternal twins than with singleton pregnancies. It all began in 1966 with an article by Stevenson, et al.[346] In that seminal study they found a high statistical relationship (P< 0.01) between DZ twinning and the incidence of anencephaly and spina bifida. They observed that the "phenomenon has not been demonstrated previously and it is difficult to suggest an explanation except that in some way there are predisposing factors in common."

Later non-ART studies have simply reported on the association between multiple births and NTDs without identifying the ova as DZ or MZ. Windham et al. found an incidence of 1.6 NTDs per 1,000 births among twin deliveries compared to a rate of 1.1 per 1,000 for singletons, but did not have access to information on their zygosity.[347] Only 3.7% of the twins had a co-twin with an NTD.

An international study by Kallen et al., published in 1994, included data from Australia, Denmark, France, Italy, Norway, South America and Sweden.[348] Their statistics were drawn from 3,584 infants with anencephaly, 4,906 with spina bifida and 1,041 with encephalocele. When compared with the twinning rate of the general population (approximately 2%), the percentage of twins among anencephalics (4.3%) was significantly higher (95% CI, 3.6-5.0), as were infants with encephalocele (3.3%; 95% CI, 2.1-4.4). The data for spina bifida were only slightly elevated (2.2%; 95% CI, 1.8-

2.6). Only ten out of 279 (3.6%) sets of twins with NTDs were concordant (e.g., each twin had the same anomaly). In other words, 96.4% of the co-twins lacked an NTD.

In a major study involving 75,844 twin deliveries and 3,789,821 singleton births in England and Whales between 1979 and 1985, Doyle, et al. (1990)[349] found a significant increase in the incidence of anencephaly in twins over singletons (OR 3.47; 95% CI, 2.73-4.36). A similar increase was not found for spina bifida (OR 1.08) or encephalocele (OR 1.16). And a recent paper by Ben-Ami, et al. (2005)[350] also found a significant correlation between anencephaly and fraternal twinning (OR 4.85; 95% CI, 1.86-12.63; P=0.001).

A case-control study by Whiteman, et al. (2000)[351] compared the incidence of multiple births among 694 NTD cases (2.02%) with 694 controls (0.58%) and found a significant odds ratio of 3.5 (95% CI, 1.2-10.6). Infants with NTDs were three and a half times more likely to come from a multiple birth than non-NTD controls.

In 2001, Lancaster and Hurst reported on NTD data out of Australia for the period between 1991 and 1997.[352] For anencephaly, the rates per 10,000 births were 4.4 for singletons, 10.4 for twins and 14.9 for triplets; for spina bifida, 6.1 for singletons, 8.3 for twins and 5.0 for triplets; for encephalocele, 1.2 for singletons, 2.5 for twins and no documented cases for triplets; and for all NTDs combined, 11.7 for singletons, 21.2 for twins and 19.9 for triplets.

Beyond the Stevenson study, a definitive answer about the association between NTDs and DZ twinning seems to be lacking. But there is further evidence to support the hypothesis. Only thirty percent of spontaneously conceived twins are MZ.[353] One can thus reasonably assume that a large majority of the above-studied twins were from dizygotic pregnancies. The real strength of the relationship, however, is seen following ART, where about 99% of the multiple conceptions are from two or more eggs. *At least half of the NTDs following assisted reproductive technology procedures arise out of twin pregnancies.*[354]

When fraternal twinning occurs, whether in the general population or following ovulation-inducing drugs, there appears to be a significant increase in the incidence of NTDs. The process by which multiple ova are produced and evolve as embryos would thus seem to be causally related to inhibiting closure of the neural tube.

The Infertility Factor

The jury is still out on the question of whether a history of prior spontaneous abortions increases the risk of delivering a child with a neural tube defect. Studies have gone both ways. Some have demonstrated an increased risk for NTD after an earlier pregnancy resulting in a spontaneous abortion,[355] whereas others have not supported this hypothesis.[356] At least one study reported on a *decreased* risk of NTD following spontaneous abortions, prompting the authors to suggest that "prior spontaneous abortion has a protective effect in relation to subsequent NTD development rather than being a major risk factor in the aetiology of NTDs."[357]

There would appear to be little uncertainty, however, regarding women who have had a difficult time conceiving, especially those faced with some degree of ovulatory dysfunction. As previously expressed in Chapter 14, studies by Cuckle and Wald (1989), Mills, et al. (1990) and Ghazi, et al. (1991) have demonstrated that a history of subfertility is not a risk factor for NTD in women who subsequently achieve unassisted conceptions. This conclusion is supported by more-recent studies as well.

The case-control paper by Shaw, et al. (1995)[358] examined the subfertility history of their cases and controls and found "no increased NTD risk associated with conception delay." Their data included 47/538 (8.74%) NTD cases and 55/539 (10.20%) normal controls (OR 0.86). Each group conceived without the use of fertility drugs after attempting conception for more than a year. Whitemen, et al. (2000) also studied the subfertility history of their NTD cases and controls. Twenty-two out of 655 (3.4%) of their cases had a history of subfertility prior to the subject pregnancy compared to sixteen out of 616 (2.6%) of their controls. Neither group used fertility drugs to conceive; the difference was not significant. They concluded that the existence of subfertility did not appear to be a risk factor for NTD.

An article by Wennerholm, et al. (2000)[359] provides support for the conclusion that ART procedures themselves (exclusive of the fertility drugs used) are not causally related to the higher rate of NTDs – or any other congenital anomalies – associated with assisted reproductive technology. They found that the incidence of congenital abnormalities with multiple pregnancies was significantly higher than singletons (OR 1.75, 95% CI, 1.19-2.58), even though both subsets used the same procedures to

384

conceive. I have also yet to see one paper which points the finger at those procedures as a risk factor for birth defects.

Given all of the above, I would suggest that human epidemiology studies overwhelmingly support the conclusion that *fertility drugs are a cause of NTDs*.

Other Congenital Anomalies

Fertility drugs (including clomiphene citrate), either alone or with the use of ART, have also been associated with a statistically significant increase in the incidence of other congenital anomalies. Procedures have involved ICSI and gamete intrafallopian transfer (GIFT), along with IVF. The anomalies include cardiovascular defects, digestive tract defects, genitourinary defects, musculoskeletal defects, orofacial defects and central nervous system (non-NTD) defects. [Table 2] Clomiphene citrate and other fertility drugs are thus associated with a *wide variety* of congenital anomalies, based upon human epidemiology studies.

Table 2
_____

- **Cardiovascular Defects**
  Lancaster (1987): 567% increased risk of *Transposition of the Great Vessel* (TGV) following IVF and GIFT (P = 0.0034).[360]
  Lancaster (1991): significant increased risk of *TGV* following IVF and GIFT (P< 0.05).[361]
  Kurinczuk (1997): 299% increased risk of major *cardiovascular defects* following ICSI (OR 3.99; P< 0.05).[362]
  Hansen (2002): 200% increased risk of *cardiovascular defects* following IVF (P< 0.001).[363]
  Ludwig (2002): 91% increased risk of *cardiovascular defects* following ICSI (OR 2.89, 95% CI 1.47-2.43; P< 0.05).[364]
  Koivurova (2002): 300% increased risk of *cardiovascular defects* following IVF (OR 4.0, 95% CI 1.4-11.7).[365]
  Anthony (2002): 56% increased risk of *cardiovascular defects* following IVF (OR 1.56, 95% CI 1.10-2.22).[366]
  Kallen (2005): 107% increased risk of major *cardiovascular defects* following IVF (OR 2.1, 95% CI 1.6-2.8).[367]
  Olson (2005): 90% increased risk of *cardiovascular defects* following IVF (P< 0.002).[368]
  Walker (2007): 125% increased risk of *cardiovascular defects* following IVF (90 per 10,000 vs. 40 per 10,000).[369]

- **Digestive Tract Defects**
  Lancaster (1990): significant increased risk of *tracheo-esophageal fistula* following IVF and GIFT (P< 0.01).[370]

Mili (1991): 239% increased risk of *atresia or stenosis of the colon, rectum or anus (imperforate anus)* following the use of clomiphene citrate (OR 4.6, 95% CI 1.01-21.19).[371]

Lancaster (1991): significant increased risk of *imperforate anus* and *esophageal atresia* following IVF and GIFT (P< 0.05).[372]

Kurinczuk (1997): 84% increased risk of *gastrointestinal defects* following ICSI (OR 1.84; P< 0.05).[373]

Bergh (1999): 290% increased risk of *esophageal atresia* following IVF (OR 3.9, 95% CI 1.4-8.5).[374]

Ericson (2001): 249% increased risk of *esophageal atresia* following IVF (RR 3.5, 95% CI 1.5-6.9); and 246% increased risk of *anal atresia (imperforate anus)* following IVF (RR 3.1, 95% CI 1.3-6.1).[375]

Kallen (2005): 283% increased risk of *esophageal atresia* following IVF (OR 4.0, 95% CI 2.6-6.3); 476% increased risk of *small gut atresia* following IVF (OR 6.4, 95% CI 4.2-9.6); and 342% increased risk of *anal atresia (imperforate anus)* following IVF (OR 4.7, 95% CI 3.2-6.9).[376]

Midrio (2006): 1,231% increased risk of *anorectal malformations* following ART (OR 13.31, 95% CI 4.0-39.6).

Walker (2007): 733% increased risk of *gastrointestinal defects* following IVF (1 per 200 vs. 6 per 10,000).[377]

- **Genitourinary Defects**

    Lancaster (1990): significant increased risk of *urinary tract* malformations following IVF and GIFT (P< 0.01).[378]

    Macnab (1991): 360% increased risk of *hypospadias* following IVF (P< 0.01).[379]

    Werler (1994): increased risk of *hypospadias* following the use of clomiphene citrate (OR 1.94, (95% CI 1.02-3.68).[380]

    Silver (1999): 441% increased risk of *hypospadias* following IVF (P< 0.001).[381]

    Wennerholm (2000): 233% increased risk of *hypospadias* following ICSI (OR 3.0, 95% CI 1.09-6.50).[382]

    Hansen (2002): 86% increased risk of *urogenital defects* following IVF (P< 0.01).[383]

    Ludwig (2002): 54% increased risk of *internal urogenital defects* following ICSI (OR 1.54, 95% CI 1.47-2.43; P< 0.05).[384]

    Kallen (2005): 69% increased risk of *hypospadias* following IVF (OR 1.7, 95% CI 1.4-2.1).[385]

    Meijer (2006): 508% increased risk of *penoscrotal hypospadias* following the use of clomiphene citrate (OR 6.08, 95% CI 1.40-26.33).[386]

- **Musculoskeletal Defects**

    Czeizel (1983): significant increased risk of *limb-reduction defects* following the use of fertility drugs, including clomiphene citrate (P< 0.05).[387]

    Lancaster (1990): significant increased risk of *vertebral defects* following IVF and GIFT (P< 0.01).[388]

    Lancaster (1991): significant increased risk of *prune belly syndrome* and *exomphalos* following IVF and GIFT (P< 0.05).[389]

    Ericson (2001): 233% increased risk of *omphalocele* following IVF (RR 3.3,

95% CI 1.3-6.9).[390]

Hansen (2002): 200% increased risk of *musculoskeletal defects* following IVF (P< 0.001).[391]

Reefhuis (2003): 280% increased risk of *craniosynostosis* following the use of clomiphene citrate (OR 3.8, 95% CI 1.1-12.3).[392]

Olson (2005): 83% increased risk of *musculoskeletal defects* following IVF (P< 0.007).[393]

- **Orofacial Defects**

  Czeizel (1989): 609% increased risk of *cleft lip/palate* following the use of clomiphene citrate (P< 0.05).[394]

  Mili (1991): 383% increased risk of *anophthalmia and microphthalmia* following the use of clomiphene citrate (OR 6.98, 95% CI 1.46-33.4).[395]

  Kurinczuk (1997): 411% increased risk of *cleft palate* following ICSI (OR 5.11, 95% CI 1.26-20.80; P= 0.023).[396]

  Kallen (2005): 139% increased risk of *orofacial clefts* following IVF (OR 2.4, 95% CI 1.9-3.1); and 367% increased risk of *choanal atresia* following IVF (OR 4.6, 95% CI 1.9-9.5).[397]

- **Central Nervous System (Non-NTD) Defects**

  Mili (1991): 93% increased risk of *central nervous system defects* following the use of clomiphene citrate (OR 2.48, 95% CI 1.11-5.55); 404% increased risk of *microcephaly* following the use of clomiphene citrate (OR 9.70, 95% CI 2.58-36.51); and 195% increased risk of *hydrocephaly* following the use of clomiphene citrate (OR 3.66, 95% CI 1.20-11.20).[398]

  Bergh (1999): 483% increased risk of *hydrocephaly* following IVF (OR 5.7, 95% CI 2.3-11.8).[399]

Mutagenicity Studies

A drug that has demonstrated to be a human mutagen has a high probability of being a human teratogen as well. *"A compound that is a direct cytotoxic agent* (mutagenic) *is more likely to have a developmental toxic* (teratogenic) *effect than one that does not (depends on reaching a cytotoxic threshold dose)."* [Rule 98] Schreiner and Holden presented a paper for peer review at the Teratology Society convention in June 1984, relative to a survey and analysis of the available literature on the relationship between mutagenicity and teratogenicity. "Mutagenesis data was subdivided into two major categories of genetic alteration: chromosomal damage and gene mutation." The survey results indicated that an agent that produced chromosome structural aberrations in-vivo and in-vitro or numerical changes by chromosomal disruption was also likely to be teratogenic, with correlations of 85%, 80% and 64% respectively. "(T)hese correlation studies demonstrate that any compound capable of damaging DNA has a high probability of also being teratogenic (as well)."

There is persuasive evidence that clomiphene citrate is mutagenic in *humans*. Its ability to damage DNA was demonstrated in-vitro by Ohnishi, et al. (1986)[400] when they used the drug to induce DNA-strand breaks in bacteria (e.coli). Ohashi (1986)[401] took it a step further when he treated human lymphoblastic leukemia cells with clomiphene citrate and was able to inhibit cell growth. "The inhibition of the cell growth by clomiphene citrate appeared to be ascribable to its potent DNA-damaging effect."

The strongest evidence for mutagenicity, however, is in Clomid's ability to cause chromosomal damage. In an in-vivo study performed by Charles, et al. (1973), measurements were taken from the uterine endometrium of women before and after use of Clomid (100 mg. x 7 days). [See Chapter 10] Structurally abnormal chromosomes were found to occur at a highly significant increase in rate (P<0.01). "Thus the karyotypic aberrations encountered in this study must be considered in relation to therapy. * * * We feel that the findings of the study reflect a highly specific action of clomiphene at the cellular level."

Epidemiology Studies

Human epidemiologic studies also support the argument that Clomid can cause chromosomal abnormalities in the fetus of women using Clomid and other ovulatory-stimulating drugs. Oakley and Flynt (1972) reported an increased incidence of two and a half times the expected rate of Down syndrome (trisomy 21) in women following ovulation-inducing agents, primarily Clomid. These statistics were later strengthened when he updated them in 1979. An odds ratio of 1.92 (95% confidence interval 1.02-3.59) for all chromosomal anomalies in pregnancies following ovulation induction was reported by Goujard, et al. in 1992.[402] Hansen, et al. (2002) looked at the potential risk of chromosomal defects following ART procedures and found a significant increase (OR 3.19; P = 0.03). While some epidemiology studies have failed to duplicate these findings, they have either lacked adequate numbers or have not been designed to gather all data on fetuses surviving beyond the first trimester. Many second trimester pregnancies with chromosomal anomalies are either spontaneously aborted or terminated by choice. Others are missed at birth, even children with Down syndrome.[403] The incidence of gross chromosomal abnormalities in the human newborn population has been estimated to be 0.5%.[404] Thus, only a study that is comprehensive in scope will pick up a significant increase in pregnancies carrying a fetus or infant with chromosomal defects.

Spontaneous Abortions

The evidence involving *first trimester* spontaneous abortions (SAs) would seem unchallengeable. As has been frequently discussed, SAs occurring during the first trimester of pregnancy are associated with a high percentage of abnormal chromosomes and/or structurally abnormal embryos. Approximately 60% of all first trimester SAs have abnormal chromosomes (Boue, et al., 1975). Boue and Boue (1973) found a statistically significant increase in abnormal chromosomes in abortuses from women who conceived with induced ovulation during a treatment cycle (83%) and abortuses from women who conceived one cycle after last taking fertility drugs (86%), compared to abortuses from women who conceived two or more cycles after last using ovulatory-stimulating agents (61%) and women who had not been exposed to ovulatory-stimulating drugs at all (60%).

Honore, et al. (1990)[405] examined 21 abortuses following use of fertility drugs, including 18 with clomiphene only. Only two (9%) were structurally normal, compared to 55% in their control population. Five of the 21 (24%) were partial hydatidiform moles; four times the rate found in their controls (6%). A partial "mole" is an abnormal mass containing embryonic tissue, and is generally associated with abnormal chromosomes. Thirteen cases had severe abnormalities of the embryo (growth disorganization or growth retardation and severe malformations) and/or placenta. "This small series suggests that abortions in pregnancies following ovulation induction have a higher incidence of partial moles and 'blighted ova' than abortions in spontaneous ovulators."

Clomid and other ovulatory-stimulating agents cause abnormally high levels of endogenous (internally produced) estrogen.[406] There now appears to be solid evidence that this side effect has either a direct or indirect relationship with an increased incidence of first trimester SAs. This has been demonstrated in several studies.

A significant association has been found between higher *pre-treatment* endogenous estrogen levels and the frequency of early SAs following ovulation induction.[407] They apparently exacerbate *distinct* pre-treatment levels of estrogen over women with *negligible* pre-treatment readings of the hormone. Women who conceive while using ovulatory stimulants likewise are exposed to higher estrogen concentrations than subfertility patients who later achieve unaided pregnancies. Garcia, et al. (1977) found 25.4% of their clomiphene patients experienced SAs, contrasted with 10.5% of their subfertility patients who later conceived without assistance; Toshinobu, et al. (1979) had similar numbers (23.6% - 8.9%); Ben-Rafael, et al. (1981) reported on comparable SA rates (29.4% - 8.8%); and I calculated consistent rates when comparing SAs for women who conceived during a treatment cycle, without hyperstimulation (21.4%), with women who conceived two or more cycles after treatment (12.4%). [See Chapters 11 and 12]

Another known side effect of clomiphene citrate, hMG and other fertility drugs is ovarian hyperstimulation syndrome (OHSS), which involves painful and enlarged ovaries. In its severe form it can cause nausea, vomiting, diarrhea, shortness of breath, blood clots, bloating and ascites (fluid accumulation in the abdomen), and frequently requires hospitalization. OHSS is also associated with even higher levels of endogenous estrogen.[408] In fact, detection of elevated estrogen has been used in the diagnosis of OHSS.[409] As will be seen, the SA rate skyrockets in the presence of OHSS – and the estrogen that accompanies it.

Caspi, et al. (1976)[410] were one of the first researchers to evaluate the incidence of SAs in the face of OHSS. Their population included patients treated with hMG (Pergonal) and hCG. "The incidence of abortion was not related to maternal age and was 17.5% in pregnancies without hyperstimulation as against 35 per cent and 33.3 percent with mild and severe hyperstimulation respectively." They did not know what to make of these numbers, but appeared to be on the right track. "The causes of the high rate of abortion (are) not understood. Brown et al. (1969) suggested that *abnormal ovarian steroid patterns* might be responsible and though the differences did not attain statistical significance, it is interesting to note that patients with hyperstimulation had the highest abortion rate." [Emphasis added.]

Five years later, Lunenfeld, et al. (1981)[411] published preliminary findings of another study, again looking at the incidence of SAs following the use of hMG and hCG. They were similarly drawn to the possible effects of OHSS on the human embryo.

"Although the factors leading to the relatively high abortion rate following induction of ovulation with hMG/hCG have not been fully elucidated, severe hyperstimulation seems to be at least one factor, as 8 of 16 patients with severe hyperstimulation aborted." Their updated report (Ben-Rafael, et al., 1983) painted a much clearer picture. "The influence of grade 2 and grade 3 hyperstimulation on the abortion rate is even more prominent when one considers all pregnancies after hMG/hCG-induced ovulation. In the first and second (groups of) pregnancies taken together, 5 of 27 women (18.5%) with grade 1 hyperstimulation aborted, while 11 of 22 women (50%) with grade 2 or grade 3 hyperstimulation aborted. This abortion rate was found to be highly significant (P<0.01)." They also established that the rate of multiple births increased with hyperstimulation. "Thus, we have *demonstrated* that the three main complications of hMG/hCG treatment, i.e., high abortion rate, multiple pregnancy, and ovarian hyperstimulation are *interrelated*." [Emphasis added.]

These earlier papers only focused on total abortions, whereas my study (Chapter 11) specifically evaluated the rate of *early* (first trimester) SAs. Recall that such spontaneous terminations occurred at the rate of 4.7% (11/236) in pregnancies conceived two or more cycles after last exposure to Clomid; 13.6% (27/199) one cycle after treatment; 14.7% (224/1,519) during a cycle of treatment without OHSS; and 22.9% (25/109) during a treatment cycle with OHSS.

Recent literature supports these findings and strengthens the hypothesis. Chen, et al. (1997)[412] reported a SA rate of 23.5% following severe OHSS among their IVF patients compared to 15.1% in pregnancies without severe OHSS, and Abramov, et al. (1998)[413] documented similar numbers: a 29.8% (31/104) SA rate in their IVF patients experiencing severe OHSS, compared to a range of 18-22% generally reported for other IVF populations; 25.0% (26/104) of their study group experienced early abortions.

But the study by Raziel, et al. (2002)[414] really brought home the point. Twenty-three out of 60 (38.3%) of their IVF pregnancies experiencing severe OHSS resulted in SAs. The abortion rate of patients with severe OHSS was significantly higher than the rate of IVF patients without OHSS during the same period of time [14.8% (169/1138), P<0.001]. Of the sixty pregnancies, 19 (31.6%) were early losses and only 4 (6.7%) occurred during the second trimester. "It (has been) hypothesized that OHSS may have a possible detrimental effect on the quality of the oocytes (ova). If so, it may have detrimental effects on the quality of the embryos and the developing pregnancy at its early stages and thus may cause pregnancy loss."

One might ask whether the ART procedures themselves (exclusive of fertility drugs) are producing ova with chromosomal anomalies. It would seem not. It is a well-accepted fact that clomiphene, hMG and other fertility drugs can cause OHSS. When it occurs following IVF or other measures, it is the drugs that are producing the enlarged and painful ovaries, not the procedures used in extracting and inseminating the ova. It would also follow that the choice of fertility drug used during ART would not have an influence on the SA rate of the subsequent pregnancies if they are unrelated. Yet, that appears to be the case. Saunders, et al. (1992)[415] explored that very question when they reviewed the obstetrical histories of 2,457 IVF and GIFT patients who conceived with clomiphene (CC) and 694 of those patients who became pregnant with the use of gonadotrophin-releasing hormone (GnRH). Comparing the total SA rate, there was a significant difference: 23.8% for CC and 19.5% for GnRH (P<0.05). When they broke out the first trimester SAs, the statistical significance became even stronger: 14.8% for CC and 10.1% for GnRH (P<0.01). Conversely, the incidence of late abortions was approximately the same with both drugs (3.4% and 3.2%, respectively).[416] Although they did not involve ART pregnancies, Radwanska, et al. (1988)[417] found similar disparities when comparing the SA rate of spontaneous ovulators (13%) with conceptions following clomiphene (19%) and hMG (31%). The differences were significant (P<0.05). Aono, et al. (1983)[418] found significant differences in the SA rate among women who conceived without the aide of fertility drugs (10.7%), bromocriptine (10.1%), clomiphene (13.8%) and hMG/hCG (22.0%).

Allow me a few rhetorical questions.

If the underlying subfertility condition is responsible for the elevated SA rate, why would there be significant differences between the choices of fertility drugs? Why would the SA rate dramatically increase in the presence of OHSS if the pathological condition producing ovulatory dysfunction was the culprit? Why would the incidence of SAs of subfertility patients conceiving without the use of fertility drugs be substantially lower than stimulated conceptions, if the drugs were unrelated to the pregnancy loss?

These studies are *presumptive* evidence of the hypothesis that fertility drugs can cause elevated levels of endogenous estrogen and OHSS, which in turn produce chromosomal abnormalities in the resulting embryo, leading to first trimester spontaneous abortions.

Direct evidence, such as the 1973 study by Boue and Boue, is rare only because of the lack of such studies. With the advent of ART over the past two plus decades, one would think that science has been presented with an excellent opportunity to reach a firm conclusion on this issue. Earlier studies either lacked control groups and/or had difficulties with the techniques used to examine and record chromosomal anomalies.[419] The study by Gras, et al. (1992)[420] took a stab at using a control group. Thirty-five percent of the ova obtained after superovulation with clomiphene and hMG/hCG had aneuploidy (abnormal number of chromosomes) compared to 20% of non-stimulated oocytes. The increase was not significant (P>0.20) due to inadequate numbers – apparently an ongoing problem. Extensive research efforts failed to turn up any studies where cytogenetic deficiencies in ova following ART procedures were compared with chromosomal anomalies in oocytes from women of normal fertility.

Animal Studies

Ovulatory-stimulating drugs have also demonstrated to be mutagenic in animals. Superovulation of *rabbits* can cause development of abnormal chromosomes in pre-implantation blastocysts (embryo prior to implantation on uterine wall). [Fujimoto, et al. (1974);[421] 9.7% of superovulated blastocysts with chromosomal anomalies vs. 0.0% for controls] Chromosomal anomalies have also been caused by superovulation in *mice*. [Takagi and Sasaki (1976);[422] 24.0% of superovulated blastocysts with chromosomal anomalies vs. 7.7% for controls; P<0.005]; [Maudlin and Fraser (1977);[423] a dose-response to drug (PMSG) used to stimulate ovulation, with percentage of chromosomal anomalies in embryos ranging from 8.0% to 20.8%]; [Luckett and Mukherjee (1986);[424] one strain of mice with 14.9% chromosomal anomalies in superovulated embryos vs. 10.7% in controls (P = 0.05); and second strain with 22.0% and 11.9%, respectively, (P<0.005)]; and [London, et al. (2000);[425] exposure of clomiphene citrate to mice oocytes resulted in significant (P<0.05) increases in chromosomal anomalies using both in-vitro and in-vivo methods].

In view of all of the above-mentioned studies and the clear demonstration of mutagenicity in Clomid, there is thus between a 64% and 85% likelihood, on this evidence alone, that Clomid is also a human teratogen.

Animal Teratology Studies

The more animal species in which a drug is teratogenic, the more likely it is to be teratogenic in humans. In a study conducted by Jelovsek, et al. (1989),[426] a list of drugs with known, suspicious, unknown or negative teratogenic capabilities were compared with animal teratology studies, using the same drugs, to evaluate their predictive capabilities and to determine whether or not the results could be extrapolated to humans. It was found that the animal studies had a positive predictive value of 75%. "This study indicated that 75% of positive human developmental toxicants can be predicted on the basis of animal study results alone."

It is also the consensus among noted teratologists within the United States that animal teratology studies do have some predictive value. *"The more animal species in which a compound has a developmental toxic effect, the more likely that compound is to have an effect in humans, but it is not a directly linear relationship (e.g., 1 positive result amounts to 1.0, 2 or more positive results counts for about 1.67)."* [Rule 14] *"If a positive...developmental toxic effect occurs across more than one animal order, that compound is more likely to have an effect...in humans than if it were just across more than one animal genus within an order (rat and mouse effect less important than rat and rabbit effect)."* [Rule 26] *"Animal studies do not need to be concordant with the pattern of malformations or other developmental toxicity in human studies in order to be counted in their evaluation."* [Rule 57] The types and nature of congenital anomalies seen in animals do not need to be the same as seen in humans in order to apply their predictive value.

Clomiphene has been found to be teratogenic in *rats*. This was initially established through in-house studies performed by Merrell Dow in 1962 [Merrell Dow nos. E-62-47, E-62-48 (enlarged heads, shortened mandible, hematomas, and soft tissue deviations of limbs), E-62-49 (soft tissue deviations of limbs, absence of tibia, head malformations, long snout, abnormal rump, hydrocephalic head, severely stunted with cartiligenous nasal appendage and umbilical hernia), E-62-51 (abnormal limb alterations, elongated snout)]. See also Diener and Hsu, 1967,[427] (hydronephrosis, hydroureters, deformed tails, missing phalanges, exencephaly, fused kidneys and severe growth retardation); Eneroth et al.,1971,[428] (hydramnion, cataracts, palatoschisis); Clark and McCormack, 1980,[429] (abnormalities of female reproductive tract); and Nyitray and Druga, 1991,[430] (edema of the neck region, hydrops fetalis, cataracta, alterations of the genitourinary tract – dilatation pelvis renalis, dystopic gonads, hydronephrosis – and abnormalities of the whole skeleton). Study E-62-51 and the published studies by Diener/Hsu and Nyitray/Druga are given added weight because the route of administration (oral) is the same route of exposure in humans and the absorption of the drug is similar. [Rule 24]

Clomiphene has been found to be teratogenic in *rabbits*. This was also initially established through in-house studies performed by Merrell Dow in 1962 [E-62-50 ('turning under' of distal portion of hind feet, bent and shortened tails, and abnormal sternal bones) and E-62-32 (similar limb abnormalities)]. These two studies are given added weight because the route of administration (oral) was the same route of exposure used in humans and the absorption of the drug is similar. [Rule 24] Lopez-Escobar and Fridhandler, 1969,[431] also found clomiphene to be teratogenic in the rabbit (protrusion of bowels and liver lobe through abdominal wall, absence of cranial vault); as did Morris, 1970,[432] (gastroschisis, cranioschisis, absence of eyelids, stunted limbs, cleft palate and hydrocephalus).

Clomiphene has been found to be teratogenic in *mice*. See teratology studies by Cutter Laboratories [Merrell Dow no. O-67-66, August 1967 (facial hemangiomas, under-developed kidney, fragmented sternum, incomplete ossification of clavicle, under-development of axis, absence of sterrebra)]; Cunha, et al., 1987,[433] (female genital tract abnormalities)]; and Dziadek, 1993,[434] (fetal growth retardation and exencephaly).

Clomiphene has been found to be a developmental toxicant in *guinea pigs*. As used by Jelovsek, et al., "developmental toxicity" includes structural and functional teratogenicity and "embryo toxicity (abortion, stillbirth, intrauterine growth retardation)." Although not specifically testing for teratogenicity, after administering clomiphene on day one of pregnancy, Motta and Hutchinson (1991),[435] found a statistically significant reduction in implantations and growth retardation in the embryos. Since there is a relationship between an increased rate of growth retardation and congenital malformations (Dziadek, 1993), this study is at least presumptive evidence that clomiphene is teratogenic in guinea pigs as well.

In any event, using the model of the Jelovsek study, there are at least *four different species* (rat, rabbit, mouse and guinea pig) in which clomiphene is developmentally toxic. Out of the *84* drugs and chemical compounds listed by Jelovsek et al. as not human teratogens (Table 1), only *three* were found to be developmentally toxic in four or more different species of animals. Thus, "on the basis of animal study results alone," it is more likely than not that clomiphene is a human teratogen.

This conclusion finds further support from the *Dziadek* study. Although given subcutaneously, the clomiphene was administered prior to conception, as it is given therapeutically to humans, and was given at a dose (mg/kg of bodyweight) comparable to the conventional dose given to women. [See Rules 76 and 77] And although it is not necessary to have concordance between the animal congenital anomalies and those seen in humans (Rule 57), it is of considerable value when it does. Dziadek found that by administering clomiphene prior to conception, she was able to induce *neural tube defects* in the offspring (exencephaly), as well as growth retardation.

Animal In-Vitro and In-Vivo Studies

Studies have also been conducted with clomiphene involving its exposure to tissue in the test tube (in-vitro) and in the bodies of various species of animals (in-vivo). These studies have demonstrated clomiphene's ability to inhibit cell growth in fetal tissue of animals – and *humans* as well. Cunha et al. (1987) conducted a study in which *human* fetal female reproductive tracts were grafted to female mice, which were thereafter exposed to clomiphene, tamoxifen and DES, all of which are chemically related, being derivative of triphenylethylene. All three drugs produced similar anomalies in the reproductive tract tissue, including abnormalities of the vagina, as well as endometrium, cervix, and fallopian tubes. "On the basis of the data presented here, antiestrogenic triphenylethylene compounds are potent estrogens in the human fetal genital tract and have the distinct potential for eliciting teratogenic change." Interestingly, when Clark and McCormack (above) administered these same compounds to pregnant rats, many of the same anomalies in the female reproductive tract were found in the embryos as were found by Cunha.

Additionally, administering clomiphene to developing animal ova and embryos, both by in-vivo and in-vitro methods, produces decreased embryonic growth rates and increased degeneration of ova and embryos. See Laufer, et al. (1983);[436] Schmidt, et al. (1985);[437] Schmidt, et al. (1986);[438] and Yoshimura, et al. (1986).[439]

All of the above in-vitro and in-vivo studies are supporting evidence of the proposition that clomiphene citrate is capable of inhibiting fetal cell growth, both in animals and in humans, when exposed directly to the drug.

Similar Chemical Structure

"In general, if a compound has a structural similarity, i.e., one side chain difference, to a known human teratogen, and if that compound's mechanism of action is similar to the known human teratogen and the known effect of that teratogen is through its pharmacologic action, then that compound is more likely to have a teratologic effect in human...." [Rule 91] Diethylstilbestrol (DES) is a known and widely-accepted human teratogen. It is also structurally similar to clomiphene citrate, both being triphenylethylene derivatives. In humans, DES causes adenosis and clear cell adenocarcinoma and structural abnormalities of the vagina, cervix, uterus and fallopian tubes in the *female* offspring exposed to the drug during pregnancy; and epididymal cysts, hypotrophic testes, microphallus, vericocele, and hypospadius in the *male* offspring. [Herbst, et al. (1971);[440] Henderson, et al. (1976);[441] Bibbo, et al. (1977);[442] Cosgrove, et al. (1977);[443] Gill, et al. (1979);[444] Whitehead and Leiter (1981).[445]]

Animal studies have demonstrated that DES and clomiphene both exert a similar pharmacologic action in producing congenital anomalies. In the study by Cunha, et al. (above), DES and clomiphene were introduced to human fetal female reproductive tracts grafted into female mice. Both demonstrated similar *estrogenicity* in the mothers. Similar findings were observed in the human fetal reproductive tracts grown to a gestational age of 16 weeks or greater. Both drugs also demonstrated similar *teratogenicity*. Comparable anomalies were found in the fetal vaginas, uteri, and fallopian tubes. As mentioned above, these same organs undergo structural changes in *human* female embryos exposed to DES. As stated by the authors, "Human fetal genital

397

tracts grown in the presence of DES, tamoxifen or clomiphene exhibit abnormalities of mesenchymal morphogenesis, which probably relate to the spectrum of structural anomalies seen in the vagina, cervix, uterine corpus, and fallopian tube of women exposed in utero to DES. * * * On the basis of these considerations, it is prudent to consider that the therapeutic use of clomiphene as a fertility drug for anovulatory women *may be associated with some degree of risk to the developing fetus* as suggested earlier by Clark and McCormack, Gorwill, et al., and Taguchi and Nishizuka." [Emphasis added]

In the study performed by Gorwill, et al. (1982),[446] clomiphene and DES were both administered to neonatal mice at the time of vaginal formation (which occurs in the human in the late first and early second trimesters). Both drugs caused *vaginal adenosis* (abnormal cells of the vagina lining), which is also caused by DES in humans. Another study involving rats by Clark, et al., published in 1982,[447] reported on the female and male offspring of the mothers injected with clomiphene on days 0, 5 and 12 of pregnancy. "The (vaginal and cervical abnormalities) of the offspring is reminiscent of the vaginal adenosis which has been observed in young girls whose mothers had received diethylstilbestrol during pregnancy. These abnormalities...were also observed in the uterus and oviduct of both offspring and rat mothers." One of 9 male pups had testicular abnormalities involving epididymal cysts and impaired spermatogenesis, which have also been reported in human male offspring exposed to DES in utero.

Given the structural chemical similarity between DES and clomiphene, and the obvious pharmacologic similarities substantiated by the above-mentioned studies, this likewise provides substantial evidence that clomiphene citrate is a human teratogen capable, at the very least, of producing anomalies similar to those caused by DES. It is thus *probable* that clomiphene is a human teratogen on the basis of these studies alone.

Biologic Plausibility

As indicated by Shepard in a Letter to the Editor in 1994,[448] this is not a required criterion. "Another criterion which is comforting to have but often not fulfilled is biologic plausibility for the cause. We have no biologically plausible explanation for Thalidomide embryopathy. Without going into detail here, I would suggest that at least one-half of all human teratogens do not fit this criterion."

However, clomiphene would appear to meet the test of biologic plausibility. Because of the importance of this criterion, elevated by recent discoveries, it will be discussed at length in the next chapter.

* * * * *

CHAPTER 19

Cause and Effect

How does a drug or other teratogen physically produce the anomaly? What biologically occurs in the mother and/or embryo that produces the malformation? What was the mechanism of action? This has always been one of the great mysteries in teratology. As surprising as it might be, science has yet to figure out how most human teratogens alter or malform an otherwise normal organ in an embryo. We might know that a given teratogen can produce a given anomaly; we just don't know *how*. Even thalidomide – one of the most potent pharmaceutical teratogens of all time – has escaped detection when it comes to understanding how it inflicted its devastation on thousands of nascent infants.

This is why it is such a major discovery when science is able to shine a spotlight on an actual means of producing a birth defect, be it a syndrome or a single anomaly, or via an environmental insult or the familial passing of a defective gene. It is the first step in possibly eliminating a tragedy facing otherwise unsuspecting parents; and, as is usually the case in science, one discovery can beget another.

Such was the case on an evening not that long ago.

It was late at night and I was updating my medical research for this book. I had been sitting in front of my laptop for several hours, inputting variations of key words to a research source on the internet, hoping to get some meaningful feedback. At the moment, it was well past my bedtime. Janet had preceded me to bed by at least an hour and a half – and I was sure to hear about it in the morning.

Suddenly a page appeared on my screen that provided a moment of enlightenment that will be etched in my memory for many years to come. To this day I have no idea what question I had posed, but sitting in front of my face was a statement from an unauthored article that provided a key to answering the question of the decade: How does clomiphene prevent closure of the neural tube? It simply stated:

"Recent studies have shown that cholesterol synthesis is critical for neural tube closure and that both dietary and genetic perturbations in the cholesterol synthesis pathway can lead to neural tube defects."

For a moment I only stared at the revelation, uncertain I was reading it correctly. I rubbed my weary eyes and read it again. The article was entitled "The Ecogenetics of Neural Tube Closure," and appeared to be dated around 1995 or 1996. The concept it conveyed was quite simple: when something blocks or inhibits the synthesis of cholesterol, prior to formation of the neural tube, it can result in an NTD. I quickly read the article, which was no longer than a page and a half. Another statement jumped out at me.

"Roux (1964) has shown that Triparanol, a drug that blocks cholesterol synthesis, is teratogenic to mice and if given to pregnant females, will cause neural tube closure defects in the embryos. Therefore, it appears that abnormalities of cholesterol production can have major effects on neural tube development."

Why did this have such an impact on me? Due to my long history with Clomid, I was in possession of certain knowledge that only a few others could claim. For example, I was aware that Triparanol was a drug that had been manufactured by Merrell back in the 1960s. I was also well-acquainted with the fact that "clomiphene citrate is related to other triarylethylene compounds such as...the cholesterol inhibitor, Triparanol," as stated in Merrell's package insert for Clomid, dated May 1991 (and all earlier editions). The two drugs were chemical cousins. But I also vaguely recalled the presence of one other statement in the same product labeling, which I shortly verified.

"Analysis by gas liquid chromatography (GLC) of serum sterols from patients on prolonged, continuous administration of Clomid yields a peak compatible with an elevated level of desmosterol. This peak is *indicative of an interference with cholesterol synthesis*." [Emphasis added.] [449]

In other words, depending upon the individual sensitivity of a given patient, and a sufficient quantity of the drug, Clomid interferes with the body's ability to synthesize (create) cholesterol. Though not as potent, *clomiphene citrate is a cholesterol inhibitor*, just like its cousin, Triparanol.

Cholesterol is synthesized through a series of conversions via enzyme reactions on various precursors, one of which is desmosterol. If one partially blocks a stream of water, it will back up and form a pond. This is why an elevated level of desmosterol is indicative of "interference with cholesterol synthesis." It is not converting to cholesterol in its conventional manner and rate and thus accumulates.

I was even familiar with the Roux article and had in fact cited it in my papers to the FDA advisory committee in 1975;[450] although for different reasons. To rebut arguments that drugs were only teratogenic when administered during the period of organogenesis, I pointed out that Roux was able to induce them with Triparanol as early as day 4 post-conception. Organogenesis begins in the rat on day eight. Along with neural tube defects (craniorachischisis, iniencephaly, etc.), he was also able to produce microcephaly, vertebral malformations, urinary anomalies and malformations of the extremities, including shortened digits. Doses were administered as late as day 10, and the timing would dictate the type of anomaly produced.

The anonymous article also cited a number of studies, which I would need to locate and read. But that would have to wait. If I took any longer to get to bed, I would find a blanket and a pillow outside the bedroom door.

The discovery year of 1993 occurred on two fronts, as also often happens in the field of science. First, a group of networking scientists, led by Dr. G. Stephen Tint, discovered that a rare hereditary syndrome (Smith-Lemli-Opitz syndrome or SLOS) was caused as a result of a deficiency in the embryo's ability to synthesize cholesterol.[451] It was considered to be the first true *metabolic* malformation syndrome. The multiple malformations included microcephaly (smaller than normal brain and cranium), facial anomalies, growth retardation, and abnormalities of the limbs and genitalia.

One of the earlier papers on SLOS presented an interesting observation: some SLOS patients are born with craniosynostosis, an anomaly involving premature fusion of the cranial sutures (fibrous joints between bones of the skull).[452] Left untreated, this condition can result in microcephaly and mental retardation. A recent study found that exposure to clomiphene citrate resulted in a significantly increased risk (OR 3.8; 95% CI, 1.1-12.3) of infants being born with this rare congenital defect.[453] Is it possible that Clomid can produce craniosynostosis via the mechanism of inhibiting the synthesis of cholesterol?

About the same time as the SLOS discovery, others were conducting studies on rodents. By the manipulation of genes, they were able to produce mice with modification of the apolipoprotein B (apoB) gene, which is instrumental in the synthesis of cholesterol.[454] The researchers were seeking to produce mice that might be protected from coronary vascular disease. But they were presented with a surprise. Although they found significant lowering in the plasma concentrations of cholesterol, many of the mice embryos with modified apoB were born with hydrocephalus and exencephaly, a neural tube defect. These findings were duplicated in later studies.[455]

SLOS is attributed to cells of intended organs receiving deficient signaling from the Sonic hedgehog (Shh) gene. [That's what it's called, I swear. But I've named it the "be-quiet gene."] The Shh gene and its proteins are dependent upon cholesterol to telegraph how certain organs should form, and are regulators for the development of the brain, limb and genitals.[456] Embryos conceived with a specific hereditarily defective enzyme (7-DHCR), fail to provide sufficient cholesterol to the Shh gene, which in turn produces the SLO syndrome.[457]

Many SLOS patients suffer from holoprosencephaly (HPE), a central nervous system defect where the brain fails to divide into two hemispheres. This same anomaly can be reproduced in embryonic rats exposed to AY9944 and BM15766, cholesterol-reducing drugs that act on the same enzyme that denies adequate cholesterol to the Shh gene found with SLOS.[458] It can also be caused in rat embryos by Triparanol, although acting on the last enzyme of another biosynthetic pathway. There are two different, though parallel, enzymatic routes leading to cholesterol. AY9944 and BM15766 act on the last enzyme (7-DHCR) of one pathway and Triparanol acts on the last enzyme (Delta 24-DHCR) of the other. Impairment of cholesterol production on either route by these three drugs can lead to HPE in rat embryos.[459] These findings and other evidence have led scientists to conclude that it is the low cholesterol rather than the backup (elevation) of the precursors that causes these congenital abnormalities.[460]

Drugs can thus impair an enzyme with the same effectiveness as heredity.

When administered to pregnant rats on gestational days 3 or 4, AY9944, BM15766 and Triparanol all deny adequate cholesterol to the Shh gene and its transmitting proteins, resulting in disruption of the normal formation of the early developing brain. These cerebral anomalies are manifested in different forms and severity: from lack of formation of the pituitary gland and/or corpus callosum (structure that joins the two cerebral hemispheres), to narrowing of the forebrain (frontal) hemispheres, to full-blown holoprosencephaly; or, in its more severe form, narrowing of the cranial end of the neural tube and even a full neural tube defect of craniorachischisis (anencephaly with exposure of upper spinal cord) and inienchephaly (extreme backward bending of the head).[461] Because the deficient signals from the Shh gene are acting primarily on the frontal/cranial end of the neural tube, a number of facial anomalies are also involved. These include micrognathia (underdeveloped lower jaw), anophthalmia (absence of eyes), cyclopia (centrally located single eye), and proboscis (elongated nose).[462] SLOS features in humans include microcephaly, absence of the corpus callosum, HPE, and facial abnormalities, including micrognathia. There have also been cases of cyclopia with associated proboscis reported.[463]

Feminization of male SLOS patients is another clinical trait seen in embryonic rats exposed to deficiencies in cholesterol synthesis. When AY9944 is administered to pregnant rats on gestational day 11, feminized male genitalia occur in embryos similar to those seen with SLOS.[464]

Finally, it has been demonstrated that AY9944 and Triparanol can reproduce SLOS-type limb anomalies. The clinical (human) features of SLOS limb abnormalities include club feet, syndactyly (parallel fusion of digits), usually of the 2nd and 3rd toes, polydactyly (extra digit) and shortened and absent digits.[465] Exposure from either of these drugs to pregnant rats on days 9 or 10 results in either delayed ossification (hardening and calcification) or outright lack of development of the affected bones. Observed anomalies include clubfeet, syndactyly of the 2nd and 3rd digits, polydactyly and ectrodactyly (absence of digits).[466]

The rat has thus been found to be a useful model for reproducing defects seen in humans that are occasioned by deficiency in cholesterol biosynthesis.

The organs affected would thus be dictated by the timing of administration of the drugs. Early exposure has a major impact on the central nervous system and later exposure can malform male genetalia and the distal limbs. Without question, cholesterol synthesis is a key element in the development of the embryo, be it animal or human.

"Deficiencies in cholesterol during embryogenesis and organogenesis cause severe abnormalities. The role of cholesterol in cell biology has been known for years. It is a key constituent of the cell membrane, the structure of which is obviously important in cell-to-cell interactions, which are essential in embryonic differentiation." [467]

The Chemical Cousin

Enter clomiphene citrate. The similarity between Triparanol and clomiphene is so widely accepted that they have often been used together in the same studies. As far back as 1970, Blohm, et al.[468] compared the two clomiphene isomers with Triparanol. All three were administered to rats for 10 consecutive days and measurements taken of the subsequent levels of desmosterol in various bodily tissues. They found that the *trans* (aka "zuclomiphene" or "Z") isomer was 10 times more potent in suppressing cholesterol than the *cis* (aka "enclomiphene" or "E") isomer, and that the trans isomer was slightly less effective than Triparanol. [Note that this study was conducted by the Department of Biochemistry, The Wm. S. Merrell Company, Division of Richardson-Merrell, Inc.]

The Z isomer, of course, is the same one that hung around for over a month in the half-life studies performed by Mikkelson, et al. (1986). Using zuclomiphene in another rat study, Ramsy, et al. (1975)[469] found significant levels of desmosterol in the central nervous system, along with another cholesterol precursor, zymosterol. Two years later, a couple of papers by Ramsey and Fredericks[470] expanded on these findings. When used on four-day-old rats, the Z isomer had a profound effect on inhibiting cholesterol synthesis in the brain and other CNS tissue.

Once someone turned on the lights about the association between NTDs, limb defects and cholesterol deficiency, two teratology studies involving clomiphene citrate became critically important – one early paper and another more recent.

The Diener and Hsu Study

The first study was conducted by Diener and Hsu (1967),[471] and involved clomiphene, Triparanol and two other drugs. All four compounds were administered orally to pregnant rats at three different dose levels. Clomiphene was administered only on days 6 through 14 at all three levels because implantation would be completely inhibited earlier than day six. It was thus commenced at least two days prior to the onset of organogenesis (day eight). Half of the pregnant females were sacrificed on day 20 and the other half allowed a normal delivery. Anatomic defects included cleft palates (opening in roof of mouth), deformed tails, missing phalanges (absent toes), and exencephaly – a neural tube defect. Significantly, the defects included abnormal bone formation and/or inhibition of skeletal ossification, a process requiring the biosynthesis of cholesterol.[472] Of the pups exposed to the low and medium doses of clomiphene, 13% and 14% had such anomalies of the skull, 13% and 5% of the vertebrae, 83% and 68% of the ribs, 9% and 23% of the metacarpals (front paws) and 0% and 4% of the metatarsals (rear paws), respectively. Triparanol-exposed pups had similar defects of the skulls, vertebrae, ribs, metacarpals and metatarsals.

> "In the present study, the most consistently observed disorder of the offspring from medicated dams was a retardation and/or malformation of the skeletal system. This was manifested by the presence of a *reduced amount of ossified tissue* in various parts of the skeleton such as the ribs, vertebrae, metacarpals, metatarsals, and skull. Whether this inhibition of ossification was *the result of an enzyme inhibition* or some other factor has not been determined." [Emphasis added.]

This study is significant for a few reasons. First, although the incidence rates differed, clomiphene and Triparanol caused similar central nervous system and skeletal anomalies in rat offspring exposed to the two drugs during the same gestational period. Due to the similarity of their chemical structures, both drugs inhibit cholesterol synthesis by acting on the same last-step enzyme (Delta 24-DHCR) that precipitates an increase in the precursor, desmosterol. This study substantiates that the two compounds act in a similar manner on the rat embryo – a model for evaluating how cholesterol deficiency influences the developing human.

Second, the study demonstrated that clomiphene could cause a neural tube defect (exencephaly) when administered two days prior to the onset of organogenesis.

Third, the shared anomalies included not only NTDs, but also *lack of ossification* and alteration of the bones. The ossification and alteration anomalies of the skeletal system discovered in 1967 were similar to those described following Triparanol and AY9944 in papers published three and a half decades later;[473] anomalies, the authors concluded, that were *precipitated by a deficiency in cholesterol synthesis.*

The Dziadek Study

The second paper was published by Marie Dziadek in 1993.[474] Her study was ground-breaking in that all prior teratology studies with clomiphene citrate exposed the animals to the drug post-conception, usually during the period of organogenesis. Dziadek chose to expose female mice to clomiphene *prior to ovulation*, similar to the timing of treatment actually employed by women. One of her treatment protocols also used a dose level (at mg/kg of body weight) comparable to a female patient receiving 100 mg/day for five days. Female mice were injected with clomiphene for two consecutive days, using 13 different protocols covering a period from 5 days prior to ovulation to ten days after conception. Three different dose levels were administered for each protocol.

The results were a reduction of embryo (blastocyst) implantations in the uterus, and of those that attached to the uterine wall, there was an increased incidence of growth retardation and exencephaly. The critical period for producing the neural tube defect was days two and three prior to ovulation and conception.

One of the reported findings that caught my attention was that all of the exencephalic fetuses in this treatment group came from separate females. In other words, even though the fetuses came in litters, *there was only one NTD in each set* that included this malformation. This coincides with what is seen among twins in humans: only about 4% of NTD twins are concordant (both with the same anomaly).[475] Almost always (96% of the time), the co-twin is normal or, on occasion, born with a different anomaly. This is an important consideration when theorizing the mechanics of how NTDs are produced (see below).

The second major observation made by Dziadek related to transferring four-day old blastocyst/embryos from pregnant rats to foster females. When unexposed (to clomiphene) blastocysts were transferred and implanted in foster mothers previously exposed to the drug prior to implantation, they had a reduced rate of implantation, and resulting fetuses showed a retardation in growth and development. Conversely, when they transferred exposed blastocyst/embryos and implanted them into unexposed foster mothers, the rate of implantation was the same as controls and there was growth retardation in only one treatment protocol. These findings implied to Dziadek that the primary problem was in *maternal support after implantation.*

"The results of these studies suggest that clomiphene citrate does not have a direct effect on embryonic tissues during the stage of neural tube closure, but that defects may arise indirectly by a *disturbance in the normal maternal support of pregnancy* which causes a progressive retardation in embryonic growth." [Emphasis added.]

The early rodent embryo has a limited ability to synthesize cholesterol. In fact, as late as days 12 to 13 of gestation, 60-70% of cholesterol is of maternal origin.[476] Although the rat embryo has exhibited the capacity to produce its own cholesterol at least as early as gestational-day ten,[477] there is little question that the early post-implantation embryo is dependent upon the maternal support system for the majority of its cholesterol. I would thus suggest that the "disturbance in the normal maternal support of pregnancy," surmised by Dziadek, was the denial of a sufficient level of cholesterol for effective signaling from the Shh gene to the preliminary structures of the neural tube – all provoked by the pre-ovulatory exposure to clomiphene.

Can these findings be translated to humans? I would ask, "Why not?" Rats and mice have demonstrated to be role models for exploring the mechanism by which deficient cholesterol production can produce congenital malformations in humans; in particular, those related to the neural tube and brain, not to mention skeletal and genitourinary defects. When Kirillova, et al. (2000)[478] compared the genetic markers in humans born with craniorachichisis and spina bifida, with those of mice embryos born with NTDs, they found similar patterns originating from the Shh gene. More importantly, *clomiphene citrate inhibits cholesterol biosynthesis at the earliest stages of gestation*, a time during which the embryo is dependent upon its production for the proper functioning of the genes telegraphing the shape and growth of embryonic organs. Its prolonged half-life and ability to continue reaching the developing embryo further down stream would also assure its biological influence on later-developing organs.

Twins with Discordant NTDs

When neural tube defects occur with twins, it is rare when both are affected. One twin will develop an NTD, while its co-twin will slip by unscathed or, on some occasions, with a different anomaly. It is rare that NTDs show up with twins that are concordant. From the studies mentioned above, only about 4% of twin pregnancies that resulted in a neural tube defect had a co-twin with the same anomaly. An article by Little and Elwood (1992)[479] brings better focus to this issue. They pooled all existing epidemiology studies that had looked at concordance by sex of the twins; an effort to factor in zygosity (whether identical or fraternal). To do this they broke out incidence rates for unlike-sex and like-sex twins. The former involve dizygotic (DZ) twins, whereas the latter include DZ and monozygotic (MZ) twins. For unlike-sex (DZ) twins with NTDS, 4.0% were concordant, whereas like-sex (DZ/MZ) twins with NTDs were concordant at a rate of 7.7%. The almost-doubling of the incidence of concordance would suggest that identical twins are much more likely to share NTDs than fraternal twins. This might imply a genetic or hereditary component to MZ twins with neural tube defects. Yet even MZ twins with NTDs have a high percentage of discordance. Whether the twins originate from two separately fertilized eggs or from an impregnated ovum that splits into two developing embryos, only a small percentage of those pregnancies have shared NTDs.

Why is that?

Not one to hold back on my views, I will share my thoughts on the subject. Call it the "Shared-Cholesterol Hypothesis." My take on the literature, including the above papers, is that at some early stage of gestation – probably shortly after commencement of implantation (day 6) – the twins begin competing for available cholesterol. When it is in limited supply, one of the twins assimilates a disproportionate share and continues with normal development and growth. Denied sufficient cholesterol, the remaining twin develops a neural tube defect.

Who wins or loses the battle over cholesterol may be dictated by the difference in genetic strength of the individual twin, a factor more likely with dizygotic embryos and less likely with monozygotic twins. This might explain the above statistical difference in the discordance of twins. Identical twins would be more likely to have a similar ability to acquire cholesterol and thus equally disposed to developing an NTD.

Another potential factor might relate to the timing of implantation. It may be as simple as "first come, first served," when it comes to distributing cholesterol. Although an early embryo is capable of synthesizing cholesterol,[480] upon attachment to the endometrium of the uterus *the mother is the primary source of the product* during the first weeks of gestation. Thereafter, the embryo becomes increasingly dependent upon its own capacity to synthesize. The first twin to the well may be the one to walk off with most of the water. It seems unlikely that both DZ twins would implant simultaneously; that more likely, one would be preceding the other down the fallopian tube into the uterine cavity. Even MZ twinning can occur prior to implantation. When it happens, one might likewise see a disproportionate sharing of cholesterol.

Utilizing clomiphene citrate to conceive can thus introduce two competing functions of the drug: multiple ovulation and inhibition of cholesterol biosynthesis. When the ovaries are at a higher level of stimulation, they are more likely to expel multiple ova, two or more of which may become impregnated with sperm. At this point they become zygotes and then begin to divide exponentially into multiple cells as blastocysts (days 4-6). Assuming we are dealing with a twin pregnancy, during the implantation process (days 6-10) by both blastocysts, there is a demand for maternal cholesterol – which, unfortunately, now is not available in sufficient quantity to accommodate both embryos.

About the same point in time, clomiphene has been working over the Delta 24-DHCR enzyme, restricting its production of cholesterol. Given its extended half-life and studies demonstrating it to be biologically active for up to 54 days after ingestion,[481] it should be unquestioned that 11 to 14 days after a round of five-to-ten tablets, the circulating clomiphene citrate would be impacting the biosynthesis of maternal – even embryonic – cholesterol. Further, it appears that impairment of the subject enzyme can be extended beyond the date of drug exposure. In a study in which Triparanol was administered to a pregnant rat with a *single dose* on day 10 of gestation, twelve days later her cholesterol level was still less than half of that found in the control.[482] Triparanol and clomiphene, of course, are chemically related and impair the same enzyme.

On days 17 through 20, the elongated neural plates of both embryos are formed and begin developing a groove down the middle with folds on either side. But at about days 21 and 22, *something is not going according to the DNA-prescribed agenda* – at least with regard to one of the twins. Lacking sufficient cholesterol, the Shh proteins are unable to signal proper closure and fusion of the folds into a neural tube for the one deficient embryo, while the co-twin develops normally. By day 24, the cranial end of the neural tube is fully closed with the more-fortunate of the two, followed by closure of the caudal (spinal) area by days 25 to 26. But although the caudal portion also closes for the unfortunate twin, the cranial end never fully forms, leaving the developing brain exposed. The mesenchyme, which has covered the enclosed portion of the neural tube, gradually hardens to form the vertebrae and skull – except for the co-twin with the exposed brain. Over the ensuing weeks, the brain is gradually destroyed through mechanical compression and disruption of its vasculature. By the second trimester, the brain is nothing more than a small vascular mass of tissue. The resulting fetus is anencephalic, and is later delivered with a normal sibling.

That's the way I see it.

Need more convincing? Compare the incidence of twinning among anencephalics and other NTDs in the general population with the same anomalies seen following IVF and other ART procedures.

When Lancaster and Hurst compiled their data on NTDS in Australia for the years 1991 through 1997,[483] they found 11.1% (38/305) of anencephalics, 4.4% (32/724) of spina bifidas, 6.7% (11/165) of encephaloceles, and 6.6% (81/1,232) for all NTDs combined, to be from twin pregnancies. Little and Elwood (1992)[484] reviewed the world literature on NTDs and twinning covering the period from 1958 through 1989. When they combined all of the various studies, their data indicated that 2.6% (266/10,089) of anencephalics, 2.1% (129/6,157) of spina bifidas, and 3.3% (12/361) of encephaloceles, were from twin pregnancies. Incidence rates varied depending upon the gestational cut-off date and whether the statistics included terminated pregnancies.

Now consider the percentage of NTDs from twin pregnancies following ART. Many such studies do not include data on the frequency of twinning among NTDs. However, those that do tell a dramatic story: Lancaster (1987) reported on three of 6 cases (50%) with spina bifida from twin pregnancies; FIVNAT (1995) reported on four of 8 (50%) NTD cases; Bergh, et al. (1999) reported on seven of 10 (70%) NTD cases (all four with anencephaly and 3 of six with spina bifida); Ericson and Kallen (2001) reported on nine of 12 (75%) NTD cases; and Kallen, et al. (2005) reported on twelve of 25 cases (48%) NTD cases (all five with anencephaly and 7 of twenty with spina bifida).

The rate of twin pregnancies among NTDs explodes from a range of 2-7% for the general population up to a range of 48-75% – and up to 100% for anencephalus –

411

following ART procedures. How is this possible? Better question: How is it possible to see such a profound increase without the two events being inextricably tied together? Although some infertility patients might be so desperate as to allow a twin pregnancy, with one anencephalic and one normal sibling, go to delivery (rather than terminate it), it is highly unlikely that this practice alone would explain such an eruption in statistics.

Other Fertility Drugs

Clomiphene citrate inhibits the synthesis of cholesterol. But what about other fertility drugs? Pergonal (hMG) and chorionic gonadotropin (hCG) are used frequently in IVF and other ART procedures – as are other fertility drugs, often without the assistance of clomiphene. Exclusive of assisted reproductive technology, pregnancies following use of the hMG/hCG combo have also shown an excess of NTDs, usually with (fraternal) twin pregnancies. I thus explored whether such drugs might likewise affect the synthesis of cholesterol – and one more piece of the puzzle fell into place.

Although non-clomiphene fertility drugs do not appear to be cholesterol inhibitors per se, they still can *suppress cholesterol* levels in early pregnancy – apparently mediated via their ability to elevate estrogen production. Studies have established that following hyperstimulation of the ovaries by fertility drugs, the resulting elevated estrogen during the luteal (post-ovulation) phase of the cycle suppresses the level of total cholesterol.[485] In fact, there is an *inverse correlation* between concentrations of estrogen and the level of total cholesterol;[486] namely, the higher the level of estrogen, the lower the concentration of total cholesterol. Add a greater number of ova – also seen with enhanced estrogen levels – and you have a prescription for another NTD tragedy: a twin pregnancy without sufficient cholesterol to go around.

IVF and other ART procedures use fertility drugs – frequently clomiphene citrate alone or in combination with other fertility drugs – to produce the multiple ova for insemination. When successful, *one out of every 4 pregnancies involves multiple conceptions.* With two or more embryos, the need and demand for available maternal cholesterol is high, especially in early gestation when the neural tube is forming. Compound the problem with a drug that at the same time restricts its production and you have a high risk for NTDs.

Some researchers believe that when a neural tube defect appears in a singleton pregnancy, it is the surviving member of an early twin conception. The fetus-fetus interaction hypothesis was first introduced by Knox in 1970.[487] He theorized that when the outermost layers of two implanting blastocysts come in physical contact with each other, the layers effectively become damaged. As a consequence, there is a genetic-driven interaction in which one embryo is destroyed and the other left with a neural tube defect.

When the deficient cholesterol level is more pronounced, something similar might occur between two competing blastocysts. The most-deprived might be destroyed and abort, while the remaining twin develops an NTD. Recall the Diener and Hsu study (above) in which the authors commented that "(t)he progeny from the dams medicated with 54 mg/kg of clomiphene were so severely retarded in growth that detailed examination was not feasible." A similar event might occur with one of two embryos in humans, which would thereafter abort and leave a co-twin behind with a neural tube defect.

Of course, a neural tube defect could arise from a single embryo as well. We are all genetically unique. The maternal response to a cholesterol-inhibiting drug is going to vary, not just from the dose level of the ingested clomiphene citrate, but also the woman's individual genetic makeup and her ability to metabolize the drug. The genetic program of each embryo would also differ. Some will require more cholesterol for normal development than others. Although it would seem that multiple pregnancies would be at a higher risk for an NTD – as a consequence of cholesterol deprivation – there is no reason to believe that all singleton conceptions would escape a similar fate.

It is generally accepted that there are many causes of neural tube defects. Heredity is certainly one of them. NTDs have been known to appear in family members of fetuses delivered with such a defect. Most scientists agree that there are environmental factors as well, and perhaps 5-7% of NTDs are caused by abnormal chromosomes, including trisomy 18. The question explored here has been whether clomiphene citrate and other fertility drugs are one of the multiple etiologic factors in producing NTDs.

As a drug that inhibits cholesterol biosynthesis and is administered only a few days before conception, clomiphene has both the capacity and opportunity to prevent closure of the neural tube. It also has the capability to produce trisomies and in laboratory

413

studies has evidenced an ability to damage DNA. As a clastogen, clomiphene citrate may even be capable of asserting a direct teratogenic effect on developing embryonic organs. But be it as a cholesterol inhibitor or all of the above, epidemiology studies support the argument that this drug is in fact causing neural tube defects.

To me it all made sense – to a point.

There still remained the lingering argument that women using ART, similar to those using only ovulatory-stimulating drugs, have a physiological abnormality producing their infertility; the ever-present "bad egg" pitch: many of these women haven't been able to conceive in years and are carrying around old and defective ova. As a group, they are also older and thus at greater risk for birth defects. Then, of course, there are the various physical procedures of removing multiple ova from a patient, dropping them in a Petri dish, fertilizing them in vitro – including via intracytoplasmic sperm injection (ICSI) into the egg – which after a few days is then inserted back into the uterus.

How does one counter that any or all of these factors play a direct role in producing an increased incidence of congenital anomalies following ART?

The answer turned out to be quite simple.

Following the use of fertility drugs, whether alone or as part of IVF procedures at a fertility clinic, *twin and higher order multiple pregnancies have a greater incidence of congenital anomalies than do singleton pregnancies.*[488] So why is this important? Because women carrying singleton and multiple pregnancies following ART all have the same general background: they are all infertility patients who have undergone the same ART procedures. In other words, ART women carrying singletons are of the same average age as ART women carrying multiple fetuses; and have gone through similar periods of infertility; and have had similar fewer pregnancies; and, of course, have gone through the same procedures – and even used the same drugs – to get pregnant. *The only meaningful distinction between the two groups is that one set of women is carrying a single embryo/fetus and the other set carrying two or more of them.*

To me, this of necessity implicated either the twinning process (e.g., the physiological means by which multiple eggs are produced, inseminated and evolve) or the drugs that are producing them – or both. A higher incidence of congenital anomalies with multiple births in this cohort of women has nothing to do with their infertility or their use of ART procedures.

This led to the next logical question: Does the twinning process itself produce maternal conditions that are hostile to a developing embryo? If so, then there should also be an excess of congenital malformations when twins or triplets are produced through natural conceptions in the general population – and would establish at a minimum that fertility drugs *indirectly* produce birth defects by stimulating the ovaries to expel multiple ova, leading to twins and higher order births. Actually, the evidence is quite overwhelming that *naturally occurring multiple births carry a higher risk of birth defects.*[489] Indeed, the higher the order of multiple births, the greater the frequency of birth defects. Li and colleagues (2003)[490] found in a study of 922,791 singletons and 24,032 infants from multiple births that singletons had an incidence of congenital anomalies of 4.823%; twins an incidence of 9.220% (1.9 RR; 95% CI, 1.8-2.0); triplets an incidence of 13.000% (2.7 RR; 95% CI, 2.3-3.2); and quadruplets and higher an incidence of 22.222% (4.6 RR; 95% CI, 2.9-7.3). See also Kato and Fujiki (1992),[491] who found a birth defect rate in singletons of 1.47%; twins at 2.17% (P< 0.05); and triplets at 3.70%; and Olson, et al. (2005),[492] who recorded an increased rate for twins (OR 1.29, 95% CI 1.05-1.58, P= 0.014) and triplets (OR 2.12, 95% CI, 1.44-3.11, P< 0.0001) over singleton pregnancies.

But do twins following fertility drugs have a higher incidence of birth defects than naturally conceived twins? This very question was explored by Kuwata, et al. (2004),[493] who calculated the incidence of congenital anomalies following three distinct procedures used in ART – namely Intracytoplasmic Sperm Injection (ICSI), Gamete Intrafallopian Transfer (GIFT) and conventional In Vitro Fertilization (IVF) – along with ovulation induction without ART (e.g, using fertility drugs alone), and compared the birth defect rates to the incidence occurring with naturally conceived twins. The answer was a resounding "yes." After making epidemiologic adjustments for maternal age, they found an increased risk for all four categories using fertility drugs, namely an incidence of 13.1% for ICSI (OR 6.7, 95% CI 2.1-21.9; P< 0.01); 8.4% for GIFT (OR 3.7, 95% CI 1.2-11.8; P< 0.05); 7.4% for IVF (OR 3.6, 95% CI 1.1-11.5; P< 0.05); and 4.9% for fertility drugs alone (OR 2.3, 95% CI 0.7-7.3), compared to 2.1% for twins conceived without the use of drugs. Although the birth defect rate for fertility drugs alone did not reach statistical significance, they still demonstrated more than a 100% increased risk.

To me this answered all of the mentioned arguments of the critics. But my venture was not yet complete. Aside from neural tube defects, my research to this point had focused only on the combined number of birth defects associated with twinning; I had not been considering the specific individual anomalies that appeared in excess in the presence of twinning. I knew that NTDs occurred more frequently with twins, but what about other defects?

I was about to open a door to a surprising discovery.

* * * * *

CHAPTER 20

The Epiphany

As one approaches the twilight of his career, he is often given to pause and reflect on what good has come of his time on earth, not so much in personal accomplishments and gains but in what he has contributed to the society which has been an integral part of his life. What mark has he left? What has he given back? Perhaps no more than a ripple on a placid lake, displaced ever so slightly by a dropped pebble for the briefest moment, only to return as if nothing had ever taken place.

Most, of course, do their best just to survive, content to live a somewhat quiet existence with family and friends, grabbing what they can of life's little pleasures, before turning to dust to join the billions who preceded them. Others through effort or happenstance find themselves with the opportunity to help others and, if fortunate, see as George Bailey did that their labors and actions have benefited their fellow man, perhaps not in grand numbers but in a meaningful way to deserving souls in dire need of rescue and assistance.

By the nature of my profession and selected specialty, I have spent a considerable number of years trying to help the diseased and disabled find a better life than the one they were experiencing when they first came through my door. Although my efforts have fallen short at times, I like to believe that I have made a better life for many others and in some small way made an impact of some consequence. There have even been a few occasions when I have gone after an appreciable splash on that lake, only to find disappointment as the water receded without so much as a water mark on the nearby shore. Such a futile effort took place in Rockville in 1975 – and again in 1994 – when, alas, the FDA once again capitulated to the will of the drug industry that controls it.

The purpose of this book, of course, was to make yet another run at that shoreline, this time bypassing the FDA and charged with a commitment to succeed. Nothing short of success would be acceptable this time around. Once published, this book would represent a beacon to the uninformed of the risks of birth defects associated with the use of fertility drugs. But there was more to offer – a lot more.

Little did I know that this literary effort would take on the force of a tsunami.

Individual Anomalies in Multiple Births

In order to verify that twins and other multiple births in the general population were at a higher risk of birth defects than singleton pregnancies, I initially focused my research efforts on six separate studies, all occurring between 1990 and 2006.[494] Although the papers varied in scope, design and population studied, they each shared a common goal of assessing the possible increased risk of *individual* anomalies in multiple over singleton pregnancies. Some compared the rates in singletons with only twins, while others included all multiple births; some studies looked only at live births, while others evaluated both live births and stillbirths; two studies gathered their respective data from a single state (Virginia and Florida), while another drew statistics from multiple countries (England/Wales, Finland, France, Hungary, Israel, Italy, Mexico and South America); at one end was a study of 116,686 singletons and 1,990 infants from multiple births, while at the other was a study of 11,818,354 singletons and 260,856 twins. But for each congenital malformation studied, all 6 papers set out in tables the complete statistics for each defect, including their respective relative risks and statistical significance.

It was when I began comparing these tables that something struck me – at first generating an appreciable level of interest, but within minutes prompting my jaw to drop onto my lap. Notwithstanding the individual differences in each study, I was witnessing a pattern: study after study the same individual anomalies were escalated in frequency in multiple births compared to singletons – and the majority of them were at a statistically significant level. Understand that many studies refer to similarities in statistics of previous efforts to compare data between singleton and multiple births. My observation in that regard was not unique. What struck me was not just the consistency of seeing the same defects at an elevated risk study after study – it was the *nature* of those anomalies.

Without exception, *each congenital defect had been reproduced in animal studies by the use of cholesterol-inhibiting drugs or by "knocking out" the Sonic hedgehog gene (Shh) and/or one or more of its transmitting proteins.*

Table 3 sets out the data from the six mentioned studies – and a few others – and the corresponding animal studies. Each paper did not include an identical set of the same anomalies as the others, but all included many of them. Each study is identified by the name of the lead author and the date of publication. Where given, I have included the

95% confidence interval. But in the smaller studies only the statistical probability was reported by the researchers. Recall that a relative risk of 1.00 indicates that the recorded incidence in both groups is equal. Thus, for example, a relative risk of 2.69 equates to a 169% increased risk.

Table 3

COMPARISONS BETWEEN ANIMAL AND HUMAN STUDIES
(SINGLETONS VS. TWIN/MULTIPLE PREGNANCIES)

Animal Anomalies	Epidemiology Studies	Human Anomalies	Relative Risk (95% CI)
Central Nervous System:			
Exencephaly/	Myrianthopoulos (1975):[495]	Anencephaly	2.69 (P> 0.05)
Craniorachischisis[496]	Doyle (1990):	Anencephaly	**3.47 (2.73-4.36)**
	Ramos-Arroyo (1991):	Anencephaly	**3.71 (P< 0.01)**
	Kato (1992):	Anencephaly	2.09 (P> 0.05)
	Mastroiacovo (1999):	Anencephaly/ Craniorachischisis	* * * * *
	England/Wales		**16.38 (12.34-21.75)**
	Finland		**21.63 (6.34-73.83)**
	France-Paris		**7.77 (3.17-19.08)**
	Hungary		**2.67 (1.70-4.19)**
	Israel		**Significant Increase**
	Italy (1)		**52.56 (3.29-840.09)**
	Italy (2)		**5.23 (3.22-8.50)**
	Mexico		1.28 (0.86-1.90)
	South America		**1.61 (1.19-2.17)**
	Li (2003):	Anencephaly	**2.64 (1.23-5.67)**
	Tang (2006):	Anencephaly	**7.44 (5.39-10.25)**
	Myrianthopoulos (1975):	Encephalocele	**9.82 (P< 0.001)**
	Doyle (1990):	Encephalocele	1.16 (0.50-2.29)
	Ramos-Arroyo (1991):	Encephalocele	**5.83 (P< 0.01)**
	Mastroiacovo (1999):	Encephalocele	**2.21 (1.66-2.96)**
	Li (2003):	Encephalocele	1.71 (0.41-7.03)
	Tang (2006):	Encephalocele	1.55 (0.94-2.56)
	Doyle (1990):	Spina Bifida	1.08 (0.83-1.38)
	Ramos-Arroyo (1991):	Spina Bifida	1.93 (P> 0.05)
	Mastroiacovo (1999:	Spina Bifida	1.17 (0.97-1.41)
	Li (2003):	Spina Bifida	1.04 (0.57-1.90)
	Tang (2006):	Spina Bifida	**2.09 (1.74-2.52)**
Hydrocephaly[497]	Myrianthopoulos (1975):	Hydrocephaly	2.38 (P> 0.05)
	Kallen (1986):[498]	Hydrocephaly	**4.51 (P< 0.01)**
	Doyle (1990):	Hydrocephaly	**1.95 (1.54-2.44)**
	Ramos-Arroyo (1991):	Hydrocephaly	**3.81 (P< 0.001)**
	Kato (1992):	Hydrocephaly	2.89 (P> 0.05)
	Li (2003):	Hydrocephaly	**3.39 (2.63-4.36)**
	Tang (2006):	Hydrocephaly	**3.43 (3.06-3.84)**
Reduct. Defects/Brain[499]	Mastroiacovo (1999):	Reduct. Defects/Brain	**1.91 (1.25-2.93)**
Gastrointestinal Defects:			
Tracheoesophageal	Myrianthopoulos (1975):	Tracheoesoph. Fistula	**7.26 (P< 0.001)**
Fistula/Esophageal	Kallen (1986):	Esophageal Atresia	**2.33 (P< 0.05)**
Atresia[500]	Doyle (1990):	Tracheoesoph. Fistula/	

		Esophageal Atresia	1.85	(1.16-2.80)
	Ramos-Arroyo (1991):	Esophageal Atresia	3.70	(P< 0.01)
	Kato (1992):	Tracheoesoph. Fistula	7.43	(P< 0.05)
		Esophageal Atresia	7.53	(P< 0.01)
	Mastroiacovo (1999):	Tracheoesoph. Fistula/		
		Esophageal Atresia	2.56	(2.01-3.25)
	Li (2003):	Tracheoesoph. Fistula/		
		Esophageal Atresia	2.26	(1.19-4.27)
	Forrester (2005): [501]	Tracheoesoph. Fistula/		
		Esophageal Atresia	4.28	(1.39-10.00)
	Tang (2006):	Tracheoesoph. Fistula/		
		Esophageal Atresia	2.64	(2.11-3.30)
Anal Atresia/	Kallen (1986):	Anal atresia	1.91	(P< 0.05)
Anal Stenosis[502]	Doyle (1990):	Atresia/Stenosis Large		
		Intestine/Rectum/Anus	1.92	(1.35-2.65)
	Kato (1992):	Anal Atresia	3.23	(P< 0.05)
	Mastroiacovo (1999):	Atresia/Stenosis Large		
		Intestine/Rectum/Anus	2.05	(1.71-2.45)
	Li (2003):	Atresia/Stenosis Large		
		Intestine/Rectum/Anus	2.89	(1.86-4.50)

Pulmonary Defects:

Agenesis/Hypoplasia	Myrianthopoulos (1975):	Hypoplasia of Lungs	1.28	(P> 0.05)
of Lungs[503]	Mastroiacovo (1999):	Agenesis/Hypoplasia/		
		Dysplasia of Lungs	2.21	(1.52-3.21)
	Li (2003):	Agenesis of Lungs	4.11	(2.62-6.45)

Genitourinary Defects:

Hypospadias/Indeter-	Doyle (1990):	Hypospadias/Epispadias	1.06	(0.88-1.26)
minate Sex/Pseudo-		Indeterminate Sex/		
hermaphroditism[504]		Pseudohermaphroditism	3.71	(2.30-5.67)
	Ramos-Arroyo (1991):	Hypospadias	1.55	(P< 0.05)
	Mastroiacovo (1999):	Hypospadia/Epispadias	1.25	(1.13-1.38)
		Indeterminate Sex/		
		Pseudohermaphroditism	2.13	(1.54-2.93)
	Li (2003):	Hypospadias/Epispadias	1.99	(1.63-2.45)
	Tang (2006):	Hypospadias/Epispadias	1.33	(1.23-1.45)
Renal Hypoplasia/	Kallen (1986):	Renal Agenesis/Hypopl.	2.50	(P< 0.05)
Dysgenesis[505]	Mastroiacovo (1999):	Renal Agenesis/Dysgen.	2.17	(1.66-2.85)
	Li (2003):	Renal Agenesis	2.33	(1.38-3.93)
	Tang (2006):	Renal Agenesis/Hypopl.	1.29	(1.01-1.66)

Musculoskeletal Defects:

Omphalocele[506]	Doyle (1990):	Omphalocele	2.21	(1.55-3.06)
		Anomalies of		
		Abdominal Wall	1.32	(0.82-2.02)
	Kato (1992):	Omphalocele/		
		Gastroschisis	5.13	(P< 0.01)
	Mastroiacovo (1999):	Anomalies of		
		Abdominal Wall	2.03	(1.69-2.43)
	Li (2003):	Omphalocele/		
		Gastroschisis	1.72	(0.88-3.35)
	Tang (2006):	Omphalocele/		
		Gastroschisis	1.53	(1.27-1.84)
Vertebral/Spinal	Kallen (1986):	Spinal Malformations	3.53	(P< 0.05)
Anomalies[507]	Kato (1992):	Scoliosis	52.0	(P< 0.01)

		Supernumer. Vertebra	**52.0**	**(P< 0.01)**
	Mastroiacovo (1999):	Deformities of Spine	**2.86**	**(1.40-5.85)**
		Anomalies of Spine	**2.78**	**(2.06-3.76)**
Anomalies of Ribs/ Sternum[508]	Mastroiacovo (1999):	Anomal. Ribs/Sternum	1.42	(0.89-2.27)
Diaphragmatic Hernia[509]	Myrianthopoulos (1975):	Anomal. Diaphragm	**3.88**	**(P< 0.05)**
	Doyle (1990):	Anomal. Diaphragm	0.92	(0.44-1.69)
	Mastroiacovo (1999):	Anomal. Diaphragm	**1.33**	**(1.02-1.74)**
	Li (2003):	Anomal. Diaphragm	1.83	(1.00-3.35)
	Tang (2006):	Diaphragmatic Hernia	**2.28**	**(1.83-2.11)**
Distorted Long Bones[510]	Mastroiacovo (1999):	Bowed Long Bones	**1.86**	**(1.13-3.06)**
Craniofacial Defects: Micrognathia[511]	Kato (1992):	Micrognathia	**4.90**	**(P< 0.01)**
Cleft Palate[512]	Myrianthopoulos (1975):	Cleft Palate	**3.70**	**(P< 0.01)**
		Cleft Lip	**3.19**	**(P< 0.01)**
	Doyle (1990):	Cleft Lip/Palate	1.04	(0.89-1.24)
	Ramos-Arroyo (1991):	Cleft Palate	1.00	(P> 0.05)
		Cleft Lip/Palate	1.47	(P> 0.05)
	Kato (1992):	Cleft Palate	1.63	(P> 0.05)
		Cleft Lip/Palate	2.04	(P> 0.05)
	Mastroiacovo (1999):	Cleft Palate	1.11	(0.92-1.34)
		Cleft Lip/Palate	**1.35**	**(1.19-1.52)**
	Li (2003):	Cleft Palate	1.49	(0.93-2.38)
		Cleft Lip/Palate	0.98	(0.62-1.57)
	Tang (2006):	Cleft Palate	1.13	(0.91-1.41)
		Cleft Lip/Palate	**1.44**	**(1.25-1.67)**
Other Facial Anomalies[513]	Doyle (1990):	Nose/Face/Skull Anom.	1.15	(0.86-1.50)
	Mastroiacovo (1999):	Skull/Face/Jaw Anom.	1.38	(0.94-2.04)
		Skull/Face Bone Anom.	**1.30**	**(1.01-1.68)**
	Li (2003):	Skull/Face Bone Anom.	**1.93**	**(1.40-2.66)**
Cardiovascular Defects: Congen. Heart Defects[514]	Kallen 1986:	Cardiovascular Defects	**2.42**	**(P< 0.01)**
	Doyle (1990):	Cardiovascular Defects	**1.59**	**(1.36-1.84)**
	Ramos-Arroyo (1991):	Cardiovascular Defects	2.12	(P> 0.05)
	Kato (1992):	Congen. Heart Defects	1.91	(P> 0.05)
	Mastroiacovo (1999):	Congen. Heart Defects	**1.48**	**(P< 0.01)**
	Li (2003):	Cardiovascular Defects	**3.50**	**(3.20-3.70)**
	Tang (2006):	Congen. Heart Defects	**1.65**	**(1.59-1.71)**

The significance of the above data becomes even more impressive when one considers that in each study the incidence of birth defects in the cohort of multiple births was calculated from the total number of *infants delivered* rather than the total number of *pregnancies* from which the twins or other multiples were born. [See Chapter 18, under the subheading *Neural Tube Defects*.] For example, recall that only about 4% of twin deliveries with anencephaly are concordant. Thus, the actual relative risk for anencephaly per pregnancy in the above studies would be closer to double the reported numbers. Since these studies do not give the percentage of concordance for each of the individual anomalies,[515] it is impossible to make an accurate calculation of the true relative risk for twin and multiple pregnancies. However, Li, et al. (2003) found that 81% of all twins (71% for triplets; 56% for quadruplets and higher) in their study group were discordant for all birth defects combined; and Ramos-Arroyo (1991) found that 79% of like-sex twins and 94% of unlike-sex twins were discordant in his study group. It would thus seem that the relative risk (and statistical strength) would likely increase for *individual* congenital anomalies in the above studies in a general range of 60-95% if one was comparing the outcome of all pregnancies instead of all delivered infants.

Cholesterol-Deficient Syndromes

There are at least 6 known syndromes[516] associated with an inherited impairment of the embryo's ability to synthesize cholesterol.[517] They include Smith-Lemli-Opitz syndrome (SLOS), desmosterolosis, CDPX2, CHILD syndrome, lathosterolosis, and Greenberg dysplasia.[518] My next step was to compare the anomalies from these syndromes – that are *known* to be caused by a deficiency in the embryo's ability to produce cholesterol – with the elevated anomalies from multiple pregnancies.

It was almost a match across the board!

With only a few (explainable) exceptions, virtually every congenital anomaly that occurred at a consistently higher frequency among twins and higher-order multiple births also occurs in one or more syndromes attributed to a deficiency in cholesterol synthesis. Consider the following:

- *Neural Tube Defects*:

  Human syndromes: SLOS (lumbar spina bifida);[519] lathosterolosis (lumbosacral spina bifida); [520] CHILD syndrome (spina bifida).[521] Although spina bifida can occur in some cholesterol-deficient syndromes, anencephaly and encephalocele are never seen. It would seem that this exception relates to the *source* and *timing* of the low cholesterol (see below).

  Animal studies: Administering cholesterol-inhibiting drugs to pregnant rats or "knocking out" cholesterol-carrying proteins in mice produce exencephaly (nonclosure of the cranium with exposed intact brain) and craniorachischisis (exencephaly with contiguous spina bifida). *Exencephaly* is considered an early stage of anencephaly, and in rodents is the equivalent of the latter condition. *Encephalocele* is exencephaly with some extrusion of the brain.

- *Hydrocephaly*:
  Human syndromes: SLOS.
  Animal studies: Impairment of Shh activity by "knocking out" cholesterol-carrying proteins in mice produces hydrocephaly (abnormal accumulation of cerebrospinal fluid on the brain).

- *Reduction Defects of the Brain*:
  Human syndromes: SLOS; desmosterolosis; CHILD syndrome.
  Animal studies: Administering cholesterol-inhibiting drugs to pregnant rats and mice or impairment of Shh activity by "knocking out" selected downstream proteins in mice produce holoprosencephaly (failure of brain to develop into two separate hemispheres), forebrain and hindbrain hypoplasia (incomplete development of the front and rear of the brain) and pituitary agenesis (failure to develop the pituitary gland).

- *Anal Atresia (Imperforate Anus)*:
  Human syndromes: SLOS.
  Animal studies: Impairment of Shh activity by "knocking out" selected downstream proteins in mice produces imperforate anus (lack of anal opening).

- *Agenesis/Hypoplasia/Dysgenesis of Lung*:
  Human syndromes: SLOS; desmosterolosis; CHILD syndrome; Greenberg dysplasia.
  Animal studies: Impairment of Shh activity by "knocking out"selected downstream proteins in mice produces agenesis (failure of development), hypoplasia (incomplete development) and dysplasia (abnormal development) of the lungs.

- *Hypospadias*:
  Human syndromes: SLOS; lathosterolosis.
  Animal studies: Impairment of Shh activity by "knocking out" selected downstream proteins in mice produces hypospadias (where urethral opening of the penis is located beneath the shaft rather than the tip).

- *Indeterminate Sex/Pseudohermaphroditism*:

Human syndromes: SLOS; desmosterolosis; lathosterolosis.

Animal studies: Administering cholesterol-inhibiting drugs to pregnant mice and rats or "knocking out" downstream Shh proteins in mice produce feminized males and ambiguous genitalia.

- *Renal Agenesis/Hypoplasia/Dysgenesis*:

  Human syndromes: SLOS; desmosterolosis; CDPX2; CHILD syndrome.

  Animal studies: Impairment of Shh activity by "knocking out" selected downstream proteins in mice produces renal hyoplasia (underdeveloped kidney) – a variant of renal agenesis (absence of kidney) – and renal dysgenesis (malformed kidney).

- *Omphalocele and Gastroschisis*:

  Human syndromes: Greenberg dysplasia.

  Animal studies: Impairment of Shh activity by "knocking out" selected downstream proteins in mice produces omphaloceles (extrusion of a part of the intestines at the umbilicus). Gastroschisis involves an extrusion of a part of the intestines through an opening in the abdominal wall at a site other than the umbilicus. Both conditions involve a defect in the muscles of the abdominal wall.

- *Vertebral and Spinal Anomalies*:

  Human syndromes: SLOS; CDPX2; CHILD syndrome; lathosterolosis; Greenberg dysplasia.

  Animal studies: Impairment of Shh activity by "knocking out" selected downstream proteins in mice or administering cholesterol-inhibiting drugs to pregnant rats produce vertebral (individual bones of the spine) and other spinal abnormalities.

- *Rib and Sternum Anomalies*:

  Human syndromes: SLOS; CHILD syndrome; Greenberg dysplasia.

  Animal studies: Impairment of Shh activity by "knocking out" selected downstream proteins in mice or administering cholesterol-inhibiting drugs to pregnant rats produce rib and sternum (breastbone) abnormalities.

- *Diaphragmatic Hernia*:

  Human syndromes: SLOS.

  Animal studies: Impairment of Shh activity by "knocking out" selected downstream proteins in mice produces diaphragmatic hernias (extrusion of abdominal organs into the chest cavity as a result of an abnormal opening in the diaphragm: a muscular and membraneous partition between the abdominal and chest cavities).

- *Distorted/Bowed Long Bones*:

  Human syndromes: CHILD syndrome.

  Animal studies: Administering cholesterol-inhibiting drugs to pregnant rats produces bowing and other distortions of the long bones (legs).

- *Micrognathia*:

  Human syndromes: SLOS; desmosterolosis; CDPX2; CHILD syndrome; lathosterolosis; Greenberg dysplasia.

  Animal studies: Administering cholesterol-inhibiting drugs to pregnant rats produces micrognathia/mandibular hypoplasia (underdeveloped lower jaw).

- *Cleft lip/palate*:

  Human syndromes: SLOS; desmosterolosis.

  Animal studies: Administering cholesterol-inhibiting drugs to pregnant rats or impairment of Shh activity by "knocking out" selected downstream proteins in mice produce cleft palate (opening in the roof of the mouth).

- *Other Facial Anomalies*:

  Human syndromes: SLOS; desmosterolosis; CDPX2; Greenberg dysplasia. Additional severe facial anomalies include cyclopia (one eye in the middle of the face), proboscis (tubular appendage for a nose), and midface/maxillary hypoplasia (underdeveloped upper jaw)

  Animal studies: Administering cholesterol-inhibiting drugs to pregnant rats or impairment of Shh activity by "knocking out" selected downstream proteins in mice produce other facial anomalies, including cyclopia, proboscis, and maxillary hypoplasia.

- *Cardiovascular Defects*:

  Human syndromes: SLOS; desmosterolosis; CHILD syndrome. The cardiovascular defects seen in these syndromes include a wide variety of anomalies.

  Animal studies: Impairment of Shh activity by "knocking out" selected downstream proteins in mice produces a variety of cardiovascular defects.

Out of 18 categories of congenital malformations occurring at a consistently higher incidence among multiple pregnancies, only *one* has not appeared in any of the literature on the described cholesterol-deficient syndromes; namely, tracheoesophageal fistula (TEF) and esophageal atresia (EA). This absence may relate to the possibility that it occurs infrequently and the complete spectrum of anomalies associated with the six described syndromes has not yet been described in the literature. Tracheoesophageal fistula involves an abnormal passageway (e.g., fistula) between the trachea and esophagus; esophageal atresia occurs when the esophagus fails to open. They are two of the earlier forming organs and, for reasons expressed below, TEF and EA would be expected to occur only rarely in syndromes associated with embryos incapable of producing normal levels of cholesterol.

Yet there can be little question that TEF and EA can be caused by deficient levels of cholesterol. Shh fails to properly function in its absence, and impairment of Shh and/or its signalling proteins produce TEF and EA in "knockout" mice[522] – one of the animal models used to recreate anomalies resulting from the above human syndromes. Indeed, TEF and EA are considered components of the VACTERL syndrome, to wit: the Vertebral-Anal-Cardiac-Tracheo-Esophageal-Renal-Limb group of anomalies. In 2001, Kim, et al.[523] demonstrated that the complete spectrum of the VACTERL syndrome can be produced in mice by disarming three of the Shh proteins (Gli1, Gli2 and Gli3) – a study that caught the attention of some doctors at the National Institutes of Health. In 2004, citing Kim, et al., Edison and Muenke published a letter-to-the-editor on a preliminary study[524] they had conducted involving the statin drugs, lovastatin, cerivastatin, atorvastatin and simvastatin. Statin drugs are used to *reduce cholesterol* as a prophylaxis against cardiovascular disease. Among 54 studied cases reported to the FDA involving exposure to statin drugs during the first trimester, the authors found twenty reports of congenital malformations. Included were cases of holoprosencephaly and anomalies associated with the VACTERL syndrome, not to mention two cases of neural tube defects (spina bifida). They concluded, "Holoprosencephaly and the VACTERL association have been linked to inhibition of cholesterol biosynthesis, down-regulation of the cholesterol-dependent sonic hedgehog morphogenic pathway, or both." In a follow-up letter involving a minor correction, Edison and Muenke added, "We still believe that the preponderance of the evidence supports the hypothesis that early gestational exposure to statin drugs may be teratogenic and that prospective studies should be initiated."

This view is apparently shared by the FDA. Since at least 2001, the package inserts on statin drugs have contraindicated use during pregnancy. The current patient labeling for Vytorin (simvastatin) states that:

"This medication must not be used during pregnancy. If you become pregnant or think you may be pregnant, inform your doctor immediately. It is recommended that young girls and women of child-bearing age use effective birth control to prevent pregnancy while taking this drug. One of these drugs (simvastatin) may cause harm to your unborn child."

[One might ask, if women are urged to use effective birth control methods while taking statin drugs, how does the FDA reconcile allowing the use of clomiphene without so much as a warning? *They are both cholesterol inhibitors.* Yet drugs that are unlikely to be taken by younger women of child-bearing age get warnings and the older women who might have a cholesterol-inhibiting drug coursing through their veins during early pregnancy are told nothing. Go figure!]

In any event, except for limb defects, all of the other six categories comprising the VACTERL syndrome occur at a greater frequency in multiple pregnancies, namely vertebral anomalies, anal atresia and stenosis, cardiovascular defects, tracheoesophageal fistula and esophageal atresia, and renal agenesis and hypoplasia. In fact, as early as 1986, Kallen[525] made this very observation:

"We found an increased rate in twins of the following malformations: hydrocephaly, cardiac defects, alimentary tract atresias (notably esophageal and anal atresia), spine malformations, and (but not reaching statistical significance) limb reductions.[526] The initials of these malformations, with the exception of hydrocephaly, are V (vertebral), A (anal), C (cardiac), TE (tracheoesophageal), R (renal) and L (limb), resulting in VACTERL, a much debated syndrome developing from the VATER syndrome. * * * It can also be noted that among the 27 twins with multiple malformations, at least 9 had malformations belonging to this category (and not counted above)."

Three of my 6 principal studies did not find an inceased incidence of limb reduction defects among multiple pregnancies.[527] I thus did not include them on my list. However, three of the studies *did* find an increased risk, although only one was statistically significant: Ramos-Arroyo (1991), RR 2.12 for upper limb reduction defects (P> 0.05) and RR 2.41 for lower limb reduction defects (P>0.05); Kato and Fujiki (1992), RR 2.08 for hypodactyly (P> 0.05); and Mastroiacovo, et al. (1999) for all limb reduction defects (RR 1.83, 95% CI 1.58-2.11). Of the remaining three, Li, et al. (2003) found an increased risk for lower limb reduction defects (RR 1.27, 95% CI 0.40-4.00), but not for the upper extremities (RR 0.95, 95% CI 0.35-2.56). Doyle, et al. (1990) found no increase (RR 0.97, 95% CI 0.68-1.35); nor did Tang, et al. (2006) for lower limb reduction defects (RR 0.24, 95% CI 0.10-0.57) and upper limb reduction defects (RR 0.86, 95% CI 0.58-1.26).

Recall, however, that all of these studies calculated their incidence rates for multiples from all *infants* rather than *pregnancies* resulting in twins and higher order births. If the calculations had been made instead from pregnancies, except for Tang's lower extremity anomalies all other statistics would have shown an increased risk.

Some additional comments about limb defects. Deficient cholesterol and impairment of Shh function primarily impacts the *distal* extremities both in animals[528] and in humans.[529] Reduction defects are reflected as absent toes in animals and usually missing or shortened fingers and toes in humans, although on occasion an entire missing limb is reported with some syndromes.[530] Because the multiple birth studies likely included *all* reduction defects, to the extent that absence of long bones are generally unassociated with cholesterol deprivation, the limb reduction defects data would be diluted against an increase.

In my view, however, the primary reason that limb reduction defects do not make as strong a showing as the other anomalies associated with the VACTERL syndrome relates to the fact that defects of the *distal* extremities occur later in organogenesis when the embryo is the predominant source of cholesterol and is less dependent upon a maternal supply of lipids (see below). Development of the bones of the fingers and toes from hand plates and foot plates occurs over post-conception days 42 to 56.

The same explanation would equally apply to the weak representation of polydactyly and syndactyly in multiple pregnancies – limb defects that are frequently seen in cholesterol-deficient syndromes[531] and also producible in cholesterol-related animal studies.[532] Note the following numbers: Doyle, et al. (1990): polydactyly and syndactyly (RR 0.77, 95% CI 0.62-0.94); Ramos-Arroyo (1991): polydactyly (RR 1.54, P> 0.05); Kato and Fujiki (1992): polydactyly (RR 1.12, P> 0.05) and syndactyly (RR 2.64, P> 0.05); Mastroiacovo, et al. (1999): polydactyly (RR 1.17, 95% CI 1.04-1.31) and syndactyly (RR 0.98, 95% CI 0.82-1.16); and Li, et al. (2003): polydactyly and syndactyly (RR 0.88, 95% CI 0.68-1.13). And although incidence calculations from pregnancies would likely push most of these statistics into an elevated risk for multiple births, the numbers would be substantially lower than the other VACTERL anomalies. Again, the explanation would seem to relate to the timing, as these anomalies do not develop in humans until the latter stages of the embryonic period. Embryogenesis concludes on day 56 (e.g., at the conclusion of 8 weeks) and the fingers and toes are formed from the seventh through the eighth week.

In addition to the above 18 anomalies, there are a couple others that I believe occur more frequently with twins and other multiples, namely craniosynostosis and the anophthalmia/microphthalmia group of congenital malformations.

Craniosynostosis (premature fusion of the cranial sutures) occurs with SLOS.[533] It can also be reproduced in animals via "knocking out" cholesterol-carrying proteins (apoB) in mice[534] and administering cholesterol-inhibiting drugs (AY9944) to rats.[535] Although this anomaly is not mentioned in any of my 6 principle studies (possibly included with anomalies of the skull and face bones), the authors of at least one published study have concluded that "craniosynostosis is more likely to develop in twins compared to singletons."[536]

Anophthalmia (absence of eyes) can be induced in rats by administering a cholesterol-inhibiting drug (triparanol) on gestation day six;[537] and microphthalmia (abnormally small eye) has been produced through "knocking out" the apoB gene in mice.[538] Microphthalmia is one of the included anomalies with SLOS and CDPX2, although anophthalmia has yet to be reported with any of the 6 syndromes resulting from the impaired biosynthesis of cholesterol. This difference can again be reconciled by considering the timing of the anomalies: anophthalmia would occur earlier in gestation, whereas microphthalmia would appear later (see below).

Because of the rarity of these birth defects, it is difficult to find a large enough study group to come up with data that are statistically significant. My six studies, however, would at least suggest that these anomalies occur more frequently with twins and other multiples. Although Doyle, et al. only found a relative risk of 0.61 (95% CI 0.07-2.20) when *combining* anophthalmia and microphthalmia, Mastroiacovo and colleagues (RR 1.45, 95% CI 0.96-2.19) and Tang's group (RR 1.13, 95% CI 0.69-1.87) demonstrated a slight risk. The data from Li, et al., however, is enlightening. When looking at statistics for *anophthalmia* alone, they had only 9 reported cases out of 922,791 singleton pregnancies; a frequency of 1 in every 102,572 deliveries. But for the 24,032 infants produced from multiple pregnancies there was not one reported case. Their cohort of children from multiples was not large enough to produce a single case. But when separating off *microphthalmia* – which occurs more frequently – they found a profound increase (RR 5.24, 95% CI 2.23-12.29). Microphthalmia occurred 44 times out of 922,791 singleton pregnancies (1 in every 20,973 deliveries) and 6 times out of 24,032 infants from multiple pregnancies (1/4,005 infants). In my view these results would indicate that combining the two anomalies in the compilations tends to mask the risk factor for microphthalmia, and to get a true reading on anophthalmia one would need a study population of multiple millions.

A study by Shaw, et al. (2005)[539] is further illuminating. Pulling from 2,531,586 live and stillbirths in California over a nine-year period (1989-1997), they found an increased risk in multiple births over singletons for both anophthalmia (RR 2.3, 95% CI 0.6-9.8) and *bilateral* microphthalmia (RR 1.8, 95% CI 0.4-7.5). Bilateral microphthalmia occurs less frequently than the unilateral presentation of the condition, and it is thus not surprising that neither calculation reached statistical significance. However, when considered along with the above 6 studies, the evidence is strongly supportive of an association between multiple births and the occurrence of these two anomalies.

Source and Timing of Cholesterol

In terms of a developing embryo, there are two potential sources of cholesterol. One is maternal (e.g., exogenous) and the other is the embryo itself (e.g., endogenous). During the course of the embryonic period – the first 8 weeks of gestation – both sources play a critical role in supplying these needed lipids. In the early stages of development, the *mother* is the primary supplier of cholesterol – along with other needed nutrients – whereas in the latter stages of organ formation, the *embryo* takes over more and more of this function. In the rat, 60-70% of cholesterol is supplied by the mother on gestational days 12-13 (which corresponds to days 28-33 in humans), but only 15-20% toward the end of gestation.[540] Studies with rats have demonstrated that the lower the *maternal* plasma cholesterol levels during early pregnancy, the greater the frequency of holoprosencephaly in the resulting fetuses.[541] The researchers used a single dose of a cholesterol-inhibitor (AY9944) on different days of gestation. But whatever the day or dose of the drug, the correlation was always with the maternal cholesterol level. In a related study, it was established that none of these anomalies would occur as long as maternal levels were maintained above a certain reading.[542] *Maternal cholesterol dictated the occurrence and frequency of the produced anomalies.*

Establishing that cholesterol exogenous to the mother can be transferred to the embryo and fetus in mice, a recent paper presented a study in which labeled cholesterol was injected into pregnant mice in one protocol over days 1-8 and another over days 10-18.[543] The gestational term ends in mice in the range of days 18-21. Gestational day eight in mice corresponds to about day 16 in humans. The labeled cholesterol reached both the embryo and the fetus, although the level in the former was almost double that found in the latter. Not surprisingly, just as with the rat, the ability to transfer maternal cholesterol to the embryo/fetus declines as the period of gestation increases.

But what about humans? Can the data from rodents be extrapolated directly to man? Although comprehensive research seems to be lacking on this issue, the available papers would suggest that the human embryo and fetus follow the same general patterns established in animal studies.

There is a general consensus that maternal cholesterol plays a significant role during the period of embryogenesis in humans, but contributes little toward the latter stages of gestation. "There is very little cholesterol supply from the mother to the fetus in the end of pregnancy, but there is delivery of cholesterol from the mother to the fetus in the first 6 months when *early embryonic development* is occurring." [Emphasis added.][544] "Because it appears that maternal cholesterol can indeed be transported from the maternal

431

to the fetal circulation, fetal cholesterol concentrations can theoretically change in parallel with the quantity of both endogenous (embryonic/fetal) and exongenous (maternal) sources of sterol."[545]

Just as with the rat and holoprosencephaly, studies have shown that the severity of SLOS can be correlated to *maternal* plasma cholesterol concentrations; namely, the lower the maternal cholesterol level, the more severe the condition.[546] The influence of maternal cholesterol over the human embryo is also reflected in studies involving a gene (apoE) instrumental in transporting cholesterol to the embryo. Mothers with a defective variant (apoE2) of this gene cannot effectively transport cholesterol to embryos with SLOS, who are then born with a more severe form of this anomaly.[547] In other words, the SLOS embryo is conceived with an impaired ability to produce cholesterol, but will be born with a less-severe form of the condition if he or she can get a little help from Mom.

So what does this all mean?

Given this basic premise – that during the *early* embryonic period *maternal* cholesterol is the principle source and during the *late* embryonic and early fetal period the *embryo/fetus* is the primary source – a foundational piece of evidence exists from which one can explain the frequency of given anomalies *caused soley or principally by the lack of adequate cholesterol* among twins and higher order multiple births and the frequency of certain anomalies in cholesterol-deficient syndromes.

In a normal pregnancy, if one assumed that the percentages in humans were the same as in rats (see above), then on gestational days 28-33, 60-70% of the cholesterol would be supplied by the mother and 30-40% produced by the embryo. Indeed, this ratio might even be higher at an earlier stage of gestation. Now consider the dynamics with twins and higher order pregnancies. Under the premise of the *shared-cholesterol hypothesis*, the embryos are meeting their sterol responsibilities, but the mother is incapable of meeting hers. Conversely, with SLOS and other cholesterol-deficient syndromes, in early pregnancy the mother is normally supplying her 60-70% allotment of cholesterol and the *embryo* is falling down on his or her job. As a consequence, with twinning one would expect to see a greater incidence of anomalies that occur *early* in pregnancy *when the principle producer of cholesterol is found wanting*. But with cholesterol-deficient syndromes the primary source of these lipids generally *does* meet her quota. As a consequence, anomalies which occur early in embryogenesis will be seen more frequently with twinning and less frequently with SLOS and the other syndromes.

A few cases in point.

Anencephaly and *encephalocele*, which occur as a result of nonclosure of the cranium end of the neural tube during the fourth week of gestation (days 22-28), are seen at a very high incidence in twins and other multiples compared to singleton pregnancies. [See Table 3.] Yet to this date, neither has been reported in association with cholesterol-deficient syndromes. Among neural tube defects, only *spina bifida* has been reported – and then only as a rare event. Consistent with this premise, the spinal portion of the neural tube closes up to a *couple days after* the cranium; and spina bifida occurs as a less-frequent risk in multiple pregnancies.

As mentioned above, *tracheoesophageal fistula* and *esophageal atresia* also occur with great frequency with multiple births (RR 1.85-7.53), but have yet to be reported in association with cholesterol-deficient syndromes. In my view this is explained by the early origin of the anomalies. The esophagus (tube to stomach) begins to separate off from the trachea (windpipe) around gestational day 31, but the trachea itself originates from the primitive foregut during the fourth week (e.g., prior to day 29). By day 35 (conclusion of the 5th week) the separation is complete.

At the other end of the spectrum, when the *embryo* has taken over production and is the predominant source of cholesterol, we see later developing anomalies with cholesterol-deficient syndromes (due to the embryo's inability to meet its programmed function) and only evidence of a slight increased risk in multiple pregnancies (where the embryo is capable of working at full capacity). The prime examples of this consequence are the anomalies of *polydactyly* and *syndactyly*, and *limb reduction defects of the digits*, all of which originate during the 7th and 8th weeks of gestation (days 43-56). Polydactyly and syndactyly are seen frequently with some of the syndromes (i.e., 80-95% with SLOS Type II), but represent only a slight risk in multiple pregnancies (see above). Distal limb reduction defects occur in cholesterol-deficient syndromes (about 20% of reported cases of SLOS Type II), but are only a low elevated risk in multiple pregnancies.

The bulk of the remaining described anomalies appear both in excess with multiple births and in association with the human syndromes, and generally develop in the midrange of the embryonic period – perhaps when the cholesterol production is being split somewhat equally between the two sources. As to any anomalies that do not fit into this pattern – such as *hypospadias* and *sexual ambi*guity, which are strongly represented in both groups, but evolve late in embryogenesis – it is my opinion that cholesterol deficiency is only a contributing cause along with other etiologic factors.

A Prime Example

Now let's take a look at one of the largest studies published to date on the outcome of pregnancies produced by IVF, namely a study by Kallen, et al. (2005).[548] Professor Kallen and colleagues' study involved all infants delivered after IVF during a twenty year period (1982-2001) in Sweden, a total numbering 16,280 babies. An expectancy rate for malformations was calculated from a total of 2,039,943 infants born in the general population of Sweden over the same period of time. I selected this study because of its size and the fact that it involved *two risk factors* associated with cholesterol production during embryogenesis, namely a high incidence of multiple births and the use of fertility drugs. No less than 38% (6,192) of the 16,280 infants were from multiple births; and essentially all IVF pregnancies involve ova (eggs) produced by ovulatory-stimulating drugs. Rather than making a separate calculation of multiple birth anomalies, the researchers compiled statistics on the incidence of birth defects from a combined population of singletons and babies from twins and higher order infants following IVF. They also made a separate analysis "for some large and important groups of malformations among IVF children." Note their selected list, including the reported relative risk or odds ratio and 95% confidence interval:

Group of Malformations	RR/OR	95% CI
Anencephaly (RR)	7.6	**(2.5-7.7)**
Spina bifida	5.1	**(3.4-7.8)**
Any NTD	4.8	**(3.3-6.9)**
Hydrocephaly w/o NTD	1.7	(1.0-3.0)
Cleft palate and cleft lip/palate	2.4	**(1.9-3.1)**
Cardiovascular defects	1.7	**(1.5-2.0)**
Major cardiovascular defects	2.1	**(1.6-2.8)**
Choanal atresia (RR)	4.6	**(1.9-9.5)**
Esophageal atresia	4.0	**(2.6-6.3)**
Small gut atresia	6.4	**(4.2-9.6)**
Anal atresia	4.7	**(3.2-6.9)**
Any alimentary tract atresia	1.9	**(1.5-2.5)**

Abdominal wall defects	1.8	(0.9-3.6)
Craniosynostosis	1.5	(0.9-2.5)
Limb reduction defects	1.5	(0.9-2.5)
Hypospadias	1.7	**(1.4-2.1)**

Look familiar?

Except for choanal atresia[549] – which is not included in any of the studies – *every listed anomaly shows up as an increased risk with multiple pregnancies.* Every birth defect has also been produced in cholesterol-related animal studies and/or is a malformation included in one or more of the cholesterol-deficient syndromes. In short, there is strong evidence that an increased risk of birth anomalies following IVF is due to a shortage of cholesterol during embryogenesis.

But there is more.

Kallen, et al. also listed IVF infants delivered with *multiple malformations* (with 3 or more major defects), excluding those born with chromosomal syndromes. After I further excluded 6 infants with established syndromes,[550] there were 12 others remaining with multiple birth defects. Significantly, of those dozen babies, no less than 9 would properly qualify as suffering from the VACTERL syndrome; of which greater than 90% have only 2 or 3 of the seven described anomaly categories.[551] Consider the following:

1. Anencephaly/*cystic kidney (R)/polydactyly (L)*/female genital malformation: VACTERL syndrome;

2. Microcephaly/esophageal atresia/pulmonary hypoplasia;

3. Anophthalmia/*endocardial cushion defect (C)*/small gut atresia/*limb malformation (L)/spine malformation (V)*: VACTERL syndrome;

4. Esophageal atresia/small gut atresia/biliary malformation;

5. *Esophageal atresia (E)/anal atresia (A)/kidney dysgenesis(R)*/hypospadias/ *polydactyly (L)*: VACTERL syndrome;

6. *Esophageal atresia (E)*/microtia/cleft lip-palate/*spine malformation (V)*: VACTERL syndrome;

7. *Anal atresia (A)*/gut malrotation/*kidney agenesis (R)/spine malformation (V)/long bone dysplasia (L)*: VACTERL syndrome;

8. Anal atresia/gut malrotation/vaginal malformation;

9. *Anal atresia (A)/kidney agenesis (R)*/hypospadias: VACTERL syndrome;

10. *Anal atresia (A)/kidney agenesis (R)/VSD* (C)*: VACTERL syndrome;

11. *Anal atresia (A)/*choanal atresia*/VSD-ASD* (C)/spine malformation (V)*: VACTERL syndrome; and

12. Arthrogryposis*/VSD* (C)/spine malformation (V)*: VACTERL syndrome.

*VSD (ventricular septum defect); ASD (atrium septum defect).

Making reference to its predecessor syndrome (e.g.,VATER), the authors took special note of this nonrandom set of anomalies. "As seen from the list of multimalformed infants…, combinations of different alimentary atresia types with kidney malformations were frequent and may represent variants of the so-called vertebral, anal, tracheoesophageal, radial or renal (VATER) nonrandom association, thought to be the result of a very early disturbance of the morphogenesis." As indicated above, the VACTERL syndrome has been implicated through animal studies – and thought by many experts in the field to be associated – with *inadequate cholesterol* during the early period of organ formation. Anencephaly, of course, is clearly related to cholesterol deficiency, and anophthalmia has been produced in relevant animal studies. As to the balance of the anomalies, gut malrotation (SLOS and Greenberg dysplasia), microcephaly (SLOS, desmosterolosis and lathosterolosis), cleft palate and/or cleft lip (SLOS, desmosterolosis), pulmonary hypoplasia (SLOS, desmosterolosis, CHILD syndrome and Greenberg dysplasia), intestinal/small gut atresia (CDPX2), biliary malformation (SLOS), hypospadias (SLOS and lathosterolosis) and female genital malformations (SLOS) are all part of the spectrum of congenital abnormalities seen with the cholesterol-deficient syndromes.

There is thus strong evidence to suggest that the above 12 infants with multiple malformations, and the babies with the listed individual anomalies in the studied IVF population, represent the consequence of inadequate cholesterol during the first 8 weeks of their respective pregnancies.

Summing It Up

Exclusive of its potential to induce chromosomal errors, available evidence establishes that clomiphene citrate can cause congenital anomalies via its capacity to inhibit the biosynthesis of cholesterol. Absent sufficient levels of cholesterol, the Shh gene and its signaling proteins malfunction and fail to activate receptor genes needed to form specific organs during embryogenesis – and perhaps impede their early growth as a fetus. Based upon animal studies and the array of known anomalies from cholesterol-deficient syndromes, clomiphene has the capacity to induce neural tube defects (anencephalus, encephalocele and spina bifida), reduction defects of the brain (holoprosencephaly, agenesis of the corpus callosum, agenesis of the pituitary gland, etc.), hydrocephaly, tracheoesphageal fistula and esophageal atresia, anal stenosis and anal atresia (imperforate anus), agenesis and hypoplasia of the lungs, hypospadias and sexual ambiguity, renal hypoplasia and dysgenesis, omphalocele and anomalies of the abdominal wall, anomalies of the ribs and spine, diaphragmatic hernia, polydactyly and syndactyly, limb reduction defects, craniosynostosis, anophthalmia, microphthalmia, micrognathia, cleft palate and cardiovascular defects – not to mention all of the ingredients of the VACTERL syndrome. Human menopausal gonadotropin (hMG) and human chorionic gonadotropin (hCG) also suppress available cholesterol and can likewise induce the same congenital malformations. Not surprisingly, the majority of these anomalies have made an appearance as a statistically significant increased risk in a number of epidemiology studies assessing fertility drugs. [See Chapter 18, under the subheading *Epidemiology Studies*.]

Multiple births – *exclusive of the use of fertility drugs* – also present a risk factor for congenital malformations. Virtually all experts in the field agree that birth defects occur at a greater incidence with pregnancies carrying two or more fetuses; with an overall increased risk of combined anomalies up to 95%, depending upon the study. This risk factor is increased by about 80% if one makes the calculation based upon the total number of multiple pregnancies resulting in congenital abnormalities rather than from the total number of infants produced from them. Focusing on the *individual* anomalies that appear in excess in multiple over singleton pregnancies, almost all of them can be reproduced in animal studies in which either the cholesterol is substantially reduced by drugs or the cholesterol-dependent gene/proteins are "knocked out" by genetic manipulation. The majority of these anomalies also appear in association with cholesterol-deficient syndromes – and those that do not, or are only rarely reported, can be reconciled by their origin in early embryogenesis.

It is proposed by this author that the primary (though not exclusive) reason for an excess of congenital malformations in multiple over singleton pregnancies in the general population is an insufficient supply of maternal cholesterol in the presence of two or more embryos, otherwise described as the *Shared-Cholesterol Hypothesis*.

A Solution to the Problem

It is an inescapable fact of life that sometimes the most obvious opportunities escape detection by our conscious thoughts. Most often it's when our brain is on overload, when our mental faculties are so inundated with facts and data that it is next to impossible to step back and see the bigger picture. For me the escape from this quagmire occurs in the early morning, shortly before daybreak, after the gray matter has had a chance for a few hours of rest and before it's engaged again for the challenges of the day.

Such was the case a few months before wrapping up this book.

As often happens with men of my vintage, my bladder had awakened me and insisted that it be relieved. Dawn had not yet arrived, and after trying to ignore its persistent pressure for a few minutes, I arose, completed the ritual and returned to bed – only to be confronted by the light-but-nevertheless-audible snoring of my lifetime mate. For a few moments I had contemplated a slight push on her shoulder, which usually functions like a button and prompts her to role over onto her side. But light was starting to filter through the drapes and I was concerned I might awaken her. Besides, the snoring wasn't that loud and maybe I might just be able to get back to sleep.

Not a chance.

Thirty minutes later I had given up on the idea. My mind, over which it seemed I had little control, drifted to my recent research. I had been reading a series of papers involving animal studies testing the premise that it was the deficiency in cholesterol, and not the buildup in its precursors, that was causing the pattern of birth defects associated with holoprosencephaly.

A particular study by Gaoua, et al. (2000)[552] had really captured my attention. One group of pregnant rats had been administered a single dose of a cholesterol inhibitor (AY9944) on day 3 of gestation (GD 3). This particular drug acts on the same enzyme that malfunctions in babies born with SLOS, 7-dehydrocholesterol reductase (7DHCR), and the fetuses were born with severe growth retardation, pituitary agenesis, reduction in brain size, hydrocephalus, cleft palate, mandibular hypoplasia (micrognathia), microcephaly, craniosynostosis, and monorhinia (a protruding nose above a single eye in the middle of the face). These are all anomalies that have been seen in babies born with SLOS (with a wide range of frequency and severity). A second group of pregnant rats, which were likewise fed AY9944 on GD 3, also received a *dietary supplement of cholesterol* over GDs 3-14. In other words, they were concurrently fed a cholesterol inhibitor and cholesterol. The results were significant – very significant.

All fetuses were delivered without any of the congenital anomalies.

Although the AY9944 was introduced with a single dose on GD 3, the drug did not reach its maximum capacity until GD 11 (human GD 22), when maternal cholesterol was reduced by 76%; and by GD 14 (human GD 40) was only back up to 56% below normal. The concurrent use of cholesterol in group 2 thus coincided with the period that AY9944 would otherwise have been effective. Yet the teratogenic effect of the drug was totally eliminated through the use of dietary cholesterol during embryogenesis.

I almost sat upright in bed as it finally sank in.

If clomiphene and other fertility drugs are producing congenital anomalies via their capacity to reduce maternal and embryonic cholesterol (as does AY9944), then the *concurrent use of dietary cholesterol tablets* ingested during the period of embryogenesis would likely eliminate the same birth defects which would otherwise be produced. Just as some patients today take folic acid tablets to reduce the risk of neural tube defects,[553] OB/GYNs or fertility specialists prescribing fertility drugs or initiating ART procedures might also order the use of cholesterol prior to the anticipated date of conception.

In fact, prenatal treatment with dietary cholesterol to possibly eliminate or reduce the severity of SLOS was one of the considerations discussed by Gaoua and his coworkers. They suggested "that supplementation of the diet of pregnant women of (an) affected fetus may have preventative activity. Under physiological conditions a 'safe' maternal excess in cholesterol exists for most mammalian species." They proposed possible treatment during the "first 2 months of pregnancy," but quickly pointed out that the amount of cholesterol which would be safe and effective was unknown, and the *quantity* used on rats could not be directly extrapolated to humans.

Others have also suggested the use of dietary cholesterol as a means of treatment both during pregnancy (upon detection by lab studies) and after delivery of an SLOS baby. At its May 28, 1998 meeting on the Role of Cholesterol and Lipids in Embryonic Development and Congenital Disease, members of the National Heart Lung and Blood Institute (NHLBI) discussed the then recently-discovered evidence related to the association between SLOS and low cholesterol. Referring to earlier teratology studies involving animals, they stated, "Some of these teratogenically induced anomalies *could be prevented by cholesterol supplementation to the mother*." [Emphasis added.] Dr. Laura Woollett, a noted expert in the field, has observed that a number of SLOS patients could benefit from an increase in maternal cholesterol, and that the "most dramatic benefits would occur if the exogenous cholesterol supply increased in early gestation, such as during the first trimester."[554] As of this writing, there are at least two studies being conducted by the National Institute of Child Health and Human Development testing the effectiveness of post-delivery treatment of of SLOS with dietary cholesterol.[555]

These efforts, however, relate to SLOS, which only occurs in a range of 20,000 to 40,000 births.[556] This would equate to about 100 to 200 cases out of about 4,000,000 births per year within the United States.[557] Delivered infants with other cholesterol-deficient syndromes are even rarer.

What I am suggesting could potentially save *thousands* of infants from severe and catastrophic birth defects each year within the United States, and possibly tens of thousands world wide.

During the year 2004, 49,458 infants were born out of 36,760 live birth deliveries following IVF and other ART procedures within the United States.[558] The Center for Disease Control, the source of this information, (curiously) does not give the incidence of congenital anomalies from these deliveries. But depending upon the study, the rate of birth defects following ART procedures can be as high as 8.6-9.35%.[559] Since we are exploring the *potential* benefits of using cholesterol therapy during early pregnancy, I will use these numbers, which would calculate out to between 4,253 and 4,624 babies with major birth defects following ART in the United States during 2004. *What if these numbers could be cut in half with the use of dietary cholesterol?* Assuming that administering fertility drugs in these studies doubled the risk – which occurred in two of the cited papers – such a result is achievable.

Now consider the use of fertility drugs outside the ART clinic setting. The vast majority of women using ovulatory-stimulating drugs do so by ingesting them at home pursuant to a physician's prescription (i.e., clomiphene citrate) – or receive injections in a doctor's office (i.e., hMG/hCG) – followed by insemination the old-fashioned way. Exclusive of ART, there are approximately 695,000 women per year using drugs to stimulate ovulation.[560] According to the Clomid package insert, clomiphene has a pregnancy rate of 30% and a spontaneous abortion rate of twenty percent. The American Society for Reproductive Medicine states in its Guide for Patients on Ovulation Drugs that the hMG/hCG combo has a pregnancy success rate of 20-30%. Since clomiphene is by far the drug of choice in this cohort of female patients, it would be fair to say that 25-30% of the women taking these drugs get pregnant (between 173,750 and 208,500 pregnancies). If these numbers were reduced by a spontaneous abortion rate of 20%, the number of induced pregnancies that are delivered each year in the United States would range from about 139,000 to 166,800. If we used a conservative birth defect rate of 5%, between 6,950 and 8,340 are born each year in the U.S. with major congenital anomalies following the use of fertility drugs outside of IVF clinics. *What if these numbers could be cut in half with the use of dietary cholesterol?*

Now take a look at numbers from twinning and higher order multiple births. According to the CDC National Vital Statistics Reports for 2003,[561] there were 136,328 (128,665 twins, 7,110 triplets and 553 quadruplets+) multiple live births in the United States that year. I could not locate any national data for anomaly rates among multiple births, but the paper by Li, et al. (2003) based their study on statistics from the state of Virginia, where they reported rates of 4.82% for singletons, 9.22% for twins, 13.00% for triplets and 22.22% for quadruplet and higher order multiples. This would equate to 11,863 twins with major birth defects, along with 924 triplets and 123 quadruplets plus; a total of 12,910. *What if this number could be cut in half with the use of dietary cholesterol?*

But what about birth anomalies in *singleton* pregnancies?

The same birth defects that occur more frequently with multiple births also occur in singleton pregnancies – they just occur more often when there are two or more embryos. Although there may be up to a six-fold increase in tracheoesophageal fistula (TEF) and esophageal atresia (EA) in multiple pregnancies, these same anomalies also occur with singletons. If the majority of these birth defects are caused by inadequate cholesterol during early embryogenesis, it may well be that in a given singleton pregnancy neither the mother nor the embryo are supplying their required proportions of lipids. Each embryo will vary in its capacity to synthesize cholesterol and each mother will vary in her own lipid profile, perhaps due to her diet, metabolism or other factors. There unquestionably will be varying combinations of these two conditions. But when they both come up short, there exists a strong probability that a cholesterol-related anomaly will result.

This is not to say that every birth defect described above occurring in singleton births is also a product of lipid deprivation. The wide array of congenital anomalies produced by inadequate cholesterol during the embryonic period can also be brought about by other causes. TEF and EA are also related to chromosomal abnormalities, including trisomies 18 and 21.[562] Heredity may also be involved in some cases. But to assume that TEF and EA anomalies are unrelated to cholesterol problems simply because they appear in singleton pregnancies would be an unfortunate example of programmed ignorance. For example, both of these defects occur in the VACTERL syndrome, which has a strong association with low cholesterol and is seen usually in singleton deliveries.

As my wife often says, "You need to think outside the box." Of the 4,000,000 plus live births every year, 97% are from singleton pregnancies.[563] Of this subgroup there are in excess of of 120,000 babies born with major congenital anomalies. *What if only 10-20% of these birth defects could be eliminated each year through the daily use of a small dietary tablet of cholesterol?*

The benefits world wide could be staggering.

To avoid any misunderstanding here, *I am not advocating self-medication.* Any use of cholesterol tablets – or a high choloric diet – by a woman contemplating pregnancy, should be done under the supervision of her physician. What you have just read is on the cutting edge of science, and safe and effective doses need to be determined through properly-designed epidemiology studies – studies that have not yet been launched. And unless the embryo is plagued with a defective enzyme – as with SLOS – or otherwise incapable of producing an adequate supply of cholesterol, dietary treatment with lipids should *only be ingested during the first two months of pregnancy.* This is the period during which organs are being formed; thereafter, they are in a growth mode. There is also research to support the premise that excessive maternal cholesterol (hypercholesterolemia) during the *post-embryonic* period may produce fatty streaks in fetal coronary arteries and lead to an early onset of atherosclerosis.[564] [There is preliminary evidence, however, that treatment with an antioxidant (vitamin E) can potentially offset this risk factor.][565] It would also seem unlikely that women with already high cholesterol levels would need treatment to enhance those levels – and further dictates the need for physician involvement to monitor lipids throughout the first trimester, and possibly even the entire pregnancy.

So where does this leave us? Through the ground-breaking work of the scientists I have cited, we have been blessed with an incredible opportunity to eliminate a large number of the major congenital anomalies occurring throughout the world – literally tens of thousands of them. Science is also awakening to the fact that impairment of its production can create anomalies beyond those suffered by babies conceived with a defective enzyme. As recent as 3-4 years ago, genetic experts began to appreciate the association between low cholesterol and the VACTERL syndrome, and women of child-bearing age are being cautioned against use of statin drugs without taking effective steps to avoid pregnancy.

The most-immediate and practical use of this knowledge, of course, is with women who are using fertility drugs to conceive, both with and without the use of IVF. *But until such time as fertility specialists and other members of the medical profession acknowledge that clomiphene and other fertility drugs can cause birth defects via their capacity to impair the production of cholesterol, no one will step forward to initiate needed studies or even consider its use during early pregnancy.*

In the end, it will be the readers of this book who will bring about such a change.

* * * * *

CHAPTER 21

Where Are We Now?

"Damn it! Damn it! Damn it!" My burst of expletives caught Janet's attention in the kitchen. It was early spring of 2004.

"What's wrong?" Her voice sounded concerned. She knew I wasn't watching a Dodger game.

"Damn it!"

"I heard you the first time. What's wrong?" By now she was standing at the entrance to our spare bedroom. I was seated behind a desk in my improvised office.

"They did nothing, absolutely nothing." In front of me I was holding a current package insert for Clomid.

"Who did nothing? What in the hell are you talking about?"

"Merrell. The FDA. Both of them. It's the Clomid package insert," I said, waving it in the air. "They didn't do crap. In fact, it's worse."

"You talking about warnings?"

"Yeah, warnings. What there is of them. It's a joke…no, a tragedy. And like a goddamn idiot I have sat on this for over nine years. What an idiot! You would think by now I would have learned."

"I thought you sent them a letter?"

"Yeah, twenty-nine pages."

My letter of October 11, 1994 was accompanied by no fewer than 41 exhibits. The entire package was an inch thick – 1¼" to be exact. Everything stated in my correspondence was backed up with supporting documents, including copies of nine published studies. Five of the papers demonstrated a statistically significant increase in the risk of neural tube defects. The existing literature demanded some form of a warning – something, anything. Notwithstanding my earlier experiences and frustrations with the FDA, I was absolutely convinced that the presented evidence could not, and would not, be ignored.

What a fool.

In my defense, there were two factors that weighed heavily on my decision to let things take their natural course. First, a draft of the Clomid labeling had been floating around the FDA for several years that addressed some of the issues I had argued in 1975.[566] At a minimum, this implied that someone at the agency was committed to putting the medical profession on notice that the human embryo was facing some degree of risk. Maybe modifications of the language had been kicking back and forth with Merrell, but even with admittedly weak evidence, important changes were in the works. Second was the strength of the recent studies. If the Boue paper was sufficient to generate a warning about abnormal chromosomes in abortuses, why would the FDA ignore five epidemiology studies implicating fertility drugs as a cause of neural tube defects? Indeed, the early draft labeling included a reference to NTDs on the basis of a dozen or so case reports. Now that red flag was supported by statistical data.

Then, of course, there was my emotional state after the dismissal of the Lust case. When I flew off to Kauai in 1997, it was as much an escape from the disappointment of that federal court decision as to associate with a Honolulu law firm on some local litigation. My five years on the Garden Isle were a needed respite from the stresses of trial work in general and Clomid in particular. I began to readjust my priorities. I had carried the Clomid banner long enough and my October 1994 letter should have been sufficient to bring about the needed warnings.

I would later learn that the 2004 package insert was essentially the same as the June 1995 version. Very little had changed in the text of the labeling over the intervening nine years. As was explained in Chapters 13 and 15, forces that would eventually compose the future Clomid insert were already in motion when my October 11, 1994 letter and attachments hit the FDA that month.

Janet shrugged her shoulders. "Well, you know where I stand on this." She then disappeared from my doorway and shouted back at me, "When you're through cussing, you might give me a hand in the kitchen."

This literary effort had its genesis about four weeks earlier. One day, out of the blue, my wife suggested that I write a book about my experiences with the Clomid litigation. Maybe somebody might be interested in some of my discoveries. At first, the idea of taking on the task of writing a book was not that exciting. I had been through it once before[567] and my effort had almost destroyed our marriage. Moderation was a concept to which I had a difficult time adjusting.

But this time it was Janet who was pressing the idea of writing a book. My curiosity had now sufficiently motivated me to stop by a local pharmacy and secure a Clomid package insert. To put my story in print, of course, could never be justified if the labeling provided the users with an adequate warning about the risk of birth defects. Since I had never gotten a reply from the FDA, I had absolutely no idea how the agency had reacted to my written presentation. I had just *presumed* my arguments had been effective. Now I had reviewed the package insert and wasn't exactly happy with what I had read.

Five minutes later I was in the kitchen, peeling potatoes, relating my discovery to my culinary companion. "So, what do you think?" I asked, after reciting the multiple deficiencies in the labeling.

"You know what I think," was her terse reply.

"That I should write a book?"

"Of course. It's what I suggested a month ago."

"You understand that's a major undertaking."

"As if I could forget."

The reference, of course, was to the abuses I had inflicted on her with my novel – not to mention some of my work-related excesses. It was one of the reasons I was cautiously approaching this major task. "I understand," I assured.

"Do you? If you go forward with this, we have got to have an agreement. No excessive hours. You owe your wife some time as well, you know."

"I know."

"I wouldn't be endorsing this except for one reason."

"What's that?"

"You owe it to the kids, the babies. Maybe rather than helping deformed babies, you might be able to prevent them from happening."

I nodded my agreement. In two sentences, Janet brought the whole matter into perspective. This was not about telling my story; it was helping the helpless. Many women using fertility drugs, if not the majority of them, can conceive without their use during a conception cycle. If I could prevent even one child from being born with a serious congenital anomaly, it would be well worth the effort.

"Deal," I said, as I stuck out my hand.

We shook and cemented our agreement. I was now committed to a course of action I had only casually considered in the past. The very next day I would be off to our storage locker, digging through dusty boxes, turning yellowing pages, and generally making a determination of what I had to work with. But for the moment, my attention was on my wife. She was making a sacrifice, and it was not unappreciated. The evening would be spent with my lifetime companion. Tomorrow would come soon enough.

What exactly had brought my temper to the boiling point? It wasn't simply the lack of warnings. True, it was upsetting, and on that topic my anger was equally spread between the FDA and myself. My ire, however, became more profound as I began to appreciate the deceptions contained within the insert and the skill of the deceivers. This was not the work of an amateur. It had the polish of a master at the top of his craft. So much so that only someone who was privy to all of the relevant facts could ever flush out the truth and reveal the misrepresentations, distortions and concealment.

Something else was equally disturbing. For any number of reasons, the text of the Clomid package insert could only exist in its current state *with the complicity of the FDA*. This conclusion finds support from several factors.

Although the FDA was already in receipt of the information and data contained within my October 1994 letter, it had never before been packaged in such a fashion and shoved in its face. It reminded the federal agency that warnings it had previously approved had been inappropriately shelved. It again called attention to the multiple deficiencies in the pre-market clinical investigation that rendered it worthless as a measuring stick to assess Clomid's risk to the human embryo. It paraded a series of published epidemiology studies implicating Clomid and other fertility drugs as a cause of neural tube defects and other congenital anomalies. And finally, it highlighted the falsity of the misrepresentation that "no causative evidence of a deleterious effect of Clomid therapy on the human fetus has been seen." It set out all of the evidence and demanded to know what the FDA was going to do about it.

I had now been given the answer: nothing.

447

Concealment of Studies

There are currently in excess of a dozen published epidemiology studies demonstrating a statistically significant increased risk of birth defects that are not once identified in the labeling. The list of included anomalies is extensive. Neural tube defects (anencephaly, spina bifida, etc.), alimentary tract closure defects, Down syndrome and other chromosomal abnormalities, congenital heart defects, cleft lip/palate, urinary tract anomalies (hypospadias, undescended testes, etc.), limb reduction defects, vertebral abnormalities, tracheo-esophageal fistula, multiple anomalies, and others, have all been implicated in one or more studies.

But it is not just the statistical evaluation made by epidemiologists that justifies putting the medical profession and potential users on notice; it is the entire package. A teratologist does not look exclusively at epidemiology studies (although they are given the greatest weight). Also considered is the timing of exposure, animal teratology studies, in-vitro and in-vivo studies, the similarity of the chemical structure to another known teratogen, whether the drug has the capacity to be mutagenic, and the biological plausibility of the drug to cause birth defects.[568] Chapters 18 and 19 present the entire case on the teratogenic risk of Clomid, including the method of analysis and the citation of *numerous* scientific and medical studies and papers on the subject in support. Yet there is absolutely no reference to *any* of them.

One might ask, why not? Why would the FDA allow Merrell to convey that its worthless pre-market study establishes the safety of Clomid, yet exclude reference to published studies demonstrating an increased risk of birth defects? Afterall, it is well-acquainted with every study I have cited in this book.

It has recently come to light that the FDA requires proof to a 95% certainty before it will take action on post-market adverse reactions.[569] Under this standard, the FDA would have to be overwhelmingly convinced that Clomid was a human teratogen before including *any* warnings making such a suggestion. Somewhere along the way, the FDA has abandoned the standard set out in the June 26, 1979 *Federal Register* – a legal standard that exists even to this day. Yet no longer are warnings required of *potential* risks, or even *probable* ones. Before doctors and their patients are entitled to learn of an undisclosed risk, it now has to be proven to a 95% certainty.

When I first discovered this impossible standard, I realized the hopelessness of my earlier goal to bring about a change in the labeling. Neither my letter of October 11, 1994, nor any action I could have subsequently taken, would have altered the mindset of an agency demanding such a high level of proof. Not even proof that Clomid was a *probable* cause of birth defects would have been enough.

A *New York Times* editorial[570] suggested that the FDA might be relenting under public pressure in the wake of the Vioxx controversy. "The F.D.A. pledges to make information about *possible* dangers public promptly, even if the evidence is not yet conclusive. That should go a long way toward breaking the inertia that typically paralyzes the agency while it waits to accumulate conclusive evidence." [Emphasis added.]

Do prescribing doctors only want to be informed about *established* risks concerning a drug? Perhaps they might still be interested in *potential* risks, especially if they are significant and the drug being prescribed is not for the treatment of a serious or possibly fatal disease or condition. If there was scientific evidence that Clomid was a *probable* human teratogen, wouldn't prescribing physicians want to know this?

I bet their patients would.

Consider the recent publicity about Femara (letrozole); a drug used for the treatment of breast cancer in postmenopausal women. Over the past few years, many fertility specialists throughout the United States, Canada and Europe have prescribed the drug for the "off-label" use of stimulating ovulation. Its use as a fertility drug was embraced by the medical community inspite of the fact that it was never approved for such use and was contraindicated for premenopausal women, especially those who have achieved pregnancy. Animal studies had demonstrated letrozole to be teratogenic in the rat. Prescribing doctors argued that the drug was not a risk to the fetus because it was only used prior to pregnancy.

Sound familiar?

But beginning November 29, 2005, newspapers in the United States and Canada carried a story about Canadian health officials (Health Canada) issuing a warning that Femara had been associated with birth defects and spontaneous abortions. It cautioned that Femara was only approved for the treatment of breast cancer – not for its use as a fertility drug. The Swiss manufacturer, Novartis Pharmaceuticals, at the request of Health

Canada, had earlier sent a "Dear Doctor" letter throughout Canada. Among other things it stated, "There have been post-market reports of congenital anomalies in infants of mothers exposed to Femara for the treatment of infertility." The basis for the warning: a *single* study[571] involving 150 patients receiving Femara for fertility treatment. Seven (4.7%) of the patients had offspring with major congenital malformations. When compared with a control group, the data indicated a statistically significant increased risk (OR 2.9; 95% CI, 1.4-5.9; P=0.022). Novartis had also received 13 adverse reaction reports involving women who had been exposed to Femara during pregnancy. Two resulted in congenital malformations and 2 in spontaneous abortions. This was sufficient to set off a major warning effort by our neighbors to the north.

But that was Canada.

Back in the United States, an FDA spokesperson stated that the agency was looking into the matter to determine whether a warning was justified. While Canada was taking action, the FDA had to sit back and think about it. Time was not of the essence. Whatever happened to the new "possibility" standard? It no doubt surprised some bureaucrats in Rockville when Novartis announced that it would voluntarily mail out a similar warning letter within the U.S.

The FDA's oversight of Clomid exemplifies its evolution over the past decade. Concealment contemplates a conscious decision to suppress or exclude. There can be no question that the FDA made an informed choice to approve clomiphene labeling that failed to contain any reference to the outlined incriminating evidence. Twenty years ago such culpability by the FDA would have been unimaginable: slow and inefficient – yes; at times seeming indifferent – I couldn't agree more; all characteristics of a typical federal bureaucracy. But concealing and suppressing incriminating studies? Never. Not to my way of thinking, and I was as much a critic of the FDA's standards as anyone. Recall that although it was moving through the system at a snail's pace, language was evolving in the Clomid labeling that would have incorporated concerns I had expressed at the advisory committee hearing of July 18, 1975.

But the FDA of the 1990s and today is not the same entity that saved us from thalidomide. Not even close. The pharmaceutical industry is now running the show. The FDA has become more of an ally than a policing agency, largely because of the industry's power and influence over Congress. Indeed, that influence runs all the way to the White House.

The relevant events over the past few years give considerable insight into the seriousness and depth of the problem. What happened with Clomid is not unique. To paraphrase a statement made at the conclusion of each episode of an old television series, *The Naked City*, "There are ten thousand stories in the pharmaceutical industry. This has been one of them." But the problem extends well beyond the conduct of several drug companies. It is the whole system of drug testing, review and monitoring that needs fixing.

The major maladies that infest that system can loosely be grouped into four categories: (1) failure to discover disabling and fatal adverse reactions before the drugs have been marketed; (2) failure to take prompt and effective action post-marketing after they have been discovered; (3) improper marketing and promotion tactics; and (4) conflicts of interest. All have been front page news over the past few years.

Pre-Market Failures

In October 2000, the Nonprescription Drugs Advisory Committee to the FDA concluded that *phenylpropanolamine (PPA)*, the active ingredient in a number of decongestants and diet aids, was the cause of hemorrhagic strokes and declared it unsafe. The following month the FDA requested all manufacturers to voluntarily discontinue marketing their PPA-containing products. The findings of the Committee were largely based upon a Yale study that had concluded *one year earlier* that PPA was capable of causing strokes. Despite setting up the study and hand-picking its investigators, the drug industry had challenged the findings of its investigators and engaged in tactics to delay the eventual meeting of the advisory committee. During the 13 months between the conclusion of the study and the action of the FDA – while the FDA dragged its feet to accommodate the industry – it is estimated that up to 500 users of PPA products suffered strokes. Following the withdrawal from the market, neither the industry nor the FDA engaged in significant advertising or direct-mail campaigns to warn the American public that the cold medicine in their homes contained a potentially lethal ingredient. Many more suffered strokes long after the PPA products had been pulled from the shelves of their markets and pharmacies.

But the story[572] actually goes back almost two decades. As early as February 1982, an FDA report warned that PPA had "the ability to cause cardiovascular effects, cerebral hemorrhage and cardiac arrhythmias." In fact, PPA was so controversial that it was the subject of a congressional hearing in 1990. Eventually it was agreed to conduct a study to get a definitive answer to the nature and extent of the risks associated with PPA. Not surprisingly, it was to be a *long-term* study, and it was funded and designed by the industry itself. Since the industry had selected the investigators who had previously expressed skepticism about the association, you can imagine the shock in their corporate offices when the results were finally announced. Yet as a consequence of the years of delay, thousands of users had suffered needless strokes.

A *Los Angeles Times* editorial on March 30, 2004, put the story in perspective. It is quoted here at length because it underscores the problems with the whole system by which we test and monitor drugs, and even proposes a possible solution.

"The story of drug makers' two-decade struggle to keep cold medicines and diet products laced with phenylpropanolamine, or PPA, on store shelves highlights the need for Congress to create stronger firewalls between drug industry funding and research.

"As Times staff writers Kevin Sack and Alecia Mundy reported Sunday, since at least 1982 the Food and Drug Administration knew this stimulant could cause some people to suffer cardiovascular effects, cerebral hemorrhage and cardiac arrhythmias. A landmark study designed – and thereafter concealed – by the industry concluded as much in 1999.

"Still, the agency only began to take pusillanimous steps toward pulling the drug off the shelves in late 2000.

"In their defense, drug makers blame the FDA. Typical is this comment by Robert G. Donovan, the former head of Sandoz Consumer Health Care, a drug maker that knew the dangers of PPA at least as far back as 1984: 'My assumption was that if there was an issue of safety, supported by sound evidence, that the Food and Drug Administration would exercise their responsibility and take the product off the market.'

"The FDA counters that the industry hampered it. Because the agency does not sponsor research, its officials say, it must rely on the industry to investigate the safety of its own products. And because the industry managed to delay the publication of research, there was insufficient evidence of PPA's dangers to take it off the market or demand label warnings.

"Congress must step in, recognizing that people are dying while fingers are pointing.

"Congress, ideally, would create an Office of Clinical Research, a federal institute to act as an ethical buffer. Funded in part by industry dollars that now flow directly to individual scientists (thus corrupting their results), the institute would test new drugs against older ones. New drugs now are compared only with inert pills or placebos in clinical trials designed by pharmaceutical firms. As envisioned by medical policy experts such as Drummond Rennie, a deputy editor of the Journal of the American Medical Assn., the institute would reserve its seal of approval only for drugs that prove superior to existing drugs.

"Congress is unlikely to act so boldly in this election year (2004), but it should at least hold hearings to examine why the Food and Drug Administration gives drug firms such sway. Though it may be appropriate to let them help design studies, their influence should end there. And drug firms should not dictate timing of a study's release.

"Legislators also should ask why, when PPA's dangers became clear, the agency did not move it to prescription-only status. This lapse is especially troubling with a nonessential, replaceable over-the-counter drug. It's also disconcerting how this case shows the FDA lacks a sound system for doctors and hospitals to raise alarms about 'adverse events' in patients using drugs, like PPA, that long have been available over the counter.

"Whether with easily obtained drugs like PPA, or with problem prescription items like the diabetes treatment Rezulin, or with its shaky regulation of herbal nostrums, the FDA shows itself to be more industry lapdog than safety sentinel.

"That's a prescription for danger that Congress and the White House must remedy."

Well, don't look forward to any help from the White House. In fact, the current administration is part of the problem, not a candidate for its solution.

Quite troubling is a story that broke on July 14, 2004, headlined "Top FDA Lawyer Assists Drug Firms in Legal Briefs."[573] In an outrageous example of taking sides, the FDA's general counsel, Daniel Troy, following his appointment in August 2001, has filed briefs to assist several pharmaceutical companies in lawsuits that alleged that the plaintiffs had suffered adverse effects from those companies' products. One of the defendants, Pfizer, Inc., was a client of the law firm Troy had left to take the FDA's top legal post. In fact, Pfizer had paid that firm $360,000 for legal services rendered by Troy during the year of his departure. With Troy's assistance, Pfizer was successful in getting the federal drug-product case dismissed.

This change in FDA policy was apparently precipitated by directions from the Bush administration. In a story appearing in the *New York Times* 10 days later, it was revealed that in 2002, the White House had initiated plans for "FDA involvement in product liability lawsuits." As part of President Bush's position on tort reform, the FDA would be asserting that its approval of drugs and medical devices (such as IUDs and heart pumps) precludes prosecution of such cases. Any drug or device approved by the FDA should be immune from suit.

Aside from all of the obvious issues concerning the failings, failures and bias of FDA personnel, the bias of many of the investigators participating in studies, and the suppression of data and outright deception in recording and reporting by drug companies, whatever happened to the notion that the FDA was there for the protection of the public? Apparently the Bush administration is of the view that it is there for the protection of pharmaceutical companies. The contrived justification: permitting such suits would undermine public health, and intrude on the federal regulation of drugs and devices, by encouraging lay judges and juries to second-guess experts at the FDA. As the argument goes, the success of such suits would result in good products being pulled from the market, depriving patients of beneficial treatments.

Forget that the current tort system has been in existence for over a half century without any noticeable impact on the marketing of "good products." Forget that experts at the FDA *need* second-guessing. Forget that the whole system of testing drugs and devices needs fixing, and that this view is shared by leaders in the medical profession. Forget the remote possibility that such lawsuits are successful – *especially* in federal court – because the products are not so "good." Forget that many of those products *need* to be pulled from the market.

Accountability is the backbone of responsibility. If a drug company is immunized from liability by FDA approval of its drugs or devices, the focus of its studies would be only on providing data that the FDA would deem necessary to declare the product safe and effective, rather than a true assessment of the actual risks associated with use of the drug or device or whether it is truly effective in treating the diseases or conditions for which it is to be approved. PPA-containing products were approved by the FDA for marketing decades before it was determined that they were capable of causing hemorrhagic strokes. The Dalkon Shield intrauterine device had been approved for marketing by the FDA long before it was learned that its multifilamentous string could wick bacteria in the uterine cavity, causing pelvic inflammatory disease. And there are hundreds of similar stories.

The simple truth is that pharmaceutical companies generate documents that the FDA never sees. Revealing interdepartment memoranda and correspondence are not part of the IND and NDA records received by the FDA, but they are obtainable through discovery efforts in litigation. In fact, many documents I have secured through litigation I was unable to acquire from the FDA through requests under the Freedom of Information Act. Knowing that poorly designed and/or fraudulently documented studies would not only result in civil liability, but possible removal of the product from the market, encourages conducting proper studies. Well-designed studies are also the best defense to a civil lawsuit. The existing system of accountability needs to be improved, not trashed.

Another controversy involves antidepressant drugs and children. When concerns arose that there might be a link between use of the drugs by children and suicide attempts, the FDA ordered its top expert to study all of the clinical studies that had examined the issue to date. After months of research he concluded that there was *twice the risk* of suicidal behavior when children used antidepressants. But prior to an advisory committee meeting in February 2004, top officials with the FDA *suppressed the report* of their own expert, and ordered him to withhold his conclusions from consideration by the advisory committee.[574]

> [If the FDA would suppress a report about teen suicides from one of its own experts, it would have little problem concealing incriminating studies on fertility drugs. This is not the same entity I challenged in the 1970s.]

When the FDA issued watered-down warnings the following month, it publically assured that they were based only on anecdotal reports from physicians and not upon any form of scientific evidence. In truth, the FDA's top scientist on the subject had reviewed and analyzed over two dozen clinical trials. The FDA's justification for its actions: its expert's conclusion was premature and further studies were needed before unnecessarily alarming patients that might benefit from the drug.

Tag line: Seven months later, officials at the FDA acknowledged that their expert had been right.[575] In the interim, they had hired researchers at Columbia University to re-analyze the same studies. The scientists reassessing the data came up with virtually the same conclusion as the FDA expert; indeed, there was twice the risk of suicide.

Then came the Vioxx controversy.[576] The arthritis drug was pulled from the market by Merck & Co. on September 30, 2004. A recent study had shown that it doubled the risk of heart attack and stroke.[577] Internal corporate memos document the company's knowledge about these risks at least four years earlier – maybe even as early as 1996.

History records that Vioxx was in trouble almost from the moment it hit the market. Released as one of the first[578] so-called COX-2 inhibitors in May 1999, it was intended to provide pain relief without the risk of internal bleeding caused by older drugs. But in March 2000 – just 10 months later – a study involving 8,100 rheumatoid arthritis patients (designated "Vigor") reported that Vioxx users were five times more likely to experience heart attacks as those taking naproxen, another pain reliever.

Merck's official position was that the higher rate was due to naproxen having a protective effect on the heart, not from Vioxx inducing cardiovascular clotting. Internal records, however, tell a different story.[579] An e-mail written by Merck's research director on March 9, 2000, acknowledged that an elevated risk of heart attack was "clearly there." A company memorandum, dating all the way back to November 21, 1996, suggests that Merck was concerned about Vioxx's potential to cause cardiac events even back then, long before it was approved by the FDA for marketing.

Following the Vigor study, a meeting of top executives was convened in May 2000. At issue was whether to pursue another study to test the possibility that its popular drug was capable of causing heart attacks and strokes. Marketing was dead set against the idea. Vioxx was bringing in annual sales of $2.5 billion. The patents on several other Merck drugs were expiring in 2000 and 2001, opening the opportunity for generic companies to take over their market position. Vioxx was vital to Merck's continued financial health. Initiating such a study would reflect badly on the drug, so it was rejected.

But more studies followed. In 2001 a paper appeared in the *Journal of the American Medical Association* (JAMA) reporting that Vioxx, and its major competitor Celebrex, appeared to increase the risk of heart attacks and strokes. The article had *reanalyzed* data from pre-market clinical trials on the two drugs.[580] The data suggested that Vioxx was a greater risk than the other COX-2 inhibitor. Scientists from Merck had earlier tried to discourage the author of the JAMA article from publishing it. In October 2002, a study out of Vanderbilt University involving Medicaid patients found that Vioxx patients taking high doses of the drug had a higher incidence of heart attacks and strokes than patients on lower doses of the drug. In the same year, a laboratory in Massachusetts determined that Vioxx damaged lipids (fatty compounds) in the blood in a manner that made them more prone to clotting. In April 2004, yet another study reported in *Circulation* that Vioxx increased the risk of hypertension.

Finally, in August 2004, an FDA scientist, Dr. David Graham, completed a large three-year study he and his associates had been working on involving 1.4 million patients from the Kaiser Permanente health care system. He concluded that high doses of Vioxx increased the risk of heart disease 3.7 times more than his control group. He also conservatively estimated that at least 27,000 users of Vioxx may have suffered heart attacks and deaths from May 1999 through December 2003, and that the actual number could be as high as between 88,000 and 139,000. The following month Merck voluntarily removed Vioxx from the market.

Next up: Baycol (cerivastatin). No sooner had the smoke cleared on Vioxx when the *Los Angeles Times*[581] cited an article (in JAMA) reporting that just three months after Baycol was introduced onto the market in 1998, Bayer and the FDA were in receipt of reports on seven cases of rhabdomyolysis, a toxic muscle degeneration condition leading to kidney problems and death. Baycol had been pulled from the market in 2001, when it was determined that the cholesterol drug posed 10 times the risk of causing rhabdomyolysis as other statin drugs, such as Lipitor, Pravachol and Zocor. When used in conjunction with a fibrate drug – used to lower triglyceride fats – *10 percent* of the patients developed the muscle disorder. In six of the seven reported cases the patient had been taking a fibrate.

One might ask: *Why would evidence of this serious adverse reaction surface only three months after marketing but escape detection during the pre-market clinical studies?*

This question is of critical importance because it underscores some major flaws in our current system of testing drugs. They include: (1) prior to marketing, the clinical studies that evaluate the safety and effectiveness of drug products are designed, monitored, documented, compiled, analyzed and reported on by their manufacturers, *the very entities that stand to lose millions of dollars* in research and development should the drug prove to be ineffective and/or unsafe; (2) since 1992, there has existed a greater emphasis on getting pharmaceutical products to market than on discovering the nature and extent of their side effects; (3) since 1992, the FDA has become financially dependent on the drug industry to meet its budgetary requirements; (4) the post-marketing department in the FDA that oversees the safety of drugs (Office of Drug Safety) has no effective means of enforcement; and (5) objective and effective testing of drugs does not really occur until after they are marketed, thus making the general consuming public the unwitting test subjects for pharmaceutical products.

So what in the hell happened in 1992?

That was the year Congress passed the Prescription Drug User Fee Act (PDUFA). In order to expedite the approval of drugs, the FDA was authorized to charge user fees to pharmaceutical companies to cover the cost of expanding its staff and other related

458

expenses. The PDUFA has a "sunset clause" that terminates the legislation every five years unless renewed. The 2002 formula calculates to a current fee of approximately $576,000 per new drug application. The sums collected from the industry currently *exceed one half of the annual budget* of the Center for Drug Evaluation and Research (CDER),[582] the division within the FDA responsible for the review and approval of new drugs, as well as monitoring their safety post-marketing.

The legislation has been effective in reducing the lag time between filing a New Drug Application and the date of a drug's official approval for marketing. Before passage of the PDUFA, the average wait was approximately 33 months; it is currently about 13 to 14 months.[583] [It took 24 months for Clomid approval between 1965 and 1967.] Saving just one year can mean additional hundreds of millions of dollars in sales. It effectively gives more than one additional year of patent life to the drug before generics can use the formula. Not a bad return for $576,000.

But there is a tradeoff. Rushing a drug to market tends to sacrifice a thorough evaluation of its safety.

And here's the kicker. The PDUFA mandates that the additional funds be committed to expediting the review of new drug applications and that those reviews meet specified goals (shortening time) as a consideration for payment of the fees.[584] In other words, if the FDA does not meet those goals, it will be in violation of the statute. To meet this requirement, a major amount of the personnel and financial resources of CDER has been committed to the NDA approval process – including all of the user fees. As a consequence, drugs are hitting the market without the standards of risk assessment that existed in 1992.

If a serious adverse reaction to a drug (such as a stroke or heart attack) struck only one out of 10,000 users, it would be impossible to detect such a risk in pre-market studies using only two or three thousand patients. Such a rare side effect could only be detected after the drug had been marketed and exposed to hundreds of thousands, and perhaps millions, of consumers of the pharmaceutical product. But the study cited by Merck in September 2004 that prompted it to pull Vioxx from the market involved only 2,586 participants, including controls.[585] Such a study could – and should – have been conducted prior to marketing. If Merck had postponed introducing Vioxx on the market another 10 months, the results of the Vigor study (above) would have been available for consideration by CDER before it granted approval. There can also be little question that a well-designed pre-market study would have detected an increased risk of developing rhabdomyolysis before the general public was exposed to Baycol, especially if it was used in conjunction with a fibrate drug.

The FDA complains that it has little power to compel drug companies to add warnings and/or initiate further studies to investigate risks once a drug has been approved for marketing,[586] yet it was a willing participant in establishing a system that rushes more drugs to the market without adequate testing. The CDER also provides insufficient financial support for the Office of Drug Safety (ODS) and gives it no enforcement powers. The ODS falls under the umbrella of the CDER and has the obligation of monitoring and detecting post-market adverse reactions to drugs.

What goes on (or doesn't go on) at the FDA post-marketing is truly unsettling.

Post-Market Inefficiency

When Dr. David Graham testified before the Senate Finance Committee on November 18, 2004, he really opened some eyes. Not only did he recite the tragic history of Vioxx, he also painted a graphic picture of inefficiency that currently exists at the FDA. At the time of his testimony, Dr. Graham had worked for the agency for 20 years and was the Associate Director for Science and Medicine of the ODS. As an insider, he spoke from a position of knowledge and experience. His words had the conviction of a concerned scientist who wanted to right the ship.

"My experience with Vioxx is typical of how CDER responds to serious drug safety issues in general. This is similar to what Dr. Mosholder (the FDA expert on antidepressant suicides) went through earlier this year when he reached his conclusion that SSRIs (Selective Serotonin Re-uptake Inhibitors) should not be used by children. I could bore you with a long list of prominent and not-so-prominent safety issues where CDER and its Office of New Drugs (OND)[587] proved to be extremely resistant to full and open disclosure of safety information, especially when it called into question an existing regulatory position. In these situations, *the new drug reviewing division* (OND) *that approved the drug in the first place and regards it as its own child, typically proves to be the single greatest obstacle to effectively dealing with serious drug safety issues.* The second greatest obstacle is often the senior management within the Office of Drug Safety, who either actively or tacitly go along with what the Office of New Drugs wants." [Emphasis added.]

Dr. Graham is describing an organizational structure in which his division (ODS) is continually butting heads with those in CDER and OND over safety issues. He went on to describe an example.

"With Lotronex, even though there was strong evidence in the pre-approval clinical trials of a problem with ischemic colitis, OND approved it. When cases of severe constipation and eschemic colitis began pouring into FDA's MedWatch program, the reaction was one of denial. When CDER decided to bring Lotronex back on the market (after its earlier removal on November 2, 2000), *ODS safety reviewers were instructed to help make this happen.* Later, when CDER held an advisory committee meeting to get support for bringing Lotronex back on the market, the presentation on ways to manage its reintroduction was carefully shaped and controlled by OND. When it came to presenting the range of possible options for how Lotronex could be made available, the list of options was *censored* by OND. The day before the advisory meeting, I was told by the ODS reviewer who gave this presentation that the director of the reviewing office within OND that approved Lotronex in the first place came to her office and *removed material from her talk.* An OND manager was 'managing' an ODS employee. When informed of this, ODS senior management ignored it. I guess they knew who was calling the shots." [Emphasis added.]

The larger picture was then described by the FDA employee. What was portrayed to Senator Grassley (R-Iowa) and his committee was not pretty.

"The problem you are confronting today is immense in scope. Vioxx is a terrible tragedy and a profound regulatory failure. *I would argue that the FDA, as currently configured, is incapable of protecting America against another Vioxx. We are virtually defenseless.* It is important that this Committee and the American people understand that what has happened with Vioxx is really a symptom of something far more dangerous to the safety of the American people. *Simply put,*

FDA and its Center for Drug Evaluation and Research are broken. * * * * The organizational structure within CDER is entirely geared towards the review and approval of new drugs. When a CDER new drug reviewing division approves a new drug, it is also saying the drug is 'safe and effective.' When a serious safety issue arises post-marketing, their immediate reaction is almost always one of denial, rejection and heat. *They approved the drug so there can't possibly be anything wrong with it. The same group that approved the drug is also responsible for taking regulatory action against it post-marketing. This is an inherent conflict of interest.* At the same time, The Office of Drug Safety has no regulatory power and must first convince the new drug reviewing division (OND) that a problem exists before anything beneficial to the public can be done. Often, the new drug reviewing division is the single greatest obstacle to effectively protecting the public against drug safety risks. A close second in my opinion, is an ODS management that sees its mission as pleasing the Office of New Drugs." [Emphsis added.]

Dr. Graham's views appear to be shared by Dr. Janet Woodstock, Deputy Commissioner of Operations for the FDA. When Dr. Woodstock appeared before a medical advisory panel to the Institute of Medicine on June 8, 2005, her comments seemed to echo the views of her FDA colleague.[588] The FDA's drug safety program had "pretty much broken down," she reported. And when it came to discovering the dangers of drugs already on the market, there was room for a "lot of improvement." She emphasized the scope of the problem by citing the Institute of Medicine's own statistic, *namely that 100,000 deaths occur each year in the United States as a result of an adverse drug reaction.*

Dr. Graham had earlier complained that his supervisors at the FDA attempted to delay his efforts to publish his recently-completed Vioxx study, demeaned his conclusions, subjected him to a number of harassing calls, and even threatened to terminate his employment or move him to another position. To protect his job, he sought assistance from the Government Accountability Project, a public-interest group that helps whistle-blowers. Since his testimony, Dr. Graham has appeared on *Nightline,* CNN and

Good Morning America. Almost over night he became an outspoken advocate for change at the FDA.[589]

During his career, Dr. Graham has also been instrumental in the market withdrawals of Rezulin (liver failure), Fen-Phen and Redux (heart valve damage), PPA-containing products (strokes), and a number of other drugs. In some ways, he is the Frances Kelsey of his time. At the risk of losing his job, he has spoken out against his employer because of his overriding belief that changes need to be made in the interest of public safety.

Conflicts of Interest

Conflict of interest not only plagues the current structure of the FDA, it also infests other parts of the drug review system as well. As has been discussed, it starts with pharmaceutical companies conducting studies of their own drug products. What drug company is motivated to design a study that might prevent its drug from ever reaching the market? Even when studies reveal potential side effects, the drug's sponsor puts a spin on the results to avoid implicating the drug.

But conflicts are also seen at other levels.

When a panel of FDA advisors published a new set of guidelines calling for aggressive use of statins (cholesterol-reducing drugs) in 2004, they omitted mentioning that six out of the nine members had previously received grants, speaker's fees or consulting fees from the manufacturers of those drugs.[590] The companies included Pfizer (Lipitor), Bristol-Myers Squibb (Pravachol), Merck (Lovastatin) and AstraZeneca (Crestor).

Vioxx and its two competitors, Celebrex and Bextra, were back in the news in February 2005. A special advisory committee had convened to evaluate and make recommendations to the FDA on the three COX-2 inhibitors. After three days of hearings, the advisory panel – on a split vote – recommended that Celebrex and Bextra should remain on the market, *and even Vioxx could return,* if Merck was so inclined. Their continued presence in the marketplace, however, would be conditional upon strengthening their warnings.

But the real story broke a week later (February 25, 2005) when the *New York Times* reported that ten of the 32 members of the advisory committee had been consultants for the manufacturers of the three drugs. Had the 10 advisors recused themselves and not voted, the count would have gone 14 to 8 to keep Vioxx off the market and 12-8 to remove Bextra. The consultants had voted 9 to 1 to retain both. The outcome would not have been any different for Celebrex, although the majority on the panel was of the view that it should come with a "black box" warning reciting the cardiovascular risks, similar to the other two drugs.

On April 26, 2006, an article appeared in the Journal of the American Medical Association[591] in which it was reported that between 2001 and 2004, 73% of 221 advisory committee meetings included at least one member or voting consultant with a disclosed conflict of interest; and that involved *disclosed* conflicts. All combined, 28% of the consultants revealed a conflict of interest. Twenty-three percent of the conflicted participants had contracts and/or grants with pharmaceutical companies that exceeded $100,000.

> [By now it must be a tradition in Rockville. Recall that two of the 13 members of the advisory committee that I addressed on July 18, 1975, not only had an earlier association with Merrell, but actually had been participants in the Clomid clinical study that I was criticizing. Thirty years later, conflicts of interest are still the standard of the day.]

Not even the National Institutes of Health (NIH) are immune from this infestation. This is particularly disturbing. When a drug company conducts or sponsors a clinical study that becomes published, the medical profession is put on notice of this fact and can take it into consideration when deciding what weight and merit to give to the study. But the NIH is a part of the federal health care system and has the appearance of being objective and independent. Whenever it oversees or funds a drug study, it is presumed that it has been conducted without bias and uninfluenced by the manufacturer of that drug.

The tentacles of the drug industry, however, are long and ubiquitous. Over the five-year period ending in December 2004, at least 530 NIH scientists had received fees, stock and/or stock options from pharmaceutical companies.[592]

The value of these perks was not inconsequential. During this period of time, a laboratory director from the National Cancer Institute received $70,000 in consulting fees from a company developing an ovarian cancer test; the NIH's top blood transfusion expert accepted $240,200 in fees and 76,000 stock options from drug companies developing blood-related products; and a senior psychiatric researcher took in $508,050 from Pfizer, who at the time was marketing an Alzheimer's drug.

One of the biggest beneficiaries of corporate largess was Dr. H. Bryan Brewer, Jr., head of the National Heart, Lung, and Blood Institute's molecular disease branch, and a top authority on cholesterol.[593] Between 2001 and 2003, he was paid $114,000 in consulting fees from four pharmaceutical companies developing or marketing cholesterol drugs, including $55,500 from Pfizer (Lipitor) and $31,000 from AstraZeneca (Crestor). Lipid Sciences, Inc., another company involved in addressing cholesterol problems, paid Brewer an additional $83,000 during the same period. In September 2003, his consulting contract was converted to an annual fee of $125,000, plus stock options. Through December 2004, Brewer held 411,927 stock options in the company.

At the same time, Brewer pulled down an annual salary from the federal government of $187,305.

Was there a *quid pro quo* for all the consulting fees and stock options? Judge for yourself. In 2003, the psychiatric researcher publically endorsed Pfizer's Alzheimer drug; a study of a competitor's ovarian cancer test was dropped by the National Cancer Institute; and the blood transfusion expert spoke and wrote about the benefits of the blood-related products he had been consulting on.

Brewer, again, justifies special attention. In 2001, along with eight other experts, he proposed stricter guidelines for reducing cholesterol levels. These standard levels were further reduced in July 2004. As a consequence, the number of patients using cholesterol-reducing drugs – and the consequent sales volume – could likely double. Eight of the nine members on the panel, including Brewer, had financial ties with drug companies that stood to see financial gains from the new standards.

On August 21, 2003, an article written by Brewer appeared in the *American Journal of Cardiology,* extolling the advantages of Crestor over three other competing drugs. The publication followed by a week the drug's approval for marketing. It prominently mentions Brewer's position with the NIH, but *fails to reveal any of his financial ties with AstraZeneca.*

Brewer concluded in the paper that the "benefit-risk profile (of Crestor) appears to be very favorable." He assured that there was no cause for concern about patients developing rhabdomyolysis, the same sometimes-deadly side effect for which Baycol had been removed from the market (see above). "No cases of rhabdomyolysis occurred in patients receiving (Crestor) at 10 to 40 (milligrams)," he wrote. Unmentioned were eight cases that were reported during the Crestor clinical studies, including one patient who had taken the low dose of 10 mgs. When asked why he had failed to mention the eight cases, he defended the omission by explaining that seven of the patients had been on doses that exceeded the recommended amount and "it was not possible to definitely conclude" that the low-dose case had been caused by the drug.

During its first year on the market, the FDA received 78 case reports of rhabdomyolysis in association with use of Crestor, two of them fatal.

The practice of highlighting positions with the NIH and omitting financial ties has likewise been followed by many of Brewer's colleagues. In fact, federal employees at the NIH have been quite reticent about revealing their secondary sources of income to anyone – even their boss. In a random sampling of outside payments to NIH scientists, a July 2004 report from the United States Office of Government Ethics found that 40% had not been approved in advance or accounted for within the agency.[594]

On September 10, 2006, the *Los Angeles Times*[595] reported on an internal review by the NIH related to a Dr. Thomas J. Walsh, one of its top cancer researchers. It was discovered that Dr. Walsh had received "consulting fees" in excess of $100,000 from various drug companies, which were neither approved nor reported, in violation of established NIH rules and procedures. It was also revealed that Dr. Walsh had even appeared on behalf of a drug company (e.g., Merck) to advocate approval of its drug to an FDA advisory committee, *based upon a review of the company's data conducted by Walsh and other NIH staffers.*

The *Times* article identified yet another senior NIH researcher, likewise caught with his hand in the cookie jar – a Dr. P. Trey Sunderland III. Dr. Sunderland's area of expertise involves Alzheimer's research. His hand was caught with an even larger bundle of dough – $612,000 from Pfizer, to be exact. In June 2006, Dr. Sunderland refused to answer questions before a congressional subcommittee investigating abuses at the NIH, seeking refuge under the 5th Amendment. On December 4, 2006, he was charged by federal prosecutors with criminal conflict of interest.

Even academic medical centers are not beyond the reach of pharmaceutical companies. In all but a few of the most prestigious medical institutions, drug companies that fund the studies have contractual agreements that effectively give them control over when or if the data from such studies can be published or otherwise distributed to the medical profession.[596] Under such circumstances, it does not take much imagination to appreciate how those conducting such studies might be influenced in their conclusions. The axiom "publish or perish" has as much relevance in medical academics as anywhere.

Marketing and Promotion Tactics

Another area of abuse involves tactics employed by pharmaceutical companies in the promotion and marketing of their drug products. This practice has likewise been recently exposed by the news media.

Stories include the prosecution of 11 sales executives from TAP Pharmaceutical Products for making kickbacks to physicians, hospitals and other customers for prescribing its products. According to prosecutors, gifts included trips to luxurious golf and ski resorts, and "educational grants" used to pay for cocktail parties, office Christmas parties and travel.[597] Three years earlier TAP had agreed to pay $875 million to resolve similar charges involving another one of its drugs.

In May 2004, a small drug company was accused of promoting one of its drugs for the treatment of a condition not approved by the FDA, boosting its annual sales on the drug from $20 million to $141 million.[598] Although drug companies are prohibited from selling their drugs for "off-label" uses, physicians are not faced with a similar prohibition. The company, InterMune, was alleged to have promoted non-approved use of Actimmune for the treatment of idiopathic pulmonary fibrosis, without evidence that it could effectively treat that condition.

The same month, a similar transgression by Pfizer was reported.[599] The company paid a $430 million settlement and pled guilty to falsely promoting its drug, Neurontin, for the unapproved treatment of migraines and back pain. It has been estimated that as much as 90% of the drug's $2.7 billion in annual sales had been attributed to off-label uses.[600] The article points out that the fine would have little impact on the company. Pfizer, the largest pharmaceutical company in the world, had sales of $45 billion in 2003.

"As Doctors Write Prescriptions, Drug Company Writes a Check," is the title of a piece appearing in *The New York Times* on June 27, 2004. One doctor reported receiving an unsolicited check in the mail for $10,000 from Schering-Plough. Others described similar experiences. The article cites payments as high as "six-figure sums."

In September 2004, a warning letter was sent to Johnson & Johnson by the FDA regarding its pain patch, Duragesic.[601] The complaint was that its promotional materials sent to physicians and other health care professionals contained "unsubstantiated" claims concerning the drug's efficacy and "false and misleading claims about the drug's safety." The concern was that the subject pamphlet could encourage unsafe use leading to hypoventilation (abnormally slow and shallow breathing) and heart attacks.

The manufacturers of Celebrex (Pfizer) and Vioxx (Merck) show up in this category as well. In January 2005, they were both criticized about marketing schemes related to their two COX-2 inhibitors. "A majority of the patients who were persuaded to use prescription arthritis drugs such as Celebrex and Vioxx would have done just as well on older, cheaper medications and would have avoided the potential risks of heart attack and stroke now linked to those blockbuster drugs, according to a study of how they were marketed and used."[602] The cited study[603] found that aggressive direct-to-consumer (DTC) advertising was responsible for their overuse. As reported, more than 70% of the patients receiving these drugs could have benefited just as well with cheaper nonprescription medications. Pfizer spent $87.6 million for DTC advertising on Celebrex in 2003; Merck spent $71.7 million on Vioxx during the same year and $79.2 million during the first nine months of 2004, at which point it was pulled from the market. The U.S. is one of only two industrialized nations in the world allowing pharmaceutical DTC advertising.

And so it goes.

Fixing the System

There is a reason that drug industry controversies fill the internet and our newspapers, seemingly on a weekly basis. The steady diet of stories is a symptom of a deeply-rooted problem that is impacting virtually everyone in this country. Very few of us make it through life without seeking the assistance of pharmaceutical products. Somewhere along the line we are all affected. Add to that the exorbitant charges for medications we all pay, especially for prescription drugs.[604] Who do you think pays for all the promotion and marketing?

But we are also unnecessarily placed at risk of developing undisclosed adverse reactions, many of them severely disabling or fatal. *It has been estimated that more than 50% of all serious side effects from drugs are discovered only after those drugs have been approved by the FDA as "safe and effective."*[605] This is a tragedy. It is also a frightening reality. It would be acceptable if the adverse reaction was a rare event; it is inexcusable when it could have been detected by a properly designed pre-market study.

Such is the case with Clomid and other fertility drugs.

As long as drug companies are responsible for designing, supervising, compiling data and reporting on the very studies that will determine whether their drugs and devices are approved for marketing by the FDA, we will continue to leave the fox guarding the henhouse.

All pre-market drug studies should be supervised by an independent third-party entity, such as the National Institutes of Health (NIH). Funding would still be by the pharmaceutical company whose drug is under study, and the company would still supply its input on the design of the study and its desired goals. But the clinical investigators would report their data and findings to the third-party entity, not to the drug company, and the results would be compiled, analyzed and summarized for the FDA by the same entity. All personnel with the supervising entity involved in compiling, analyzing and summarizing would *sign a conflict of interest form*, subject to appropriate sanctions in the event of any nondisclosures. Only with true detached and objective assessment of clinical studies of drugs and devices will we ever achieve complete and candid reports on their safety and effectiveness.

This failure of our system is perpetuated by the ineptness of the FDA post-marketing, specifically the inaction of its Center for Drug Evaluation and Research (CDER). When an office within CDER is assigned the task of monitoring drugs and detecting their undisclosed side effects (e.g., ODS), but lacks any enforcement power to take action, something needs to be changed. The ODS needs to act independent of the approval division (OND) and possess enforcement powers, even independent of CDER.

On September 22, 2006, a fifteen-member panel, established under the direction of the Institute of Medicine (IOM) of the National Academy of Sciences, issued comprehensive and sweeping recommendations for a major overhaul of the FDA. Significantly, this panel had been convened at the request of the FDA following the Vioxx debacle. Going in, it thus had the seal of approval of the very entity it was evaluating. Among its many recommended changes, it was urged to (1) strengthen the FDA's safety staff, including added funding, and to give it an integral role in drug approval; (2) give the FDA authority to order drug companies to conduct post-market safety studies; (3) give the FDA greater authority to impose fines and injunctions on drug companies; (4) review the risks and benefits of all new drugs after five years; (5) require drug companies to register and post a summary of all Phase II through Phase IV clinical trials on the internet, regardless of outcome; (6) require during the first two years on the market that all new drugs carry a black triangle, or similar designation, warning that their risks and benefits have not been fully investigated; (7) restrict advertising of all new drugs during their first two years on the market; (8) implement strict policies against conflicts of interest on advisory committee panels; and (9) establish a 6-year term for the FDA commissioner.

Senators Edward Kennedy (D-Mass.) and Michael Enzi (R-Wyo.) introduced a bill on August 3, 2006, which included many of the IOM panel's recommendations. Congress was also mandated to look at user-fee legislation during 2007, which necessitated confronting the whole issue of FDA reorganization. The Kennedy-Enzi bill (S1082) ultimately became the vehicle for those changes. On May 9, 2007, S1082 came up for a floor vote before the full Senate, but not before Pharmaceutical Research and Manufacturers of America (PhRMA) – the lobbying arm of the drug industry – exercised its muscle and considerable influence over the upper house of Congress. By the time the smoke cleared, what remained was a watered-down version of the original bill, with many of its important provisions either trashed or minimized. After a few futile skirmishes, the final vote was an overwhelming 93-1. Many senators voted in favor of the measure, recognizing that something had to change and the final version was the best that could be salvaged. On July 11, 2007, similar legislation (HR2900) was passed in the House of Representatives, although at odds with a number of the provisions of the Senate version. After several conference committee meetings – with the Senate urging pro-industry amendments and the House pushing for safety measures – on September 19, 2007, an agreement was reached on compromise legislation, which was thereafter passed by the House on the same date (405-7) and the Senate on September 20, 2007 (by a unanimous consent vote). President Bush is expected to sign it into law.

But what did we end up with? Some good and some bad.

The good news: (1) members of an *advisory committee* may not participate in a meeting regarding a particular matter if that member (or immediate family member) has a *financial interest* that could be affected by the member's advice, except that a *limited* number of waivers can be provided, either as a non-voting or voting member, if the member has "essential expertise" that is necessary to consider; (2) the Director of the NIH is to maintain a *public data bank on the Internet* of any and all premarket and postmarket clinical studies conducted with drugs or medical devices, which shall include truthful, non-misleading, relevant and comprehensive information, including summaries understandable by the lay public; (3) the FDA may require *postmarket studies or clinical trials* to assess a known or suspected serious risk on the basis of "new safety information" not available at the time of approval; (4) the FDA may require *postmarket changes in labeling* when it becomes aware of "new safety information" it determines should be included as a warning, contraindication, precaution, adverse reaction or black box warning; (5) the FDA may require either a *premarket or postmarket risk evaluation and mitigation strategy* to ensure that the benefits of the drug outweigh the risks of the drug, upon making a determination that "new safety information" justifies such an evaluation; (6) the FDA may suggest changes in any television, radio or print *advertising* about a drug or require changes if it determines that it would otherwise be false or misleading; (7) the FDA is required to develop a system for *postmarket risk identification and analysis*, including safety data from at least 25,000,000 patients by 2010 and 100,000,000 patients by 2012; (8) a *substantial proportion of the user fees* paid by drug companies will be allocated to postmarket safety matters; and (9) FDA *enforcement powers* for violating the above new laws include assessing fines ranging up to

$10,000,000 and possibly higher, depending upon the circumstances, and even suspension or withdrawal of approval of the drug.

The bad news: the portion of the 427-page bill that deals with drugs is devoted almost excusively to *postmarket* safety issues. The current system for the testing of drugs prior to marketing remains intact; drug companies will continue to be responsible for designing, supervising, compiling data and reporting on the very studies that will determine whether their drugs will be approved for marketing. Further, the structure of the FDA essentially remains the same. Although the Office of Drug Safety (ODS) will have a voice on matters involving postmarket safety, the extent of its authority and influence is unclear. Determinations on the decisions to require postmarket studies and/or clinical trials, changes in the labeling and risk evaluation and mitigation strategies "shall be made by individuals at or above the level of individuals empowered to approve a drug (such as division directors within the Center for Drug Evaluation and Research)." The only division directors empowered to "approve a drug" are those who head the Office of New Drugs (OND). How this statutory language will ultimately be interpreted remains to be seen, but it appears to this writer that the FDA may still be burdened with the same conflict of interest and deficiencies complained of by Dr. David Graham in front of Congress. The ODS, which monitors the postmarket performance of drugs, remains emasculated and still must go to the director of OND or to the head of the Center for Drug Evaluation and Research (CDER) to address safety issues it discovers. The FDA may have new powers, but the ODS still has no effective means of enforcement.

So, what can you do about it?

Recognize that any additional improvement in our current system for protecting the general public from dangerous drugs will not come about through efforts of the medical profession and/or the FDA – and it most definitely will not happen due to voluntary cooperation from the drug industry. Our protection can only come from Congress; and 2008 is an election year.

We need stronger laws that are there to protect the consumer, not the special interests of the pharmaceutical industry. We need laws that separate the function and powers of the drug approval division from the function and powers of the post-market safety division. We need laws within the approval division which mandate equal

472

consideration of a drug's benefits and risks. We need laws that provide for financial independence of the FDA from the drug industry. And most importantly, we need laws that take clinical investigations of pharmaceutical products away from industry and place them into the hands of independent scientists.

Expect to see strong opposition from industry on any additional legislation. PhRMA – aka *Big Pharma* – is a powerful lobbying organization in Washington, and will twist a lot of legislative arms to defeat any law that might have futher impact on pharmaceutical sales and profits. Anticipate no help from the White House. The President has already demonstrated where he lines up when it comes to taking sides between consumers and industry.

But guess what? There is something more powerful and influential than any lobbying organization that drug companies could ever package and drag to Washington D.C. It is your individual right to vote. That's right. Remember, in politics money is only a means to an end. Without votes, no one returns to his or her important job in the U.S. Senate or the House of Representatives. All you need to do to bring about important changes at the FDA is to resolve that you are going to do something about it. You need to express it in a letter to your local senator or congressperson. Letters can make a difference. *You can make a difference.* John Donne said it so eloquently over four centuries ago.

"No man is an island, entire of itself,

every man is a piece of the continent, a part of the main,

if a clod be washed away by the sea,

Europe is the less, as well as if a promontory were,

as well as if a manor of thy friends or of thine own were,

any man's death diminishes me, because I am involved in mankind,

and therefore never send to know for whom the bell tolls,

it tolls for thee."

I wrote this book to put users of fertility drugs on notice that there are risks of birth defects associated with use of those drugs. I have presented the evidence and leave it up to you to give it what weight you deem appropriate. In that regard, I have accomplished my goal. But there is a bigger story here. It involves a major health issue that impacts all of us. We also have an opportunity to make a difference in society today and in the future. I have done everything I can to bring about needed changes in the law – and will continue to do so.[606]

The rest is up to you.

* * * * *

NOTES and REFERENCES

Introduction

[1] Unlike compensatory damages in an injury case for pain and suffering, past and future medical expenses, loss of earnings and future loss of earning capacity, *punitive damages* are awarded only for the pupose of punishment. In California they can only be awarded when the defendant's conduct has reached such a level as to constitute oppression, fraud or malice. [California Civil Code section 3294.]

[2] Toole vs. Richardson-Merrell, Inc. (1967) 251 Cal.App.2nd 689, 60 Cal.Rptr. 398.

[3] *Teratology* involves the biological study of birth defects and their causes. A drug or chemical, or any other environmental agent, is *teratogenic* if it causes malformations to the developing embryo.

[4] Daubert vs. Merrell Dow Pharmaceuticals, Inc. 113 S.Ct. 2786 (1993).

[5] The human product of a conception is considered an *embryo* during the first 8 weeks after it was conceived; thereafter he or she is considered a *fetus*.

Chapter 1
An Inroduction to Drugs

[6] "Nicholas Richards" is a fictitious name.

[7] "Rosalie Chapman" is a fictitious name.

[8] A *package insert* is the product labeling for a drug, printed by the pharmaceutical company, which accompanies the packaged drug to the pharmacy. It contains everything a prescribing physician would want to know about a drug, including its chemical composition, action, pharmacology, indications (what it is intended to treat), contraindications, warnings, precautions, adverse reactions and dosage.

[9] *Organogenesis* is the period during which the organs are formed and develop in the embryo.

[10] "Philip Chapman, M.D." is a fictitious name.

[11] A *syndrome* is a group of symptoms that collectively indicate or characterize a disease, disorder or other abnormal condition. A syndrome is usually named after the physician or scientist that discovered the pattern.

[12] The pretrial procedures during which information and records are sought from other individuals and legal entities are referred to as *discovery*. This includes the taking of depositions (pretrial testimony under oath), service of interrogatories (written questions answered under oath by a party), request for admissions (uncontested facts to be admitted by an opposing party), formal requests for the production of records served upon parties, and subpoenas served upon nonparties to the lawsuit.

[13] Merrell case nos. 15252, 17685, 19948, 20901, 21915, 21983, 21984, and 22796.

[14] The first three digits of the case number relate to the number assigned to the clinical investigator, whereas as the last three digits belong to a specific patient of that investigator.

[15] I would learn months later, directly from Judge Fredricks, that after the settlement conference he had approached Judge Stothers about assigning the case to him for trial if at all possible. Without taking sides, he found the case extremely interesting and a welcome break from all the routine cases he frequently saw.

[16] Alex Dugally would later retire from the County Clerk's office and open his own attorney service, used by law firms to file court documents and to serve lawsuits and subpoenas. One of his clients was Terence J. Mix, Attorney at Law.

Chapter 2
Clomid on Trial:
The Plaintiffs' Case

[17] This was equal to approximately $312,000 in 2005 dollars.

[18] I have often wondered what would have happened to my career if we had settled that day. One thing is for sure. I never would have seen another Clomid case and you wouldn't be reading this book.

[19] A *motion in limine* literally means a "motion at the beginning." It is a motion filed by a party at the very beginning of trial, frequently directed to issues pertaining to anticipated evidence, but also to address any number of other matters that might arise or be of use during the trial. The idea is to get a ruling from the trial judge before a jury starts hearing anything about the case.

[20] A motion for *nonsuit* usually takes place after the plaintiff has put on all available evidence and rested his or her case. The defendant, before calling one witness, can successfully argue such a motion if he or she can persuade the court that giving plaintiff's evidence all of the value to which it is legally entitled, including every legitimate inference which may be drawn from the evidence in plaintiff's favor, there is no

evidence to support a jury verdict in plaintiff's favor. Since opening statements are a showcase of the evidence expected to be introduced by a party, a motion for nonsuit can be made at that time as well if such promised evidence still would not support a verdict.

[21] Wardrop vs. City of Manhattan Beach (1958) 160 Cal.App.2nd 779, 326 P.2nd 15.

[22] Since any award of damages is in a current lump sum, including future out-of-pocket medical expenses and future loss of earnings, the total amount of such future losses must be reduced to their present value. *Present value* is the amount of money it would take today, invested at a reasonable rate of return, to equal the future costs and losses at the time they are incurred.

[23] *BAJI* is the Book of Approved Jury Instructions, and is used in all civil cases in California. These are pre-printed jury instructions approved by the Committee on Standard Jury Instructions of the Los Angeles Superior Court and Judicial Council of the State of California.

[24] A *Down syndrome* patient has a flat face, small ears and mouth, and broad hands and feet, with mild to moderate mental retardation. Heart defects are common and have a direct effect on life expectancy when present.

Chapter 3
Clomid on Trial:
The Defendant's Case

[25] A *mucaca mulatta* is a rhesus monkey.

[26] See Lab. Anim. Care 1968 June; 18(3): 339-45.

[27] See Anat. Rec. 1967 May; 158(1): 99-109.

[28] To bring the incidence of birth defects down to a lower rate, Merrell used total *pregnancies* (2,369) as its denominator, rather than total *deliveries* after deducting spontaneous abortions, hydatidiform moles, and tubal pregnancies (1,886), as is done with almost all other studies.

[29] This film had previously been viewed by me outside of the presence of the jury. I had successfully objected to certain portions of the film, but allowed the footage I felt would be informative or might tie into my arguments.

[30] See Fert. & Ster.: Proc. V World Congress, January 16-22, 1967, Excerpta Med., 68-73, 1967.

[31] A *curriculum vitae* is a professional's resume. It covers in detail not only all of his or her education, training and employment throughout his or her life, but also a complete bibliography of every professional article or book he or she has written. Although it can be a useful guideline for examining your own expert witness, since it contains references to everything the witness has ever written on his or her specialty, it also provides fertile ground for cross-examination material.

[32] I had no way of knowing if this was an accurate statement, since the ages of the patients in the Clomid clinical studies were not available to me at the time.

[33] Wilson, James G. Environment and Birth Defects. New York and London: Academic Press, 1973, p.106.

[34] Ibid, p.105.

[35] Ibid, p.103.

[36] Ibid, pp.139-140.

[37] Teratology – Principles and Techniques. Edited by James G. Wilson and Josef Warkany. University of Chicago Press (1965). "Embryological Considerations in Teratology" by James G. Wilson (pp.251-260 at p.253).

[38] Ibid, pp.252-253.

[39] Morris, et al. Fertility and Sterility. 18(1): 18-34 (1967).

[40] Dyson & Kohler, The Lancet, pp.1256-1257, June 2, 1973.

[41] My retained experts advised that to make a useful comparison with a malformation rate in the general population, one would need a group combined with all of the same countries in the same ratio as the Clomid studies – a near-impossible task. It was suggested that the Clomid clinical studies were no more than a marketing tool; used by Merrell to promote its fertility drug throughout the world.

[42] This pain may have been a symptom of *ovarian hyperstimulation syndrome*, a known side effect of fertility drugs. This would later be a significant factor in my contention of how fertility drugs can damage a fertilized egg (zygote) or embryo.

[43] This would be the last of my two trials in front of Thomas W. Fredricks.

[44] The amount of this 1974 verdict had a 2005 approximate value of $2,370,000. At the time, it was the highest jury verdict in the history of the Southwest District of the Los Angeles Superior Court.

Chapter 4
The Chromosome Factor

[45] A drug is *mutagenic* if it is capable of causing chromosomal damage or gene mutation.

[46] Am. J. Hum. Gen. 24: 20a (1972); Teratology 5: 264 (1972).

[47] Both occurred in the Clomid clinical studies.

[48] "Drug Influences on Malformations," Clin. Perinatol. 6(2): 403-414, at 409-410 (1979).

[49] A *cohort* study is a prospective study in which patients who presently have a certain condition, and/or receive a certain form of treatment, are followed over time and compared with a control group who are not affected by the condition or do not receive the treatment.

[50] *Meiosis* occurs in the ovary when a single cell with 23 pairs of chromosomes splits into two cells, with each retaining only one set of the 23 chromosomes.

[51] These numbers can vary depending upon the study, but generally convey the increased rate.

[52] Ford, J.H., The Lancet, 54, January 6, 1973.

[53] The term, *pH,* refers to the measure of the balance of acidity and alkalinity. They are equally balanced at 7.0. As that number rises, the alkalinity increases and acidity decreases.

[54] See discussion under heading, *Clinical Pharmacology.*

[55] Confidential Status Report to Clinical Investigators, dated August 1, 1964, p.13.

[56] Boue, J. et al. Teratology 12: 11-26, 1975.

[57] Ibid.

[58] Charles, D. et al. Jour. Obstet. Gynecol. Brit. Comm. 80: 264-270, March 1973. See the history on this paper in Chapter 10.

[59] Arakaki, D.T. and Waxman, S.H. Am. J. Obstet. Gynecol. 107: 1199, 1970.

[60] Lancet, 1: 1256-7, June 2, 1973.

[61] Sandler, B. Lancet, 2: 379, August 18, 1973.

[62] Barrett, C. and Hakim, C. Lancet, 2: 916-917, October 20, 1973.

[63] Case nos. 041-213 and 271-047.

[64] Case no. 108-045.

[65] See current package insert under heading, *Multiple Pregnancy.*

[66] See current package insert under heading, *Pregnancy.*

[67] Bull. Wld. Hlth. Org. 1966, 34, suppl. 81.

[68] Lancet, 1: 31, January 5, 1974.

[69] Burnell, G.M. Arch. Gen. Psychiatry 30: 183-184, February 1974.

[70] Thompson, C. et al. Fertility and Sterility 21: 844-853, 1970.

[71] Carr, D.H., Chromosomes and Abortion, 223. Advances in Human Genetics, Plenum Press, 1971, Ed. by Harris, H. and Hirschorn, K.

[72] Warkany, J. Jour. Ped. 61: 803-812, 1962; Longo, A. and Maccani, U. Aggior. Ped. 16: 311-318, 1965; Riccardi, V.M., et al. Jour. Ped. 77: 664-672, 1970; Caspersson, T. et al. J. Med. Genet. 9: 1-7, 1972.

[73] Humua, R.K. et al. Am. J. Med. Gen. 61(2): 171, Jan. 1996.

[74] Carter, C.O. J. Med. Gen. 10: 209-34, Sept. 1974; Janerich, D.T. Teratology 8: 253-256, Dec. 1973.

Chapter 5
An Invitation to Rockville, Maryland

[75] See article on Kelsey in FDA Consumer magazine, U.S. Food and Drug Administration, March-April 2001 edition.

[76] About the same period of time, a Dr. W.G. McBride in Australia made a similar discovery.

[77] On October 7, 2000, at the age of 86, Kelsey was also inducted into the National Women's Hall of Fame in Seneca Falls, New York.

[78] This had been a requirement under the Act since 1938.

[79] Catalog of Teratogenic Agents, 7th Ed., The Johns Hopkins University Press, p.xxii.

Chapter 6
Selling the Mix Hypothesis

[80] I had also discovered that *elevated* estrogen levels could likewise raise the pH in the oviduct.

[81] Vandenburg, J. Clin. Endocrin. Metab. 37: 356, 1973.

[82] *Estradiol* is the principle estrogen secreted by the ovaries.

[83] Not only did the Boues look at the possible role of ovulation-inducing drugs in causing chromosomal anomalies, they also evaluated maternal age, oral contraceptives, radiation and a number of other factors.

[84] Bull. Wld. Hlth. Org. 1966, 34, suppl. 81.

[85] I had a basal cell (skin cancer) lesion removed from my left eyelid and was still sporting a bandaid.

[86] One of the two (Merrell no. 208-033) conceived only one cycle after treatment. In the Boue study, this group had just as high an incidence of abnormal chromosomes as the group that conceived during a cycle of treatment.

[87] A *retrospective* study is one designed to look back at records already prepared from earlier examinations of patients.

[88] A *prospective* study is one designed to examine patients in the future and to record information from those examinations pursuant to the study's design.

Chapter 7
Working the System

[89] Clomid investigator no.029.

[90] Clomid investigator no.123.

[91] The following phone conversation was drawn from Merrell Interdepartment Memo, dated November 14, 1975, from Dorsey E. Holtkamp, Ph.D. to The Files.

[92] The pervasiveness of this problem, even to this day, will be addressed in Chapter 20.

[93] National Institute of Child Health and Human Development. One of the National Institutes of Health.

[94] Both Jack Chewning, a doctor/lawyer, and Fred Lamb, had been very active in the Breimhorst case, assisting Belanger and his office with pretrial discovery and the trial itself.

[95] The meeting is summarized in Merrell Interdepartment Memo, dated April 7, 1976, from John B. Chewning to Those Concerned.

[96] Brent, a prominent teratologist, had also testified on behalf of Merrell at the Breimhorst trial.

[97] Although the clinical investigations officially concluded in May 1967, Merrell continued to record the outcome of all pregnancies up until 1970, as long as the conceptions occurred prior to marketing.

[98] The submission contains only a few minor updates on March 22, 1976, 5 days after the meeting with Ortiz and his staff.

[99] Clomid Pregnancy Data printout of January 1970, p.60.

[100] The Lancet, 1: 679-680, March 24, 1973.

[101] Even Oakley found only 2 patients (not three) who did not conceive during a treatment cycle.

[102] Recorded during a personal review of records from all 2,635 pregnancies occurring during the pre-market clinical investigations.

[103] Barrett and Hakim, The Lancet 2: 916-17, October 20, 1973.

[104] Field and Kerr, The Lancet 2: 1511, December 21, 1974.

[105] Some infants had more than one type of anomaly.

[106] Two additional cases of spina bifida occurred in association with 2 of the anencephaly reports.

[107] July 18, 1975 Hearing Transcript, pp.38-39.

[108] See letter from Holtkamp to Oakley, dated May 25, 1976.

[109] CDC nos. 03112, 03638 and 04992; Merrell nos. 29349, 29353 and 29354.

[110] Warkany, J. et al. Journal of Pediatrics 61: 803-812, 1962; Longo, A. and Maccani, U. Aggiornamento Pediatrico 61: 311-318, 1965; Riccardi, V. M. et al. Journal of Pediatrics 77: 664-672, 1970; Carr, D.H., Chromosmes and Abortion, Advances in Human Genetics, Vol.2, Ed. by H. Harris and K. Hirschorn, p.223, Plenum Press, N.Y., 1971; Caspersson, T. et al. Jour. Med. Gen. 9: 1-7, 1972; Wright, Y.M. et al. Jour. Med. Gen. 11: 69-75, Mar. 1974.

[111] July 18, 1975 transcript, p.35.

[112] The Lancet, 1: 679-680, March 24, 1973.

[113] Boue, J. et al. Teratology 12: 11-26, 1975.

[114] Boue, J. and Boue, A. Rev. Fr. Gynecol. Obstet. 68: 625-643, 1973.

[115] Emphasis added, The Lancet, at p.680; Teratology, at p.20.

[116] Emphasis added, Merrell's translation (#7802) of Rev. Fr. Gynecol. Obstet. 68: 625-643, 1973.

[117] Teratology, at p.11.

[118] Schumacher vs. Merrell Dow Pharmaceuticals, Inc. (Los Angeles Superior Court No. C472802); Responses to Plaintiffs' Interrogatories Propounded to Merrell Dow Pharmaceuticals Inc. (First set), dated January 16, 1985; no.77.

Chapter 8
Ancient Knowledge

[119] 6th Acta Endocr. Congr. Suppl. 119 (1967) 224.

[120] See reference to the Triparanol story in the Introduction.

[121] Fertility and Sterility 19: 351-62 (1968).

[122] Clomid Pregnancy Data printout of January 1970, pp.28-34.

[123] Obstet. Gynecol. 30: 699-705 (1967).

[124] Clomid Pregnancy Data printout of January 1970, p.114.

[125] Conn. Med. 31: 695-697, October 1967; Amer. J. Obstet. Gynecol. 98: 1037-1042, August 15, 1967.

[126] Clomid Pregnancy Data printout of January 1970, pp.75-76.

[127] British Med. J. 4: 446-449, November 25, 1967.

[128] Clomid Pregnancy Data printout of January 1970, p.110.

[129] Sanpu Chiryo 17(2): 185-198, 1968.

[130] Clomid Pregnancy Data printout of January 1970, p.111.

[131] Gynaecologia (Basel) 165: 221-232, 1968.

[132] Clomid Pregnancy Data printout, p.113.

[133] Breimhorst partial trial transcript of April 2, 1974, pp.26-27.

[134] Clomid Pregnancy Data printout of January 1970, pp.51-55.

[135] The Gandy vs. Merrell Dow Pharmaceuticals, Inc. (LASC No.C703146) trial took place in Los Angeles, California between May 2, 1994 and May 16, 1994. It settled just prior to closing arguments.

[136] For the handsome price of $28,800; Gandy trial transcript of May 13, 1994, pp.972-973.

[137] Gandy trial transcript of May 13, 1994, pp.1003-1010.

[138] A *double blind* study involves two groups of patients, one using the drug under study and the other a placebo (an inactive substance such as a sugar pill). The study is "double blind" when neither the patient nor the investigator knows which product any patient is using until conclusion of the study. See Inter-Department Memo, dated August 14, 1963, from Hoekenga to Werner.

[139] Hoekenga memo, dated September 1, 1965.

[140] Interdepartment Memo from Hoekenga to Schwab, dated September 9, 1965.

[141] Because Clomid was chemically related to Triparanol, the FDA was concerned about possible cataracts.

[142] Three babies were born with congenital heart defects.

[143] Breimhorst deposition of Hoekenga, dated February 5, 1974, p.55.

[144] FDA Memorandum from Berliner to Bennett, dated December 13, 1965, p.2.

[145] Interdepartment Memo from Johnson to Bunde, dated May 27, 1966.

[146] Inter-Department Memo from O'Dell to Schwab, dated June 1, 1966.

[147] Interdepartment Memo from Hoekenga to Levin, dated July 14, 1969.

[148] This comment may have been motivated by the fact that during the pre-market studies, there were 8 infants born with congenital heart defects.

[149] Schumacher vs. Merrell Dow Pharmaceuticals, Inc. (LASC No.C472802); Responses to Plaintiffs' Interrogatories propounded to Merrell Dow Pharmaceuticals, Inc. (First Set), dated January 16, 1985, No.77.

Chapter 9
Feathering the Nest

[150] Interdepartment Memo from Lindsay to Schwab, dated February 22, 1967.

[151] Interdepartment Memo from Hoekenga to Schwab, dated February 24, 1967.

[152] Gandy vs. Merrell Dow Pharmaceuticals, Inc. (LASC No. C703146); Goddard depos. transcript of April 22, 1994, pp.108-109.

[153] Ibid, pp.13-30.

[154] Before leaving Ormont, Goddard was already spending 10-15% of his time consulting for other pharmaceutical companies; Ibid, p.17.

[155] Gandy trial transcript for May 13, 1994, pp.972-973.

[156] Gandy vs. Merrell Dow Pharmaceuticals, Inc.; Goddard depos. transcript of April 22, 1994, pp.32-35.

[157] Ibid, p.972.

[158] Gandy trial transcript of May 13, 1994, p.1025.

[159] Goddard deposition transcript of April 22, 1994 re Gandy, p.28.

[160] Gandy trial transcript of May 13, 1994, pp.1024 -1026.

Chapter 10
Controlling the Controls

[161] Toxic. Appl. Pharmacol. 10: 565-76, May 1967.

[162] Proc. Europ. Soc. Study Drug Tox. 12: 299-306, 1971.

[163] Fertility and Sterility 20: 697-714, Sept.-Oct. 1969.

[164] Contraception. 2: 85-97, August 1970.

[165] Interdepartment Memo from Holtkamp to The Files, dated January 7, 1972.

[166] Charles was also conducting investigations on Bendectin on behalf of Merrell.

[167] Correspondence from Charles to Holtkamp, dated January 14, 1972. See also Interdepartment Memo from Holtkamp to The Files, dated January 25, 1972.

[168] Ibid.

[169] Correspondence from Charles to Heming, dated January 14, 1972.

[170] Interdepartment Memo from Hoekenga to Levin, dated February 1, 1972.

[171] Interdepartment Memo from Holtkamp to The Files, dated January 28, 1972.

[172] Interdepartment Memo from Holtkamp to Hoekenga, dated February 22, 1972.

[173] Interdepartment Memo from Holtkamp to The Files, dated March 9, 1972, p.2.

[174] Handwritten note, dated Octber 11, 1973.

[175] J. Obstet. Gynaec. Brit. Comm. 80: 264-70 (1973).

[176] Ibid, at p.264.

Chapter 11
A Homemade study

[177] Out of my four new post-Breimhorst cases, one had already settled.

[178] *Ovarian Hyperstimulation Syndrome* is a known side effect from fertility drugs that involves swollen and painful ovaries, and in more severe cases multiple ovarian cysts and an accumulation of fluid in the abdomen.

[179] There would be one exception: the Boues never examined abortuses of patients who conceived while experiencing OHSS.

[180] Unfortunately, the majority of the case histories included only Merrell forms. Thus, in most instances I was unable to look for transposition errors.

[181] Clomid Pregnancy Data printout, dated January 1970, p.1.

[182] As indicated, these statistics were compiled from cases where Clomid was only ingested prior to conception. If I had included cases in which Clomid was consumed during a conception cycle, and after conception as well, it would not have significantly changed the numbers. This group had a first trimester SA rate of 12.5% (15/120). If both groups were combined, the SA rate would have been 14.6% (239/1,639).

[183] Fertility and Sterility 28(7): 707-717, 1977.

[184] Inter. J. Fertil. 24(3): 193-197, 1979.

[185] Vandenberg and Yen, J. Clin. Endocrinol. Metab. 37: 356-365, 1973.

[186] Fertility and Sterility 30(5): 538-544, November 1978.

[187] Excerpta Medica, p.235, 1973.

[188] Brit. Jour. Obstet. Gynecol. 83: 967-973, Dec. 1976.

[189] The *corpus luteum* is a temporary endocrine structure that developes from an ovarian follicle after it has released a mature egg. It secretes the hormone progesterone, which thickens the uterine lining in preparation for the fertilized egg.

[190] Obstet. Gynecol. 46(1): 23-28, July 1975.

[191] Fujimoto, S. et al. J. Reprod. Fert. 40: 177-181, 1974.

[192] Takagi and Sasaki, Nature 264: 278-281, 1976; Maudlin and Fraser, J. Reprod. Fert. 50: 275-280, 1977.

[193] This communication involved an early draft of my study which only looked at total abortions; I had not yet broken down the statistics for first trimester spontaneous abortions.

[194] Bityk vs. Richardson-Merrell, Inc. (LASC No. C108370); Admission of Facts, July 27, 1979.

[195] His $250,000 offer in 1979 was equal to approximately $708,000 in 2005 dollars.

[196] Although a number of records can be acquired from the FDA through the Freedom of Information Act, it had repeatedly refused to produce communications between Merrell and that government agency, claiming that they were privileged.

[197] A settlement of $450,000 in 1979 would have equaled approximately $1,250,000 in 2005.

[198] Manzo vs. Richardson-Merrell, Inc. (San Bernardino Superior Court No.168832); Responses of Richardson-Merrell, Inc. to Plaintiff's Request for Admissions of Fact, No.81, April 13, 1981.

[199] One of the National Institutes of Health (NIH).

[200] Manzo vs. Richardson-Merrell, Inc.; deposition of Gerald F. Chernoff, February 18, 1982, pp.53-55.

[201] Ibid, pp.39-45; pp.49-51.

Chapter 12
The Evidence Grows

[202] Int. J. Epidemiol. 12 (4), 445-449, 1983.

[203] It would appear that they gave no consideration to the half-life factor.

[204] Nature 246: 37-39, November 2, 1973.

[205] Diener and Hsu, Toxic. Appl. Pharmacol. 10: 565-576, 1967.

[206] Morris, Contraception 2: 85-97, August 1970.

[207] Fertility and Sterility 36(5), 560-564, November 1981.

[208] Fertility and Sterility 39(2): 157-161, February 1983.

[209] Supra, Int. J. Fertil. 24(3): 193-197, 1979.

[210] See Chapter 11.

[211] McCormack and Clark, Science 204: 629, May 11, 1979. See also Clark and McCormack, Science 197: 164, 1977.

[212] Clark and McCormack, J. Ster. Biochem. 12: 47-53, 1980. The authors supplemented their findings in Adv. Exp. Med. Biol. 138: 87-98, 1982.

[213] Am. J. Obstet. Gynecol. 144: 529-532, 1982.

[214] Am. J. Obstet. Gynecol. 147: 633-639, 1983.

[215] Am. J. Obstet. Gynecol. 153: 679-684, 1985.

[216] Published by the Canadian Pharmaceutical Association, its use is similar to the Physician's Desk Reference (PDR) in the United States.

[217] Merrell Nos. 24900, 27218 and 31368.

Chapter 13
The Check is in the Mail

[218] See correspondence from Thomas B. O'Dell (Merrell) to Mrs. Eva Castro (FDA), dated May 6, 1980; from O'Dell to Solomon Sobel, M.D. (FDA), dated May 20, 1980; and from O'Dell to the Division of Metabolism and Endocrine Drug Products, dated July 25, 1980.

[219] *Product information* includes data, reports and information on the various labeling categories, including clinical pharmacology, contraindications, warnings, precautions, adverse reactions and overdosage.

[220] The *Federal Register* is the official publication for rules, proposed rules and notices of Federal agencies and organizations. Among other things, it publicizes certain actions it intends to take concerning pharmaceutical products. Its purpose is to invite comments and suggestions from the private sector before taking such actions.

[221] 21 CFR 201.57, as revised through April 1, 2001, states in part: "Warnings. Under this section heading, the labeling shall describe serious adverse reactions and *potential* safety hazards, limitations in use imposed by them, and steps that should be taken if they occur. The labeling shall be revised to include a warning as soon as there is reasonable evidence of an association of a serious hazard with a drug; *a causal relationship need not have been proved.*" [Emphasis added.]

[222] It's interesting to note that the July 1992 Serophene package insert can be found in the FDA's Clomid file (NDA 16-131) *with the quoted language highlighted.*

[223] The text of the draft makes this clear. See language under the heading, *Clinical Studies.*

[224] Although these statistics do not appear in the current labeling, they come from a number of different sources, including discovery on various lawsuits, a review of the original records and even on earlier package inserts.

[225] Out of 2,635 total pregnancies, the outcome of 266 of them was unknown, purportedly because the physician investigators lost track of the patients.

[226] Manzo vs. Richardson-Merrell, Inc. (San Bernardino Superior Court case no.168832); Bunde deposition transcript of March 3, 1979, pp.17-19.

[227] Ibid, pp.22-23.

[228] Ibid, p.32.

[229] J. New Drugs 5: 193-198, July-August 1965.

[230] Manzo vs. Richardson-Merrell, Inc.; Answers to Interrogatories (Third Set), dated October 26, 1978, Exhibit "G."

[231] Breimhorst vs. Richardson-Merrell, Inc. (Los Angeles Superior Court case no.SWC 19125); Hoekenga deposition transcript of March 1, 1974, p.15.

[232] Manzo vs. Richardson-Merrell, Inc.; Amended Responses to Request for Admissions, dated September 25, 1978, Admission No.24.

Chapter 14
A Prophesy Validated

[233] Stevenson, A.C. et al. Bull. Wld. Hlth. Org., 1966, 34 Suppl. 81.

[234] The Lancet, 1386.

[235] The article cites a paper by a Dr. W.H. James.

[236] The Lancet, 167, July 15, 1989. The study assessed the risk for several other congenital malformations as well, which will be discussed later.

[237] The Lancet, 1530, December 23/30, 1989.

[238] Reproductive Toxicology, 5: 83-84, 1991.

[239] Teratology 42: 325, 1990.

[240] Teratology, 44(4): 477, October 1991.

[241] The Lancet, 1281, November 25, 1989.

[242] Teratology, 42: 467, 1990.

[243] The Lancet, 1392, December 9, 1989.

[244] Teratology, 45: 326, March 1992.

[245] The Lancet 335: 178, January 20, 1990.

[246] Ped. Res. 29 (4 Part 2): 70A, April 1991; Am. J. Epidemiol. 134: 748, Oct. 1991

[247] CDC case nos. 03112, 03638 and 04992, respectively.

[248] The Lancet, 336: 103-104, 1990.

[249] Mills, et al. The New England Journal of Medicine 321(7): 430-435, August 17, 1989.

[250] Stoll, et al. Proc. Reprod. Toxicol. 14:75, October 2, 1999.

[251] The Lancet, 344: 445-446, August 13, 1994.

[252] To preserve his privacy, I have chosen to keep his identity confidential.

[253] Cited as footnote 7 in the article (Am. J. Epidemiol. 134: 748, 1991).

[254] Fertility and Sterility 56: 918-922, November 1991.

[255] Teratology 49: 273-281, 1994.

[256] Because use of abnormal controls can only weaken the odds ratio, a positive association could only get stronger if they were eliminated.

[257] Supra.

[258] Fertility and Sterility 55(4): 726-732, April 1991.

[259] Erickson, J.D. Teratology 43: 41-51, 1991.

[260] Teratology 47: 263-273, April 1993.

[261] Toxic. Appl. Pharmacol. 10: 565-576, May 1967.

[262] Fertility and Sterility 20(5): 697-714, Sept.-Oct. 1969.

[263] Contraception 2: 85-97, August 1970.

Chapter 15
Back in the Saddle Again

[264] Fertility and Sterility 46: 392-396, 1986.

[265] *Isomers* are molecules within a drug or chemical that share the same formula, but in which the atoms are arranged differently, resulting in different properties or effects.

[266] Geier, et al. Fertility and Sterility 47(5): 778-784, May 1987.

[267] Acta Obstet. Gynecol. Scand. 55: 371-375, 1976.

[268] Fertility and Sterility 40(2): 187-189, August 1983.

[269] These numbers presume each multiple birth was a set of twins. But the clomiphene pregnancies would more likely result in triplets, quadruplets, quintuplets, etc. than pregnancies from spontaneous ovulators. If that did in fact occur, then the percentage of Clomid pregnancies resulting in multiple births would be even smaller.

Chapter 16
Does Anyone Really Care?

[270] See letter from Solomon Sobel, M.D. to Marion Merrell Dow, Inc., dated September 30, 1994.

Chapter 17
The Federal Court of Science

[271] State court judges in California are elected to four-year terms.

[272] Daubert vs. Merrell Dow Pharmaceuticals, Inc. 113 S.Ct. 2786 (1993).

[273] Transcript of December 5, 1994, pp.53-69.

[274] Daubert vs. Merrell Dow Pharmaceuticals, Inc. 43 F.3rd 1311 (9th Cir. 1995); after remand from the U.S. Supreme Court.

[275] Frye vs. United States, 293 F. 1013 (D.C. Cir. 1923).

[276] In particular, Rule 702.

[277] The court pointed out, however, that simply because a scientific theory or technique has been published is not controlling; that publication does not necessarily correlate with reliability, and "in some instances well-grounded but innovative theories will not have been published. * * * The fact of publication (or lack thereof) in a peer-reviewed journal thus will be a relevant, though not dispositive, consideration in assessing the scientific validity of a particular technique or methodology on which an opinion is premised." 113 S.Ct. 2786 at 2797.

[278] There can be little question that the Supreme Court intended a less stringent standard for admitting expert opinions. "Moreover, such a rigid standard would be at odds with the Rules' liberal thrust and their general approach of relaxing the traditional barriers to 'opinion' testimony." 113 S.Ct. 2786 at 2790.

[279] One might argue that the defendant's experts must meet the same standard, but since the plaintiff bears the burden of proof and must put his or her case on first, the plaintiff must successfully negotiate this mine field before a defendant is compelled to put on one witness.

[280] "For one thing, experts whose findings flow from existing research are less likely to have been biased toward a particular conclusion by the promise of remuneration; when an expert prepares reports and findings before being hired as a witness, that record will limit the degree to which he can tailor his testimony to serve a party's interest." 43 Fed.3rd 1311 at 1317.

[281] See Chapter 10.

[282] For an example of possible bias resulting from the source of a grant, see Werler, et al., The Lancet, 344: 445-446, August 13, 1994, and comments related to said study in Chapter 14.

[283] See Chapter 3, April 2, 1974.

[284] It would seem that the Ninth Circuit has ignored an important observation made by the Supreme Court in Daubert. "(R)espondent seems to us to be overly pessimistic about the capabilities of the jury, and the adversary system generally. Vigorous cross-examination, presentation of contrary evidence, and careful instruction on the burden of proof are the traditional and appropriate means of attacking shaky but admissible evidence." 113 S.Ct. 2786 at 2798.

[285] "Plaintiffs submitted their experts' affidavits while Frye was the law of the circuit and, although they've not requested an opportunity to augment their experts' affidavits in light of Daubert, the interests of justice would be disserved by precluding plaintiffs from doing so. Given the opportunity to augment their original showing of admissibility, plaintiffs might be able to show that the methodology adopted by some of their experts is based on sound scientific principles. For instance, plaintiffs' epidemiologists might validate their reanalyses by explaining why they only chose certain of the data that was available, or the experts relying on animal studies might point to some authority for extrapolating human causation from teratogenicity in animals." 43 Fed.3rd 1311 at 1319-1320.

[286] 43 Fed.3rd 1311 at 1320. The Ninth Circuit rationalized that since women unexposed to Bendectin have a rate of one limb reduction defect per thousand births (when unrelated to Bendectin), to demonstrate that plaintiffs' defects are more likely than not due to Bendectin, a rate of more than two per thousand births was required to establish *probability*. Anything less would only fall into the area of *possibility*.

[287] See Daubert footnotes 13 and 16.

[288] Citations to the relevant legal authority and text of the record before the Court have been excluded.

[289] The actual date of the last publication was 1983.

[290] More specifically, in late 1983/early 1984.

[291] These two rules from the Jelovsek article relate to assessing whether an individual case birth anomaly is associated with the ingestion of a drug. A copy of the article was attached to Done's declaration and was part of the record available for review by the appellate court.

[292] The article by Hoyme et al. [Pediatrics, Vol.85, No.5, 743-747, May 1990] involved assessing 10 individual cases with birth anomalies associated with maternal exposure to cocaine in which the "spectrum of anomalies" was "enlarged." A copy of the article was attached to Done's declaration and was part of the record available for review by the appellate court.

Chapter 18
I Rest my Case

[293] Teratology 42: 521-533, 1990.

[294] Teratology – Principles and Techniques, edited by James G. Wilson and Josef Warkany, University of Chicago Press (1965), "Embryological Considerations in Teratology," by James G. Wilson, pp.251-260, at 253.

[295] Ibid, p.253.

[296] Fertility and Sterility 46(3): 392-396, September 1986.

[297] Fertility and Sterility 47(5): 778-784, May 1987.

[298] Geier, et al. Amer. J. Obstet. Gynecol. 157: 1009, October 1987.

[299] Written by Marilynn Marchione, Associated Press Medical Writer.

[300] New England Journal of Medicine, 346(10): 725-730, March 2002.

[301] European Journal of Medical Genetics, 48(1): 5-11, Jan.-Mar. 2005.

[302] Fertility and Sterility, 84(5): 1308-1315, November 2005.

[303] Human Reproduction, 20(2): 328-338, 2005.

[304] Reproductive Toxicology 9(4): 399-400, 1995.

[305] Reproductive Toxicology 9(5): 491-493, 1995.

[306] Fertility and Sterility 64 (5): 936-941, November 1995.

[307] Greenland and Ackerman missed 4 cases of rachischisis from the paper, another neural tube defect.

[308] The Lancet 1: 167, 1989.

[309] Fertility and Sterility 56: 918-922, 1991.

[310] Nygren and Andersen Human Reproduction 17: 3260-3274, 1999; Lynch, et al. Obstet. Gynecol. 97: 195-200, 2001.

[311] Pinborg, et al. Human Reproduction 19(2): 435-441, February 2004.

[312] Windham and Sever Am. J. Hum. Genet. 34: 988-998, 1982; Windham, et Acta Genet. Med. Gemellol. 31: 165-172, 1982.

[313] Ibid.

[314] Beral and Doyle British Medical Journal 300: 1229-1233, 1990; Rizk, et al., Hum. Reprod. 6(9): 1259-1264, 1991; Bergh, et al. The Lancet 354: 1579-1585; Lynch, et al.. supra.

[315] FIVNAT, Fertility and Sterility 64(4): 746-756, October 1995.

[316] An epidemiology study was considered *relevant* if it consisted of a sufficient number of pregnancies to detect an increased risk in NTDs and was designed to look at these specific anomalies (e.g., rather than simply "congenital malformations" or abnormalities of the "central nervous system").

[317] Cornel, et al. The Lancet, 1: 1386, June 17, 1989.

[318] Czeizel, The Lancet, 2: 167, July 15, 1989.

[319] Cuckle and Wald, The Lancet, 2: 1281, November 25, 1989; Vollset, The Lancet, 335: 178, January 20, 1990.

[320] Robert, et al. Reproductive Toxicology, 5(1): 83-84, 1991.

[321] Goujard, et al. Teratology, 45: 326, March 1992.

[322] Shaw, et al. Reproductive Toxicology 9(4): 399-400, 1995.

[323] Medveczky, et al. Pharmacoepidemiology and Drug Safety, 13(7): 443-455, July 2004.

[324] Wu, et al. Birth Defects Research (Part A), 76: 718-722, 2006.

[325] Lancaster, The Lancet, 2: 1392-1393, December 12, 1987.

[326] Karabacak, et al. The Lancet, 2: 1391-1392, December 9, 1989.

[327] Cornel, et al. The Lancet, 2: 1530, December 23/30, 1989.

[328] Milunsky, et al. Teratology, 42: 467, 1990.

[329] Beral and Doyle, British Medical Journal, 300: 1229-1233, 1990.

[330] Rizk, et al. Human Reproduction, 6(9): 1259-1264, 1991.

331 Rufat, et al. Fertility and Sterility, 61(2): 324-330, February 1994.
332 FIVNAT, Fertility and Sterility, 64(4): 746-756, October 1995.
333 Westergaard, et al. Human Reproduction, 14(7): 1896-1902, 1999.
334 Bergh, et al. The Lancet, 354: 1579-1585, 1999.
335 Wennerholm, et al. Human Reproduction, 15(4): 944-948, 2000.
336 Lancaster, et al. Reproductive Toxicology, 14: 74, 2000.
337 Ericson and Kallen, Human Reproduction, 16(3): 504-509, 2001.
338 Kallen, et al. Birth Defects Research (Part A), 73: 162-169, March 2005.
339 Mills, et al. The Lancet, 336: 103-104, July 14, 1990.
340 Mili, et al. Pediatric Research, 29(4 Part 2): 70A, April 1991.
341 Werler, et al. The Lancet, 344: 445-446, August 1994.
342 Lammer, Reproductive Toxicology, 9(4): 399-400, 1995.
343 Whiteman, et al. American Journal of Epidemiology, 152(9): 823-828, 2000.
344 Kurachi, et al. Fertility and Sterility, 40(2): 187-189, August 1983.
345 Kallen, et al. Obstetrics and Gynecology, 100(3): 414-419, September 2002.
346 Bull. Wld. Hlth. Org. 34: suppl. 81, 1966.
347 See Windham and Sever Am. J. Hum. Genet. 34: 988-998, 1982; Windham et al. Acta Genet. Med. Gemellol. 31: 165-172, 1982.
348 Teratology 50: 322-331, 1994.
349 J. Epidem. Comm. Hlth. 45: 43-48, 1990.
350 Prenat. Diagn. 25: 1007-1010, 2005.
351 Am. J. Epidemiol. 152(9): 823-828, 2000.
352 Trends in Neural Tube Defects in Australia, supra.
353 Schachter, et al. Human Reproduction 16: 1264-1269, 2001; Sperling and Tabor Acta Obstet. Gynecol. Scand. 80: 287-299, 2001.
354 See discussion in Chapter 19.
355 Carmi, et al. Amer. J. Med. Genet. 51: 93-97, 1994; Evans, Br. Med. J. 1: 975-976, 1979; Clarke, et al. Br. Med. J. 4: 743-746, 1975; Whitemen, et al. Amer. J. Epidemiol. 152(9): 823-828.
356 Todoroff and Shaw Amer. J. Epidemiol. 151: 505-511, 2000.
357 Kurinczuk and Clarke Paediatr. Perinat. Epidemiol. 7(2): 167-176, April 1993.
358 Reproductive Toxicology, supra.
359 Human Reproduction, supra.
360 GIFT: gamete intrafallopian transfer; Lancaster, The Lancet, 2: 1392-1393, December 12, 1987.
361 Lancaster, Teratology, 44(4): 477, October 1991.
362 Kurinczuk and Bower, British Medical Journal, 315(7118): 1260-1265, 1997.
363 Hansen, et al. New England Journal of Medicine, 346(10): 725-730, March 2002.
364 Ludwig and Katalinic, Reproductve BioMedicine Online, 5(2): 171-178, July 2002.
365 Koivurova, et al. Human Reproduction, 17(5): 1391-1398, August 2002.
366 Anthony, et al. Human Reproduction, 17(8): 2089-2095, August 2002.
367 Kallen, et al. Birth Defects Research (Part A), 73: 162-169, March 2005.
368 Olson, et al. Fertility and Sterility, 84(5): 1308-1315, November 2005.
369 Walker, et al. (unpublished), Associated Press, February 9, 2007.
370 Lancaster, Teratology, 42: 325, 1990.
371 Mili, et al. American Journal of Epidemiology, 134: 748, October 1991.
372 Lancaster, Teratology, 44(4): 477, October 1991.
373 Kurinczuk and Bower, British Medical Journal, 315(7118): 1260-1265, 1997.
374 Bergh, et al. The Lancet, 354: 1579-1585, November 1999.
375 Ericson and Kallen, Human Reproduction, 16(3): 504-509, 2001.
376 Kallen, et al. Birth Defects Research (Part A), 73: 162-169, March 2005.
377 Walker, et al. (unpublished), Associated Press, February 9, 2007.
378 Lancaster, Teratology, 42: 325, 1990.
379 Macnab and Zouves, Fertility and Sterility, 56(5): 918-922, November 1991.
380 Werler, et al. The Lancet, 344: 445-446, August 1994 (personal communication).
381 Silver, et al. The Journal of Urology, 161: 1954-1957, 1999.
382 Wennerholm, et al. Human Reproduction, 15(4): 944-948, 2000.

[383] Hansen, et al. The New England Journal of Medicine, 346(10): 725-730, March 2002.
[384] Ludwig and Katalinic, Reproductive BioMedicine Online, 5(2): 171-178, July 2002.
[385] Kallen, et al. Birth Defects Research (Part A), 73: 162-169, March 2005.
[386] Meijer, et al. Birth Defects Research (Part A), 76(4): 249-252, 2006.
[387] Czeizel, et al. International Journal of Epidemiology, 12(4): 445-449, 1983.
[388] Lancaster, Teratology, 42: 325, 1990.
[389] Lancaster, Teratology, 44(4): 477, October 1991.
[390] Ericson and Kallen, Human Reproduction, 16(3): 504-509, 2001.
[391] Hansen, et al. The New England Journal of Medicine, 346(10): 725-730, March 2002.
[392] Reefhuis, et al. Pediatrics, 111(5): 1163-1166, May 2003.
[393] Olson, et al. Fertility and Sterility, 84(5): 1308-1315, November 2005.
[394] Czeizel, The Lancet, 2: 167, July 15, 1989.
[395] Mili, et al. American Journal of Epidemiology, 134: 748, October 1991.
[396] Kurinczuk and Bower, British Medical Journal, 315(7118): 1260-1265, 1997.
[397] Kallen, et al. Birth Defects Research (Part A), 73: 162-169, March 2005.
[398] Mili, et al. American Journal of Epidemiology, 134: 748, October 1991.
[399] Bergh, et al. The Lancet, 354: 1579-1585, 1999.
[400] Mutation Research 65: 57-61, 1986.
[401] Biochem. Biophys. Res. Comm. 138(3): 1203-1210, 1986.
[402] Teratology 45: 326, 1992.
[403] Stevenson, et al. Bull. Wld. Hlth. Org. 34: Suppl. 81, 1966.
[404] Lubs and Ruddle, Science 169: 495-497, 1970.
[405] Teratology 41(5): 566, 1990.
[406] Vandenberg and Yen, J. Clin. Endocrinol. Metab. 37(3): 356-365, 1973.
[407] Oelsner, et al. Fertility and Sterility 30(5): 538-544, November 1978; Ben-Rafael, et al. Fertility and Sterility 39(2): 157-161, February 1983; Lam, et al. Am. J. Obstet. Gynecol. 160: 621-628, 1989.
[408] Forman, et al. Ferility and Sterility 53: 502-509, 1990; Chen, et al. J. Formosa Med. Assoc. 96: 829-834, 1997.
[409] Oelsner, et al., Fertility and Sterility, Ibid.
[410] Brit. J. Obstet. Gynecol. 83: 967-973, December 1976.
[411] Advances in Diagnosis and Treatment of Infertility, Insler and Bettendorf, eds., Elsevier N. Holland, Inc., 27-31, 1981.
[412] J. Formosa Med. Assoc. 96: 829-834, 1997.
[413] Fertility and Sterility 70(6): 1070-1076, December 1998.
[414] Human Reproduction 17(1): 107-110, 2002.
[415] Human Reproduction 7(8): 1154-1158, 1992.
[416] The gestational age was unknown for the balance of the SAs.
[417] Intern. J. Fertil. 33(3): 162-167, May-June 1988.
[418] Contracept. Fertil. Sex. 11: 1301-1303, 1983.
[419] Spielmann, et al. J. IVF Embr. Trans. 2(3): 138-142, 1985; Martin, et al. J. Reprod. Fertil. 78: 673-678, 1986; Wramsby and Fredga, Human Reproduction 2(2): 137-142, 1987; Wimmers and Van der Merwe, Human Reproduction 3(7): 894-900, 1988.
[420] Human Reproduction 7(10): 1396-1401, 1992.
[421] J. Reprod. Fert. 40: 177-181, 1974.
[422] Nature 264: 278-281, November 1976.
[423] J. Reprod. Fert. 50: 275-280, 1977.
[424] Journal of Heredity 77: 39-42, 1986.
[425] Fertility and Sterility 73(3): 620-626, March 2000.
[426] Obstet. Gynecol. 74: 624-636, 1989.
[427] Toxic. Appl. Pharmacol. 10: 565-76, May 1967.
[428] Proc. Europ. Soc. Study Drug Tox. 12: 299-306, 1971.
[429] Jour. Ster. Biochem. 12: 47-53, 1980.
[430] Teratology, 44: 25A, 1991.
[431] Fertil. Steril. 20: 697-714, Sept./Oct. 1969.
[432] Contraception, 2: 85-97, August 1970.

433 Hum. Pathol. 18: 1132-1143, 1987.

434 Teratology 47: 263-273, 1993.

435 J. Reprod. Fertil. 92: 65-73, 1991.

436 Am. J. Obstet. Gynecol. 147: 633-639, 1983.

437 Am. J. Obstet. Gynecol. 153: 679-684, 1985.

438 Am. J. Obstet. Gynecol. 154: 727-736, 1986.

439 Fertility and Sterility 45: 800-804, 1986.

440 New Engl. J. Med. 284: 878, 1971.

441 Pediatrics 58: 505-507, 1976.

442 Obstet. Gynecol. 49: 1-8, 1977.

443 J. Urology 117: 220-222, 1977.

444 J. Urology 122: 36-39, 1979.

445 J. Urology 125: 47-50, 1981.

446 Am. J. Obstet. Gynecol. 144: 529-532, 1982.

447 Adv. Exper. Med. Biol. 138: 87-98, 1982.

448 Teratology, 50: 97-98, 1994.

Chapter 19
Cause and Effect

449 Since June 1995, the language has stated: "Patients on prolonged CLOMID therapy may show elevated serum levels of desmosterol. This is most likely due to a direct interference with cholesterol synthesis."

450 Arch. Franc. Pediat. 21: 451-464, 1964; I even had it translated from French to English.

451 Tint, Am. J. Med. Genet. 47: 573-574, 1993; Irons, et al. The Lancet 341: 1414, 1993; Tint, et al. New Engl. J. Med. 330: 107-113, 1994; Opitz and de la Cruz, Am. J. Med. Genet. 50(4): 326-338, May 1994; Irons, et al. Am. J. Med. Genet. 50(4): 347-352, May 1994.

452 Curry, et al. Amer. J. Med. Genet. 26: 45-57, 1987.

453 Reefhuis, et al. Pediatrics 111(5): 1163-1166, May 2003.

454 Homanics, et al. Proc. Natl. Acad. Sci. USA 90(6): 2389-93, March 15, 1993.

455 Homanics, et al. Teratology 51(1): 1-10, January 1995; Farese, et al. Proc. Natl. Acad. Sci. USA 92(5): 1774-78, February 1995; Huang, et al. J. Clin. Invest. 96(5): 2152-61, November 1995; Tozawa, et al. J. Biol. Chem. 274(43): 30843-48, October 1999.

456 Roux, et al. Amer. J. Clin. Nutr. 71(5 Suppl): 1270s-1279s, May 2000.

457 Gofflot, et al. Amer. J. Med. Genet. 87: 207-216, 1999.

458 Ibid.

459 Roux, et al. Amer. J. Clin. Nutr., supra.

460 Gofflot, et al. Hum. Mol. Genet. 12(10): 1187-1198, May 2003.

461 Kolf-Clauw, et al. Teratology 54(3): 115-125, September 1996; Dehart, et al. Amer. J. Med. Genet. 68(3): 328-337, January 1997; Kolf-Clauw, et al. Teratology 56(3): 188-200, September 1997; Gofflot, et al. Amer. J. Med. Genet. 87(3): 207-216, November 1999; Roux, et al. Amer. J. Clin. Nutr. 71(5 Suppl.): 1270s-1279s, May 2000.

462 Roux, et al. Amer. J. Clin. Nutr., supra.

463 Ibid.

464 Ibid.

465 Ibid. See also Curry, et al. Amer. J. Med. Genet. 26: 45-57, 1987; Porter, J. Clin. Invest. 110: 715-724, 2002.

466 Chevy, et al. J. Lipid Res. 43(8): 1192-1200, August 2002; Gofflot, et al. Hum. Mol. Genet. 12(10): 1187-1198, May 2003.

467 Roux, et al. Amer. J. Clin. Nutr., supra.

468 Biochem. Pharm. 19: 2231-2241, 1970.

469 Neurosci. Abs. 1: 328, 1975.

470 Biochem. Pharmacol. 26: 1161-1167, 1977; Biochem. Pharmacol. 26: 1169-1173, 1977.

471 Toxicol. Appl. Pharmacol. 10: 565-576, 1967.

472 Chevy, et al. J. Lipid Res. 43(8): 1192-1200, August 2002.

473 Chevy, et al. J. Lipid Res., supra; Gofflot, et al. Hum. Mol Genet., supra.

474 Teratology 47: 263-273, April 1993. See also the discussion in Chapter 14.

[475] Windahm and Sever, Amer. J. Hum. Genet. 34: 988-998, 1982; Kallen, et al. Teratology 50: 322-331, 1994.
[476] Chevallier, Biochem. Biophys. Acta 84: 316-339, 1964; Roux, et al. Teratology 19: 35-38, 1979.
[477] Roux, et al. Amer. J. Clin. Nutr. 71 (5 Suppl.): 1270s-1279s, May 2000.
[478] Teratology 61: 347-354, 2000.
[479] Elwood, Little and Elwood (1992), Epidemiology of neural tube defects, Monog. Epidemiol. Biostat. 20: 335-389.
[480] Diczfalsuy, In: Advances in the Biosciences, Raspe, ed. Pergamon Press, 343-366, 1970.
[481] Geier, et al. Amer. J. Obstet. Gynecol. 157: 1009, October 1987.
[482] Chevy, et al. J. Lipid Res. 43(8): 1192-1200, August 2002.
[483] Trends in Neural Tube Defects in Australia, AIHW National Perinatal Statistics Unit, Univ. New South Wales, 2001.
[484] Elwood, Little and Elwood (1992), supra.
[485] Haines, et al. Fertil. Steril. 68(2): 231-5, Aug. 1997; Tadmor, et al. Int. J. Fertil. Menopausal Stud. 39: 105-110, 1994.
[486] Tadmor, et al., Ibid.
[487] Develop. Med. Child Neurol. 12: 67, 1970.; see also Knox, Brit. J. Prev. Soc. Med. 28: 73-80, 1974.
[488] Bonduelle, et al. Human Reproduction, 11(7): 1558-1564, 1996 (1.9% in singletons, 4.8% in twins, and 6.7% in triplets); Ericson and Kallen, Human Reproduction, 16(3): 504-509, 2001; Bonduelle, et al. Human Reproduction, 17(3): 671-694, 2002; Olson, et al. Fertility and Sterility, 84(5): 1308-1315, November 2005.
[489] Kallen, Acta Genet. Med. Gemellol., 35: 167-178, 1986; Doyle, et al. Journal of Epidemiology and Community Health, 45: 43-48, 1990; Ramos-Arroyo, Acta Genet. Med. Gemellol., 40: 337-344, 1991; Kato and Fujiki, Acta Genet. Med. Gemellol., 41: 253-259, 1992; Mastroiacovo, et al. American Journal of Medical Genetics, 83: 117-124, 1999; Li, et al. Birth Defects Research (Part A), 67: 879-885, 2003; Olson, et al. Fertility and Sterility, 84(5): 1308-1315, November 2005; and Tang, et al. Maternal and Child Health Journal, 10(1): 75-81, 2006.
[490] Birth Defects Research (Part A), 67: 879-885, 2003.
[491] Acta Genet. Med. Gemellol., 41: 253-259, 1992.
[492] Fertility and Sterility, 84(5): 1308-1315, November 2005.
[493] Twin Research, 7(3): 223-227, 2004.

Chapter 20
The Epiphany

[494] Doyle, et al. Journal of Epidemiology and Community Health, 45: 43-48, 1990; Ramos-Arroyo, Acta Genet. Med. Gemellol., 40: 337-344, 1991; Kato and Fujiki, Acta Genet. Med. Gemellol., 41: 253-259, 1992; Mastroiacovo, et al. American Journal of Medical Genetics, 83: 117-124, 1999; Li, et al. Birth Defects Research (Part A), 67: 879-885, 2003; and Tang, et al. Maternal and Child Health Journal, 10(1): 75-81, 2006.
[495] Myrianthopoulos, Birth Defects (Orig. Art. Ser.) 11: 1-39, 1975.
[496] Repetto, et al. Teratology, 42(6): 611-618, December 1990; Homanics, et al. Proc. of the National Acadamy of Science USA, 90(6): 2389-2393, March 1993; Homanics, et al. Teratology, 51(1): 1-10, January 1995; Farese, et al. Proc. Of the National Acadamy of Science, 92(5): 1774-1778, February 1995; Huang, et al. Journal of Clinical Investigation, 96(5): 2152-2161, November 1995; Tozawa, et al. Journal of Biological Chemistry, 274(43): 30843-30848, October 1999; and Roux, et al. American Journal of Clinical Nutrition, 71(5 Suppl.): 1270S-1279S, May 2000.
[497] Homanics, et al. Proc. Of the National Acadamy of Science, 90(6): 2389-2393, March 1993; Homanics, et al. Teratology, 51(1): 1-10, January 1995; Huang, et al. Journal of Clinical Investigation, 96(5): 2152-2161, November 1995; and Gaoua, et al. Journal of Lipid Research, 41(4): 637-646, April 2000.
[498] Kallen, Acta Genet. Med. Gemellol., 35: 167-178, 1986.
[499] Barbu, et al. Proc. Soc. Exp. Biol. Med., 176(1): 54-59, May 1884; Repetto, et al. Teratology, 42(6): 611-618, December 1990; Huang, et al. Journal of Clinical Investigation, 96(5): 2152-2161, November 1995; Dehart, et al. American Journal of Medical Genetics, 68(3): 328-337, January 1997; Kolf-Clauw, et al. Teratology, 56(3): 188-200, September 1997; Tozawa, et al. Journal of Biological Chemistry, 274(43): 30843-30848, October 1999; Gofflot, et al. American Journal of Medical Genetics, 87(3): 207-216,

November 1999; Gaoua, et al. Journal of Lipid Research, 41(4): 637-646, April 2000; and Roux, et al. American Journal of Clinical Nutrition, 71(5 Suppl.): 1270S-1279S, May 2000.

[500] Pepicelli, et al. Curr. Biol., 8(19): 1083-1086, 1998; Motoyama, et al. Nature Genetics, 20(1): 54-57, 1998; and Litingtung, et al. Nature Genetics, 20(1): 58-61, 1998.

[501] Forrester and Merz, Public Health, 119: 483-488, 2005.

[502] Kimmel, et al. Journal of Pediatric Surgery, 35: 227-231, 2000; Kim, et al. Journal of Pediatric Surgery, 36(2): 381-384, February 2001; and Mo, et al. American Journal of Pathology, 159(2): 765-774, August 2001.

[503] Pepicelli, et al. Curr. Biol., 8(19): 1083-1086, 1998; Motoyama, et al. Nature Genetics, 20(1): 54-57, 1998; and Kim, et al. Journal of Pediatric Surgery, 36(2): 381-384, February 2001.

[504] Lanoue, et al. American Journal of Medical Genetics, 73(1): 24-31, November 1997; Roux, et al. American Journal of Clinical Nutrition, 71(5 Suppl.): 1270S-1279s, May 2000; Haraguchi, et al. Development, 128: 4241-4250, 2001; Mo, et al. American Journal of Pathology, 159(2): 765-774, August 2001; Perriton, et al. Developmental Biology, 247: 26-46, 2002; and Petiot, et al. Development, 132: 2441-2450, 2005.

[505] Kim, et al. Journal of Pediatric Surgery, 36(2): 381-384, February 2001; and Yu, et al. Development, 129: 5301-5312, 5312, 2002.

[506] Kim, et al. Journal of Pediatric Surgery, 36(2): 381-384, February 2001.

[507] Chiang, et al. Nature, 383(6599): 407-413, October 1996; Mo, et al. Development, 124(1): 113-123, 1997; Roux, et al. American Journal of Clinical Nutrition, 71(5 Suppl.): 1270S-1279S, May 2000; and Kim, et al. Journal of Pediatric Surgery, 36(2): 381-384, February 2001.

[508] Chiang, et al. Nature, 383(6599): 407-413, October 1996; Mo, et al. Development, 124(1): 113-123, 1997; and Roux, et al. American Journal of Clinical Nutrition, 71(5 Suppl.): 1270S-1279S, May 2000.

[509] Kim, et al. Journal of Pediatric Surgery, 36(2): 381-384, February 2001.

[510] Chevy, et al. Journal of Lipid Research, 43(8): 1192-1200, August 2002.

[511] Repetto, et al. Teratology, 42(6): 611-618, December 1990; Dehart, et al. American Journal of Medical Genetics, 68(3): 328-337, January 1997; Gaoua, et al. Journal of Lipid Research, 41(4): 637-646, April 2000; and Roux, et al. American Journal of Clinical Nutrition, 71(5 Suppl.): 1270S-1279S, May 2000.

[512] Wassif, et al. Human Molecular Genetics, 10(6): 555-564, 2001.

[513] Chiang, et al. Nature, 383(6599): 407-413, October 1996; Dehart, et al. American Journal of Medical Genetics, 68(3): 328-337, January 1997; Kolf-Clauw, et al. Teratology, 56(3): 188-200, September 1997; Lanoue, et al. American Journal of Medical Genetics, 73(1): 24-31, November 1997; and Roux, et al. American Journal of Clinical Nutrition, 71(5 Suppl.): 1270S-1279S, May 2000.

[514] Kim, et al. Journal of Pediatric Surgery, 36(2): 381-384, February 2001; and Gianakopoulos and Skerjanc, Journal of Biological Chemistry, 280(22): 21022-21028, 2005.

[515] Ramos-Arroyo (1991) gave discordance numbers for some selected individual birth defects.

[516] It is controversial as to whether the Antley-Bixler syndrome should be included with this list, so I have chosen to exclude it.

[517] Also described as inborn errors of cholesterol synthesis.

[518] Porter, Journal of Clinical Investigation, 110(6): 715-724, September 2002; and Herman, Human Molecular Genetics, 12: R75-R88, 2003.

[519] Curry, et al. American Journal of Medical Genetics, 26: 45-57, 1987.

[520] Herman, Human Molecular Genetics, 12: R75-R88, 2003.

[521] Herbert, et al. Arch. Dermatol., 123(4): 503-509, 1987.

[522] Pepicelli, et al. Curr. Biol. 8(19): 1083-1086, 1998; Motoyama, et al. Nature Genetics 20(1): 54-57, 1998; and Litingtung, et al. Nature Genetics 20(1): 8-61, 1998.

[523] Journal of Pediatric Surgery 36(2): 381-384, February 2001.

[524] New England Journal of Medicine 350(15): 1579-1582, April 2004.

[525] Acta Genet. Med. Gemellol. 35: 167-178, 1986.

[526] Although not reaching statistical significance, limb reduction defects had a relative risk of 1.39.

[527] Doyle, et al. (1990), Li, et al. (2003) and Tang, et al. (2006), Ibid.

[528] Chiang, et al. Nature 383(6599): 407-413, October 1996; Roux, et al. American Journal of Clinical Nutrition 71(5 Supp.): 1270S-1279S, May 2000; and Chevy, et al. Journal of Lipid Research 43(8): 1192-1200, August 2002.

[529] Curry, et al. American Journal of Medical Genetics 26: 45-57, 1987; and Porter, Journal of Clinical Investigation 110(6): 715-724, September 2002.

[530] Happle, et al. European Journal of Pediatrics 134(1): 27-33, 1980.

[531] Polydactyly and syndactyly are among the group of anomalies seen in SLOS, CDPX2, Lathosterolosis and Greenberg dysplasia.

[532] Roux, et al. American Journal of Clinical Nutrition 71(5 Suppl.): 1270S-1279S, May 2000; Chevy, et al. Journal of Lipid Research 43(8): 1192-1200, August 2002; and Gofflot, et al. Human Molecular Genetics 12(10): 1187-1198, May 2003.

[533] Curry, et al. American Journal of Medical Genetics 26: 45-57, 1987.

[534] Huang, et al. Journal of Clinical Investigation 96(5): 2152-2161, November 1995.

[535] Gaoua, et al. Journal of Lipid Research 41(4): 637-646, April 2000.

[536] Lajeunie, et al. Journal of Neurosurgery, 103(4 Suppl.): 353-356, 2005.

[537] Roux, et al. American Journal of Clinical Nutrition 71 (5 Suppl.): 1270S-1279S, May 2000.

[538] Huang, et al. Journal of Clinical Investigation 96(5): 2152-2161.

[539] American Journal of Medical Genetics 137A: 36-40, 2005.

[540] Chevalier, Biochim. Biophys. Acta 84: 316-339, 1964. See also Tint, et al. Journal of Lipid Research 47(7): 1535-1541, July 2006 (majority of cholesterol in early embryonic mice is maternal in origin).

[541] Barbu, et al. Proc. Soc. Exp. Biol. Med. 176(1): 54-59, May 1984.

[542] Roux, et al. J. Nutr. 110: 2310-2312, November 1980.

[543] Yoshida and Wada, Journal of Lipid Research 46: 2168-2174, 2005.

[544] Conference report from the NIH Conference on Holoprosencephaly and Early Embryonic Development, by Siobhan Dolan, M.D., Medscape Ob/Gyn & Women's Health 7(1): 2002.

[545] Woollett, American Journal of Clinical Nutrition 82: 1155-1161, 2005.

[546] See Woollett, American Journal of Clinical Nutrition 82: 1155-1161, 2005, citing Cuniff, et al. American Journal of Medical Genetics 68: 263-269, 1997; Tint, et al. Journal of Pediatrics 127: 82-87, 1995; and Witsch-Baumgartner, et al. American Journal of Medical Genetics 66: 402-412, 2000.

[547] Witsch-Baumgartner, et al. Journal of Medical Genetics 41: 577-584, 2004.

[548] Birth Defects Research (Part A) 73: 162-169, March 2005.

[549] Choanal atresia is a closed nasal passage, usually by an abnormal bony or membranous tissue; the anomaly can be either bilateral or unilateral.

[550] Goldenhaar syndrome, Saethre-Chotzen syndrome, Prader-Willi syndrome, Russel-Silver syndrome, Larsen syndrome and Zellweger syndrome.

[551] Ritter, et al. American Journal of Medical Genetics 63: 529-536, 1996.

[552] Journal of Lipid Research 41(4): 637-646, April 2000. See also Roux, et al. Teratology 19(1): 35-38, February 1979; Roux, et al. Journal of Nutrition 110(11): 2310-2312, November 1980; and Barbu, et al. Journal of Nutrition 118(6): 774-779, June 1988.

[553] It is recommended that women of child-bearing years routinely take 400 micrograms per day of folic acid to reduce the risk of NTDs.

[554] American Journal of Clinical Nutrition 82: 1155-1161, 2005.

[555] Simvastatin Therapy in Smith-Lemli-Opitz Syndrome (Identifier # NCT00064792); Study of Inborn Errors of Cholesterol Synthesis and Related Disorders (Identifier # NCT00046202).

[556] Lowry and Yong, American Journal of Medical Genetics 5: 137-143, 1980.

[557] CDC 2003 National Vital Statistics Reports 54(2), November 24, 2004: 4,089,950 live births and 27,970 stillbirths.

[558] CDC National Summary and Fertility Clinics Reports, December 2006.

[559] Ludwig and Katalinic, Reproductive BioMedicine Online 5(2): 171-178, July 2002 (8.6%); Hansen, et al. New England Journal of Medicine 346(10): 725-730, March 2002 (8.6%/9.0%); Merlob, et al. European Journal of Medical Genetics, 48(1): 5-11, Jan.-Mar. 2005 (9.00%/9.35%).

[560] 2002 National Survey of Family Growth (59.375% of 1,169,659 seeking treatment to conceive during the prior year; see Tables 97 and 98.)

[561] National Vital Statistics Reports 54(2): 1-116, September 8, 2005.

[562] See Forrester and Merz, Public Health 119: 483-488, 2005 and studies cited therein.

[563] Ibid, CDC National Vital Statistics Reports.

[564] Palinski and Napoli, FASEB J. 16: 1348-1360, 2002.

[565] Ibid.

Chapter 21
Where are we Now?

[566] See Chapter 13.

[567] *A Question of Judgment*, Bantam 1985.

[568] Jelovsek, et al. Teratology 42: 521-533, 1990.

[569] See testimony of FDA employee, Dr. David Graham, before the Senate Finance Committee on November 18, 2004. Dr. Graham, who works in the Office of Drug Safety, was highly critical of this standard. He equated it to "beyond a shadow of a doubt."

[570] New York Times, *Half a Step on Drug Safety*, February 17, 2005.

[571] Biljan, et al. Fertility and Sterility 84 (Supp.1): S95, 2005.

[572] Los Angeles Times, *A Dose of Denial*, March 28, 2004.

[573] See Baltimore Sun article.

[574] Los Angeles Times, *FDA Kept Suicide Findings Secret*, April 6, 2004.

[575] New York Times, *F.D.A. Links Drugs to Being Suicidal*, September 14, 2004.

[576] New York Times, *Despite Warnings, Drug Giant Took Long Path to Vioxx Recall*, November 14, 2004.

[577] Later published in the New England Journal of Medicine on February 15, 2005.

[578] Celebrex preceded it by four months, in January 1999.

[579] Reuters, *Report: Merck Tried to Bury Vioxx Concerns for Years,* November 1, 2004.

[580] Dr. David Graham testified before the Senate Finance Committee on November 18, 2004, that a Merck *pre-market* study (#090) "found nearly a 7-fold increase in heart attack risk with low dose Vioxx."

[581] Los Angeles Times, *Report: Bayer Held Back on Drug Dangers*, November 23, 2004.

[582] Washington Post, *FDA Is Flexing Less Muscle*, November 18, 2004.

[583] Chicago Tribune, *Flaws in Drug Agency Put Consumers at Risk*, February 20, 2005.

[584] On September 14, 1992 and September 21, 1992, FDA Commissioner Kessler wrote letters to Congress outlining the goals that would be met if it would authorize user fees. In passing the act, Congress expressly incorporated those goals into the PDUFA. 21 U.S.C. sec. 379g (note). See also Chicago Tribune, February 20, 2005, supra.

[585] Bresalier, R.S. et al. New England Journal of Medicine, February 15, 2005.

[586] New York Times, *Looking for Adverse Drug Effects*, November 27, 2004; Washington Post, *How to Improve Drug Safety*, December 2, 2004; Chicago Tribune, *Flaws in Drug Agency Put Consumer at Risk*, February 20, 2005.

[587] The OND is another office (along with ODS) under the CDER umbrella. The OND is directly responsible for reviewing the new drug applications within the targeted deadlines.

[588] New York Times, *Drug Safety Problem's Broken, a Top FDA Official Says*, June 9, 2005.

[589] Dr. Graham's views are largely echoed in a very telling investigative report on the FDA by the Government Accountability Office (GAO), dated March 31, 2006, and provided to Congress at that time. This GAO report, along with Dr. Graham's testimony, no doubt played a major role in securing support for the Food and Drug Administration Amendments Act of 2007, which was passed by Congress in late September 2007.

[590] Newsday, *Panel's Ties to Drugmakers Not Cited in New Cholesterol Guidelines*, July 15, 2004.

[591] Lurie, et al. JAMA, 295(16), 1921-1928, April 26, 2006.

[592] To read the full story, see Los Angeles Times, *The National Institutes of Health: Public Servant or Private Marketer?* December 22, 2004.

[593] Ibid.

[594] Ibid.

[595] Los Angeles Times, *NIH Audit Criticizes Scientist's Dealings*, p. A1, by David Willman.

[596] New York Times, *Free the Academic Drug Tests*, November 30, 2004.

[597] The Seattle Times, *Eleven Drug-Company Executives Face Trial in Kickback Case*, April 13, 2004.

[598] New York Times, *Suit Charges Promotion of Drug's Off-Label Use*, May 12, 2004.

[599] Washington Post, *Pfizer to Pay $430M Settlement*, May 13, 2004.

[600] Los Angeles Times, *When Drugs are Used Off-Label*, June 7, 2004.

[601] Newsday, *FDA Warns Johnson & Johnson Unit on Pain Patch Claims*, September 14, 2004.

[602] Washington Post, *New Study Criticizes Painkiller Marketing*, January 25, 2005.

[603] Alexander, G.C. et al. Archives of Internal Medicine, January 24, 2005.

[604] For a good book on this topic see <u>The Truth About the Drug Companies: How They Deceive Us and What to do About It</u>, by Marcia Angell, M.D., Random House (2004).

[605] Center for Health Policy Research, George Washington University, *Time to Act on Drug Safety*, JAMA, 279: 1571-73, 1998.

[606] On October 1, 2007, I sent letters to the Director of the Office of New Drugs and the Director of the Office of Drug Safety forwarding Chapters 18 and 19 of this book and requesting appropriate warnings and an assessment of clomiphene citrate under the new guidelines for risk evaluation and mitigation strategy.

EXHIBITS

INCREASED FREQUENCY OF
CHROMOSOMAL ANOMALIES IN ABORTIONS
AFTER INDUCED OVULATION

SIR,—In a study from 1965 to 1972, chromosomal examination of 1457 spontaneous abortions from the first trimester of the pregnancy showed 892 (61%) abnormal karyotypes. In 97% these chromosomal aberrations were numerical changes—trisomies, double trisomies, monosomies, triploidies, and tetraploidies.[13]

By a statistical analysis of these observations we are studying factors which may increase the probability of such chromosomal imbalance in the zygote: (1) maternal age, significant only in the determination of trisomies (especially D and G)[13]; (2) delays between ovulation and fertilisation; (3) intrafollicular over-ripeness of the ovum,

CHROMOSOME ABNORMALITIES IN ABORTIONS AFTER INDUCED
OVULATION

Group	No. of abortions	No. abnormal	Karyotypes					
			T Normal	T Trisomy	T Monosomy	T Triploidy	T Tetraploidy	T Translocation
1	47	39 (82%)	8	23	3	10	3	0
2	14	12 (86%)	2	7	1	2	2	0
3	23	14 (61%)	9	9	2	3	0	0
4	1374	828 (60%)	546	441	134	167	49	37

which may lead to triploidy; and (4) irradiation of the father or the mother, increasing the frequency of abortuses with chromosomal aberrations.[13]

We wish to point out the possible effect of drugs which induce or stimulate ovulation on the frequency of abnormal chromosomal karyotypes in abortions.

84 abortions were in women who had been treated with human menopausal gonadotrophin (H.M.G.) and human chorionic gonadotrophin (H.C.G.), with clomiphene citrate and H.C.G., or with H.C.G. alone. The frequency of chromosomal aberrations in the abortuses has been compared in four groups: group 1, 47 abortions after therapy given in the cycle during which fertilisation occurred; group 2, 14 abortions after therapy given in the cycle before fertilisation; group 3, 23 abortions after therapy given two or more cycles before fertilisation; and group 4, 1374 abortions in women who had not been treated with these drugs.

The results in groups 1 and 2 are similar (see table), which agrees with the observation that these treatments are effective during two cycles. On the other hand, there is a significant difference ($\chi^2 = 4.9$) between groups 1 and 2 and group 3. The frequency of abnormal karyotype in group 3 is similar to that in women who have never been treated for sterility. The results in groups 1 and 2 were similar whether therapy was given for amenorrhœa or anovulation, or for recurrent abortion in women of normal fertility.

The indications of induction of ovulation should be considered carefully, especially in the case of women with previous abortions. A prospective study[14] of 473 women has shown that such therapy may increase the risk of having a conceptus with chromosomal anomalies.

Centre International de l'Enfance,
Laboratoire de la S.E.S.E.P.,
Château de Longchamp,
75016 Paris.

JOELLE G. BOUÉ
ANDRÉ BOUÉ

EXHIBIT 1

NDA 16-131

DEPARTMENT OF HEALTH, EDUCATION, AND WELFARE
PUBLIC HEALTH SERVICE
FOOD AND DRUG ADMINISTRATION
ROCKVILLE, MARYLAND 20852

AUG 15 1975

Merrell-National Laboratories
Division of Richardson-Merrell, Inc.
Attention: Dr. Thomas B. O'Dell
Cincinnati, Ohio 45215

Gentlemen:

Reference is made to your new drug application for Clomid (clomiphene citrate) Tablets.

As you are aware, the Obstetrics and Gynecology Advisory Committee convened on July 17 and 18, 1975 and discussed Clomid as one of the agenda items. The Committee recommended that further prospective and retrospective data be collected by your firm regarding the occurrence of congenital anomalies, including Down's Syndrome, in children of mothers treated with clomiphene citrate.

We are requesting that your firm initiate studies to collect such data. Please submit your proposed protocols for our review and comment prior to the initiation of the studies.

Sincerely yours,

Edwin M. Ortiz, M.D.
Director
Division of Metabolism and
Endocrine Drug Products
Bureau of Drugs

EXHIBIT 2

495

NEW   *100-176*   *this outcome*   DEC 9 '66

FOLLOW-UP   ANALYSIS OF PREGNANCY IN PATIENTS TREATED WITH CLOMID *submitted in HB3 2-7-67 tab (cycle date not listed in HB3)*

Patient's Name   Investigator <u>Dr. N. Vorys</u>

Dose, duration, dates <u>last</u> Clomid course: <u>200x5 1-3-66 thru 1-7-66</u>

E. D. Conception: <u>LMP:12-30-65</u>   E. D. Confinement:_____

<u>Pregnancy and Delivery</u>

   Complications during pregnancy/delivery:___See data attached_____

_____

_____

   Single birth__x__   Multiple: Twins_____   Other (specify):_____

                Placenta: monochorionic_____ Multichorionic_____

                Blood type of multiple_____
                (when fraternal-identical status is doubtful)

<u>Outcome of Pregnancy</u> (classify by weight in grams)   Date of birth <u>9-23-66</u>

    ☐ Abortion (less than 500)   ☐ Immature (500-999)

    ☐ Premature (1000-2499)   ☒ Term (2500 grams [5-1/2 lb.] or more)

   Please include the following information where applicable:

Weight 5/8½ grams Gestation _38_ wk.   Sex___   Live Birth__x__   Stillbirth_____

Live birth with neonatal death (incl. length life)_____

<u>Relation of Clomid to Pregnancy</u>

    ☒ Attributable to Clomid therapy   ☐ Probably attributable to Clomid therapy

    ☐ Probably attributable to Clomid plus other therapy _____
                                   (specify)

    ☐ Attributable to other therapy _____
                                (specify)

    ☐ Not attributable to infertility therapy.

Congenital anomalies: _____See data attached_____

<u>Comments</u> (incl. cause for abortion, premature delivery, or neonatal death, if known)

     Del. at Lima, Ohio by /Dr. Shankland and history of del. is_____

in the data attached._____

_____   *Nichols Vorys MD*
Return to: Medical Research Department   *Anthony S. Neri, MD.*
        The Wm. S. Merrell Company
        Division of Richardson-Merrell Inc. _____
        Cincinnati, Ohio 45215   M.D.

EXHIBIT 3

496

No. 157
Bettendorf, G.
Hamburg, Germany

Final report on the tests carried out with Clomid

(clomiphene dihydrogen citrate)

1) Total number of treated patients: about 189

2) Total number of Treatment cycles: about 300

3) Dosages taken: 5 x 50 mg.   10 x 100 mg.
                   5 x 100 mg.   10 x 150 mg.
                  10 x 50 mg.   10 x 200 mg.

4) Total number of tablets given out: ?

5) Number of ovulatory cycles following treatment: 69%

6) Total number of conceptions: 40 out of 104

7) Number of Pregnancies completed: 18

8) Multiple pregnancies: 0

9) Number of abortions: 12

10) Data on side effects:

   a) cystic enlargement of ovaries: 10.8%

   b) hot flushes: 8.2%

   c) other side effects, such as visual disturbances, skin complaints,

      hair loss, etc.: 3 patients

11) Special comments: The data on the number of patients and cycles

    are actually somewhat higher because some patients did not return.

    Not included are patients who received Clomid on experimental basis

    (for example, Clomid test).

12) Time and duration of clinical trials: 1963 to 1967. Hamburg,

                                           Jan.12, 1967.

EXHIBIT 4

4407

CLOMID PREGNANCY DATA
AS OF JANUARY, 1970

SUBJECT: ALL PATIENTS

CASE NO. INV.PT.	AGE	PAI. DX.	G V D	NO. PREV. CLOM. PREG.	PREG. ABOR.	NO. DE- SIRED PREG.	HUS- BAND FER. ST.	ART. IN- SEM.	TOT. # TRI. CY.	DOSE LAST CLO. CY.	DUR. LAST CLO. CY.	DAYS CLO. TO CON- CEP.	TIME	CONCEP DATE MO-YR	PG. OUT- COME RPTD	DEL. DATE MO-YR	DEL. SEX	$ N L	R U N L	ANOM. O	GEST. LNG. DAYS	WGT. GMS.	CON. RK. PG.	SUB.ID. C O H	D E L
155-008	NS	000.0	?	0	?	9	9	9	94	15C	05	1	05	11/65	1	07/66	1	3	X		254	2350	9	13 13
155-009	NS	634.1	?	0	?	1	9	9	99	100	04	1	08	05/65	1	01/66	2	0	X		254	2630	9	13 13
155-010	NS	000.0	?	0	?	9	9	9	99	100	09	1	10	12/64	1	06/65	2	0	X		284	2900	9	13 13
155-011	NS	000.0	?	0	?	9	9	9	99	050	05	1	10	03/65	1	12/65	1	0	X		266	3100	9	13 13
155-012	NS	000.0	?	0	?	9	9	9	99	050	07	1	11	12/63	1	09/64	1	0	X		269	2950	9	13 13
155-013	NS	634.1	?	0	?	1	9	9	99	100	05	1	15	12/65	1	09/66	1	0	X		269	3000	9	13 13
155-014	NS	000.0	?	0	?	9	9	9	99	050	10	1	06	04/64	1	05/64	9	9			040	NS	9	13 13
155-015	NS	000.0	?	0	?	9	9	9	94	100	10	1	02	01/64	1	10/64	5	0	X		259	2640	9	13 13

10 TOTAL PATIENTS LISTED THIS INVESTIGATOR   10

156-004	NS	000.0	?	0	?	9	9	9	01	050	05	1	15	11/63	1	NS/NS	9	9	X		NS	NS	9	03 03
156-005	NS	000.0	?	0	?	9	9	9	01	100	03	1	09	08/63	1	06/64	1	0	X		281	3000	9	03 03
156-006	NS	000.0	?	0	?	9	9	9	01	050	05	1	03	06/64	1	03/65	1	0	X		270	2900	9	03 03
156-007	NS	000.0	?	0	?	9	9	9	71	050	05	1	10	01/65	1	10/65	1	0	X		258	3300	9	03 03

4 TOTAL PATIENTS LISTED THIS INVESTIGATOR   4

| 157-015 | NS | 000.0 | ? | 0 | ? | 9 | 9 | 9 | 94 | 100 | 10 | 3 | 15 | 08/65 | 1 | 11/65 | 9 | 9 | X | | NS | NS | 9 | 03 03 |
| 157-016 | NS | 000.0 | ? | 0 | ? | 9 | 9 | 9 | 01 | 100 | 05 | 1 | 10 | 06/65 | 1 | NS/66 | 1 | 0 | X | | NS | 3950 | 9 | 03 03 |

2 TOTAL PATIENTS LISTED THIS INVESTIGATOR   2

| 159-001 | | 634.1 | | | | 1 | / | 0 | / | | | | | | | | | | | | | | | 01 |
| 159-009 | | 634.1 | | | | 2 | / | 0 | / | | | | | | | | | | | | | | | 10 |

89

EXHIBIT 5

SUMMARY OF DR. UMBERGER'S EVALUATION OF CLOMIPHENE

After a thorough analysis of the animal studies performed using
Clomiphene, Dr. Umberger submitted a detailed pharmacologic report in
May 1963. The subsequent comments are those which are most pertinent
in the final evaluation.

Pharmacologically the properties of Clomiphene are similar to related
compounds MER-29 and Tace. It appears to have an inhibitory effect
on cholesterol synthesis at the demosterol stage. Data, although not
clear cut, suggest the drug may produce skin affections, alopecia,
and lens opacities.

There are some animal studies showing inhibition of ovulation, while
human use is recommended to induce ovulation. These findings are
somewhat at variance with each other. Future studies may prove to be
more definitive and less contradictory. The submitted human investigations are not well standardized as to criteria of use and response.

Teratogenicity has been demonstrated in animals. Human pregnancy
cases are quite limited and therefore inconclusive.

Animal fertility studies are suggestive of prolonged action of the
drug, perhaps due to deposition and sustained release from fat depots.
The drug could therefore be effective longer than the duration of its
administration. It may carry over from the phase of induced ovulation
into early pregnancy to interfere with the zygote and fetus.

EXHIBIT 6

499

In the human the excretion pattern of tagged Clomid is similar to that in the monkey, with 51% of orally administered drug being excreted in 5 days, and 37% after intravenous administration. Excretion is principally in the feces, and since it appears here for 6 weeks after administration, the existence of entero-heptic recirculation pool is suggested. The rather unexpectedly long persistence of part of Clomid-C^{14} in the system, even after single doses, must be suspected of being able to produce adverse reactions, such as the action on visual per-formance and a possible teratogenic action in instances of an initiated pregnancy.

Teratogenic Potency:

A summary of the teratogenicity tests is shown below. Rats, one treatment, s.c. on day 12 of pregnancy.

Dose (mg/kg)	Pups	Litters with Malformations	% of mal-formed pups	Resorptions	Type of Malformations
1,000	62	5/5	11.3	14	7 pups with ab-normal hind limb 1 tibia missing
200	103	11/11	28.2	14	24 with abnormal hind limbs 1 with long snou 7 with cranial anomalies
40	113	6/10	9.7	4	9 abnormal hind limbs; 1 abnor-mal rump; 1 hydroceph
8	113	5/10	5.3	4	6 abnormal hind limbs
1.6	103	1/10	1.0	4	1 stunted with nasal appendage and umbilical hernia
0	158	0/9	0	0	None

It would appear that the severity of teratogenic action is dose related. The apparently decreased action of the highest dose is explainable with the increased embryocidal action of this dose. Note also that the 1,000 mg dose did cause a skeletal anomaly.

EXHIBIT 7

DEPARTMENT OF HEALTH, EDUCATION, AND WELFARE
PUBLIC HEALTH SERVICE
CONSUMER PROTECTION AND ENVIRONMENTAL HEALTH SERVICE
WASHINGTON, D.C. 20204

FOOD AND DRUG ADMINISTRATION

NDA 16-131

JUN 4 1969

The William S. Merrell Company
Division of Richardson-Merrell Incorporated
Cincinnati, Ohio 45215

Attention: Dr. Mark T. Hoekenga

Gentlemen:

Reference is made to your communication dated August 1, 1968 reporting
experiences as required by the provisions of regulation 130.13 and section
505(j) of the Federal Food, Drug, and Cosmetic Act for the preparation
Clomid (clomiphene citrate) Tablets.

We have reviewed the report and recommend the following:

1. That all living infants conceived in association with Clomid
   therapy be followed, if possible, by competent personnel
   for a period of at least two years, and a report submitted.

2. That complete autopsies be performed, if possible, on all
   abortions, stillborns, deadborns, and neonatal deaths produced
   in association with Clomid therapy and the findings submitted.
   It is suggested that gross and microscopic anatomical studies
   be done and a search made for genetic and enzyme abnormalities.

3. That patients having severe visual disturbances during Clomid
   therapy be followed and the findings submitted.

Sincerely yours,

Edwin M. Ortiz, M. D.
Director, Division of Metabolic
and Endocrine Drug Surveillance
Office of Marketed Drugs
Bureau of Medicine

EXHIBIT 8

501

FORM No. 102

INTERDEPARTMENT MEMO

THE WM. S. MERRELL COMPANY
Division of Richardson-Merrell Inc.

To   Dr. R. H. Levin

From   Mark T. Hoekenga, M.D.

Subject MEETING WITH FDA ON JUNE 4 CLOMID LETTER
July 9, 1969

Date July 14, 1969

Copies to
CABunde
DEHoltkamp
FDLamb
JKLindsay
JSScott
RHWoodward
REWilliams (RMI)

Dr. O'Dell and I met with Drs. Edwin M. Ortiz and Leslie Dill regarding Dr. Ortiz's letter of June 4 and our reply of June 19. Dr. Ortiz had recommended that living infants resulting from Clomid therapy be followed for 2 years, and that autopsies and search for genetic and enzyme abnormalities be made on abortions, stillborns, and neonatal deaths. Our June 19 reply essentially wondered why the request was being made. For convenience, a copy of our June 19 letter is attached.

Regarding Recommendation 2:

Apparently the June 4 FDA letter was mostly Dr. Dill's idea. He did most of the talking at our meeting. His starting point related to recommendation 2, that the 30% abortion rate in one of our Clomid pregnancy categories was unusually high. He was referring to a group of 43 abortions out of 141 pregnancies that occurred when the time of Clomid administration was not stated. I have underlined these figures in red on the attached "Table 11A" taken from our February 1969 Periodic Report. Actually it would have been more appropriate for Dr. Dill to have referred to the top line on Table 11A in which it is indicated that 328 abortions occurred in 1836 patients when conception occurred during the last treatment cycle; the 328 abortions represent 18 per cent of the total pregnancies in the group, an incidence that we believe to be anticipated in the ex-infertility type of patient we are dealing with. Be that as it may, Dr. Dill has an impression that we should want to be able to show that Clomid does not increase the abortion rate. His thought is that chromosomal studies would clarify this point. It is well known, of course, that chromosomal aberrations are common in aborted human fetal material (XO aneuploidy, triploidy, tetraploidy, trisomics of Groups A, B, C, D, E, F, and G, etc.). Dr. Dill thought that if Clomid-related abortuses proved to have a 10% higher rate of chromosomal aberrations than non-Clomid ones, this would be significant. We stated that we would think about his comments but would be disinclined to initiate any kind of a chromosomal survey or study unless it could be designed to be statistically significant. It would, of course, have to be a prospective one, in a large medical center using a lot of Clomid.

Regarding an enzyme abnormality search in abortions, stillbirths, etc., I feel that we drew a complete blank. Dr. Dill spoke vaguely of

EXHIBIT 9

FORM No. 102

INTERDEPARTMENT MEMO

THE WM. S. MERRELL COMPANY
Division of Richardson-Merrell Inc.

To Dr. M. T. Hoekenga

Date **February 22, 1972**

Copies to JWNewberne

From D. E. Holtkamp, Ph.D.

Subject CLOMID/Dr. David Charles
(your memo, 2/15/72)

In follow-up of the January report from Dr. Charles, Dr. Newberne and I have been discussing the possibility of starting a pilot study for trying to evaluate the effect of Clomid (clomiphene citrate) on chromosome pattern. In response to your question, we feel that it is too early to try to start a laboratory approach _in vitro_ or in animals and that the literature be reviewed first. I have started two MEDLARS literature searches for 1964 to present.

We have reviewed the Clomid bibliography. One _in vitro_ test was reported with the use of Clomid and at high concentrations, chromosome changes were induced. On the other hand, reproduction tests using the methodology employed currently, were conducted at Merrell with the isomers and these tests failed to show problems.

Dr. Charles' former colleague, Dr. Turner, has supplied me with a "privileged document" which he has sent to Dr. Charles as principal investigator for additions and editing. This report still has insufficient detail to permit appraisal of methodology and results and we must await the additions by Dr. Charles. References to methodology in this report will be pursued. I hope to be meeting with Dr. Charles and Dr. Turner in Boston sometime next week.

Dr. Newberne and I feel that a more critical and objective type of pilot study could be designed after more opportunity to review the literature and receipt of the more detailed report. Methodology, _per se_, will be especially important and since so many approaches could be tried, we need time for selections.

EXHIBIT 10

PROTOCOL AND LEGEND

1. NO: Sequential number of case history.
2. CASE NO: Merrell number of case history.
3. AGE: Age of pt. at commencement of tx.
4. PRIOR ABORT.: No. of S/A prior to Clomid tx.
   - (a) ?: Unknown.
   - (b) 0: None.
   - (c) 1: 1 prior S/A.
   - (d) 2: 2 prior S/A.
   - (e) C: Clomid pregnancy.
5. AMT. LAST DOSE: Amount of Clomid given during last dose in relation to conception (mg./days).
6. DATE LAST DOSE: The inclusive dates during which the last dose of Clomid was ingested.
7. TX. TO CONCEP.: Timing of last dose of Clomid treatment in relation to date of conception.
   - (a) Star: last tx. during *cycle of conception* (prior to date of conception only)
   - (b) 1: Last tx. *one* cycle prior to the cycle of conception.
   - (c) 2+: Last tx. *two or more* cycles prior to the cycle of conception.
   - (d) Concep. Cycle & After: Last Clomid tx. during cycle of conception (including after date of conception).
   - (e) After Concep.: Last Clomid tx. after date of conception only (not prior to date of conception).
   - (f) Hyperstim.: Hyperstimulation of the ovaries, as a result of Clomid tx., during the cycle of conception.
   - (g) ?: Timing of tx. in relation to conception unknown.
   - (h) Timing of cycles in relation to tx. first determined by date of LMP (last menstrual period) or number of menstrual periods between date of last tx. and date of conception.
   - (i) If menstrual periods not given, then next utilize reference in the records to "cycles," including number of cycles from date of last treatment to date of conception.
   - (j) If no reference to menstrual periods or cycles, then considered tx. during cycle of concep. if date of concept. *within 30 days* of date that started last tx.; *one cycle* prior if concept. *within 31-60 days* of date that started last tx.; and *two or more* cycles prior if date of concept. *after 60 days* following start of last tx.

8. DATE CONCEP.: Date of conception.
9. DATE DEL.: Date of delivery (termination) of pregnancy.
10. OUTCOME: Outcome of pregnancy.
    - (a) L: Live.
    - (b) N: Normal.
    - (c) S: Stillborn.
    - (d) T: Term.
    - (e) P: Premature.
    - (f) I: Immature
    - (g) F: Female.
    - (h) M: Male.
    - (i) I: Infant (no sex given).
    - (j) ?: Outcome unknown.
    - (k) Abortion:
      - (1) Termination of pregnancy Where embryo or fetus weighs less than 500 gms. (1 lb., 1.6 oz.); where mult. births, weight of heaviest fetus used.
      - (2) If weight not given, then delivery of fetus that is 20 wks. Or less from date of conception.
      - (3) If weight and duration of pregnancy not given, then use description given by investigator (i.e.,"abortion," "miscarriage," etc.)
11. MISC.:
    - (a) Mult.: Multiple birth.
    - (b) ND: Neonatal death.
    - (c) SB: Stillbirth.
    - (d) Ectopic: Ectopic pregnancy.
    - (e) Hyd.: Hydatidiform mole.
    - (f) LBW: Low birth weight (38 wks. Or more gestation weighing less than 2500 gms.)

EXHIBIT 11

504

NO.	CASE NO.	AGE	PRIOR ABORT.	AMT. LAST DOSE	DA LAST DOSE	TX. TO CONCEP.	DATE CONCEP.	DATE DEL.	OUTCOME	3 MISC.
31	A 013-105	33	0	50×5	7-16-66 / 7-20-66	HYPERSTIM. *	8-4-66	9-27-66	ABORTION *	
32	A 013-106	24	0	50×5	9-5-66 / 9-6-66	HYPERSTIM. *	9-12-66	3-25-67	IMMATURE FEMALE	NEONATAL DEATH
33	013-107				1-11-67 / 1-17-67	*	1-19-67	9-67	LPF	MULT. IUD
34	A 013-108	28	1	50×7	8-26-66 / 9-2-66	HYPERSTIM. *	9-16-66	1-12-67	ABORTION	*
35	A 013-109	37	1	50×7	8-20-66 / 9-5-66	HYPERSTIM. * LMP 4-2-67 * 1	9-20-66	6-16-67	NTF	
36	013-110				2-16-67 / 3-22-67		4-67	12-29-67	NTF	
37	014-001	35	0	50×18 / 100×3	11-13-61 / 12-3-61	AFTER CONCEP.	11-11-61	8-20-62	NORMAL TERM MALE	
38	014-004	30	0	50×14	11-8-61 / 11-21-61	LMP 1-13-62 2+	1-23-62 TO 2-1-62	11-10-62	NORMAL TERM FEMALE	
39	014-008	27	0	150×3	2-16-62 / 2-18-62	2+	7-12-62	5-7-63	NORMAL TERM MALE	
40	014-009	30	0	50×9	12-26-61 / 1-3-62	2+	7-15-62	4-20-63	NORMAL TERM MALE	
41	014-010	25	0	100×7	1-8-62 / 1-14-62	2+	10-10-62	3 MOS.	ABORTION	
42	A 014-012	23	1	150×5	4-30-62 / 5-4-62	2+	2-10-63	12-19-63	BIRTH DEFECT MALE *	
43	014-013	UNK.	0	150×7	4-13-62 / 4-19-62	2+	7-2-62	5-6-63	NORMAL TERM FEMALE	
44	014-016	28	0	200×1	5-2-62	2+	12-29-62	9-20-63	NORMAL TERM FEMALE	
45	014-023	25	0	200×3	8-6-62 LMP 3-23-63	2+	4-2-63	7-10-63	ABORTION	

EXHIBIT 12

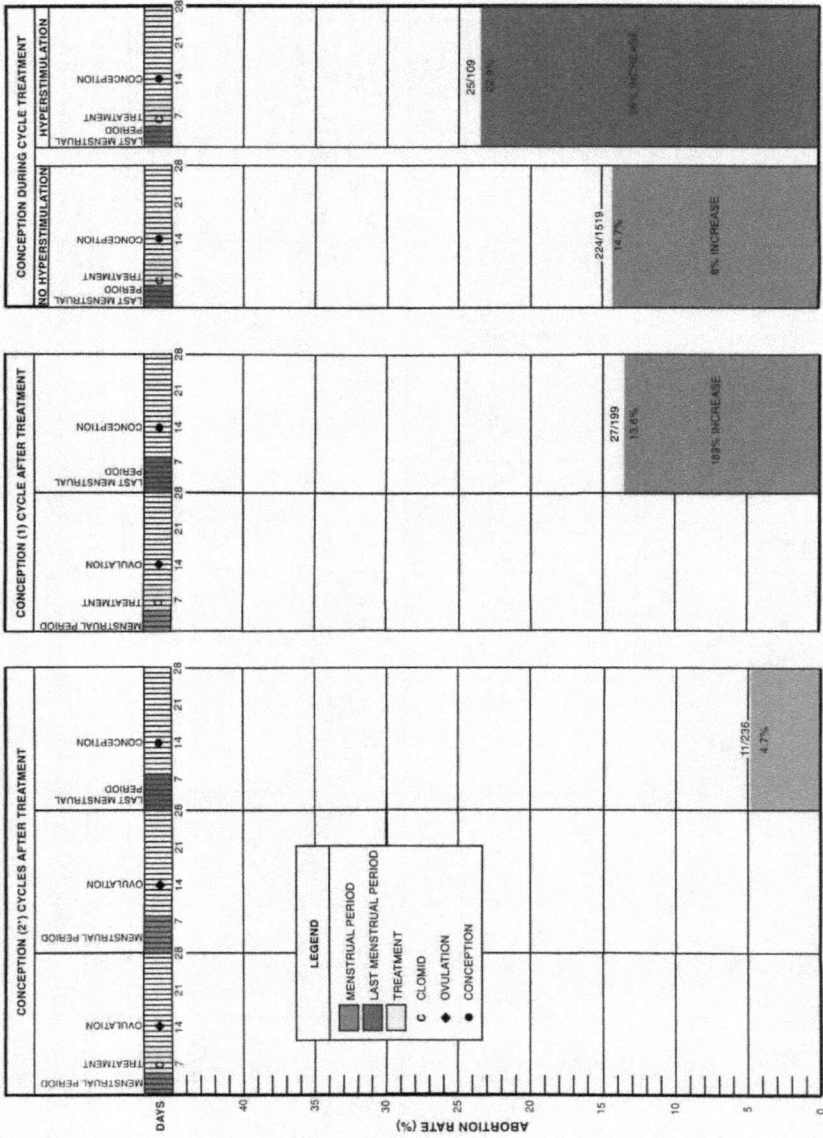

CLOMID: PREMARKETING ABORTION RATES

FIRST TRIMESTER SPONTANEOUS ABORTIONS

EXHIBIT 13

506

Clomid Prescribing Information, Copy Seria   Y451B (030581)

twin, 11 (0.5%) triplet, 7 (0.3%) quadruplet, and 3 (0.13%) quintuplet. The
outcome of these pregnancies resulting in one or more live births is listed
in Table 1.

Of the 165 twin pregnancies for which sufficient information was available,
the ratio of monozygotic to dizygotic twins was about 1:5.

After Clomid was available upon prescription in the United States in 1967,
there was a report of a sextuplet birth attributed to Clomid. None of the
sextuplets, each weighing less than 400 grams, survived, although each
appeared grossly normal.

4. Pregnancy Wastage and Birth Anomalies

The overall incidence of reported birth anomalies from pregnancies associated
with maternal Clomid ingestion during the investigational studies was within
the range of that reported in published references for the general population.
Among the birth anomalies spontaneously reported as individual cases since
commercial availability of Clomid, the proportion of neural tube defects has
been high among pregnancies associated with ovulation induced by Clomid, but
this has not been supported by data from population-based studies.

The physician should explain so that the patient understands the assumed risk
of any pregnancy whether the ovulation was induced with the aid of Clomid or
occurred naturally. The incidence of abortion, stillbirth, and other pregnancy wastage as well as incidences of neonatal deaths and birth anomalies
reported during the investigational clinical studies of Clomid is listed in
Tables 2, 3, and 4.

EXHIBIT 14a

The patient should be informed of the greater pregnancy risks associated with certain characteristics or conditions of any pregnant woman: e.g., age of female and male partner, history of spontaneous abortions, Rh genotype, abnormal menstrual history, infertility history (regardless of cause), organic heart disease, diabetes, exposure to infectious agents such as rubella, familial history of birth anomaly, and other risk factors that may be pertinent to the patient for whom Clomid is being considered. Based upon the evaluation of the patient, genetic counseling may be indicated.

Population-based reports have been published on possible elevation of risk of Down's Syndrome in ovulation induction cases and of increase in trisomy defects among spontaneously aborted fetuses from subfertile women receiving ovulation inducing drugs (no women with Clomid alone and without additional inducing drug). However, as yet, the reported observations are too few to confirm or not confirm the presence of an increased risk that would justify amniocentesis, other than for the usual indications because of age and family history.

The experience from patients of all diagnoses (Table 2) during clinical investigation of Clomid shows a pregnancy wastage or fetal loss rate of 21.4% (abortion rate of 19.0% and other loss rate of 2.4%).

ADVERSE REACTIONS

Symptoms/Signs/Conditions

Adverse effects appeared to be dose-related, occurring more frequently at the higher doses and with the longer courses of treatment used in investigational studies. At recommended dosage, adverse effects are not prominent and infrequently interfere with treatment. The incidence of symptoms and/or signs

Clomid Prescribing Information, Copy Serie   451B (030581)

EXHIBIT 14b

CONGENITAL MALFORMATIONS AFTER IN-VITRO FERTILISATION

SIR,—In analysing further data from the register of in-vitro fertilisation (IVF) and gamete intrafallopian transfer (GIFT) pregnancies in Australia and New Zealand,[1] we found more infants than expected with two types of congenital malformation—namely, spina bifida and transposition of the great vessels.

In the 1979–86 fertilisation cohort of IVF pregnancies notified to the register by sixteen IVF units, there were 1694 live births and stillbirths of at least 20 weeks' gestation, and 3 terminations of pregnancy (at 17, 20, and 22 weeks) after prenatal diagnosis of fetal abnormalities.[2]

37 fetuses and infants had major congenital malformations, an incidence of 2·2% (95% confidence interval 1·5–2·9%). Because the IVF figures included terminations of pregnancy and some infants whose malformations were diagnosed beyond the early neonatal period, they are not directly comparable with the incidence of 1·5% for major malformations in Australia.[3] Nevertheless, the national data can be used to determine the expected numbers of major malformations diagnosed at birth or in the first week.

6 infants had spina bifida compared with an expected number of 1·2 (p = 0·0015; one-sided Poisson). 2 of these infants had other malformations. 1 had trisomy 18 and an absent left auditory canal, renal dysplasia, absent urethra, and imperforate anus. There is a well-recognised association between trisomy 18 and spina bifida but even if this infant is excluded, the probability of 5 cases is still 0·0075. The other infant with multiple malformations had sirenomelia, renal agenesis, colonic atresia, and ventricular septal defect. 1 of the infants with isolated spina bifida had a twin with trisomy 18. The spinal lesion was in the lumbosacral region in all 6 infants. These 6 infants were born during a period of more than three years to women treated in three of the larger IVF units. No previous children with spina bifida had been born to these mothers. None of the 37 malformed IVF infants had other neural tube defects.

4 infants had transposition of the great vessels, compared with an expected number of 0·6 (p = 0·0034). 1 of these infants also had other malformations (gastroschisis, tracheo-oesophageal fistula, ventricular septal defect, and hypoplastic kidneys). The mothers had been treated in different IVF units and the births occurred over a period of six years.

The increased numbers of infants with spina bifida and transposition could be chance findings, but the probability for each is low. 3 of the infants with spina bifida and 2 with transposition were from multiple births, which occur frequently in IVF after transfer of more than one embryo.[4] The early management of the pregnancies resulting in these 10 malformed infants did not differ from that in other IVF pregnancies, but a more detailed study of laboratory techniques is required.

While our results show an overall incidence of major malformations in IVF births similar to that in the population, further data from other IVF groups are needed to determine whether spina bifida, transposition, and possibly other malformations occur more often than usual. There have been insufficient births in most IVF centres to examine uncommon outcomes such as congenital malformation in single units. Obtaining reliable information about these infants poses some difficulties because many women treated by IVF have their babies in hospitals other than the one associated with the IVF unit.

If the findings in respect of spina bifida are confirmed, prenatal diagnosis by ultrasound is now readily available. Indeed, ultrasound is used routinely in IVF to monitor ovarian follicular size and the appearance and number of gestational sacs. However, the ultrasound examinations in the first few months of pregnancy are usually done too early to detect spina bifida.

Since it may be some years before there are adequate numbers of births to determine conclusively if the risk of congenital malformations is increased after IVF, our findings also have implications for the current restriction of research on early embryos.

National Perinatal Statistics Unit.
University of Sydney,
Sydney, NSW 2006, Australia

PAUL A. L. LANCASTER

1. Australian In Vitro Fertilisation Collaborative Group. High incidence of preterm births and early losses in pregnancy after in vitro fertilisation. Br Med J 1985; 291: 1160–63.
2. National Perinatal Statistics Unit, Fertility Society of Australia. IVF and GIFT pregnancies, Australia and New Zealand, 1986. Sydney: NPSU, 1987.
3. National Perinatal Statistics Unit. Congenital malformations, Australia, 1981–1984. Sydney: NPSU, 1986.
4. Lancaster PAL. How many oocytes/embryos should be transferred? Lancet 1987; ii: 110.
5. Dawson K. In vitro fertilisation: Legislation and problems of research. Br Med J 1987; 295: 1184–86.

EXHIBIT 15

Here is the breakdown of clomiphene exposure by timing relative to the LMP

	#cases/#controls	MVRR (95% CI) *
−6 → −4	13/48	0.8 (0.4−1.7)
−3	13/53	0.8 (0.4−1.5)
−2	13/59	0.7 (0.3−1.3)
−1	13/62	0.7 (0.3−1.3)
1	11/48	0.7 (0.3 ch.5)
2	0/5	

Hypospadias

11	244	255	or = 1.94
85	3656	3741	(1.02, 3.68

* These RRs compare the exposed in a given time window to those unexposed from −6 to +2.

WITHOUT HYPOSPADIAS

NTD

22	1020	
85	3656	3741

As far as control subgroups go — we did our analyses of any use of a fertility drug among defect subgroups in the large pool of all subjects (i.e. before a sample was selected to reduce the control group to a more manageable size) We were looking for either a doubling or halving in rate of drug use compared to controls overall — the larger pool gave us more power to do this. Those are the numbers + rates referred to in the article. The rates for chromosomal anomalies (n=1078) was 1.6%, for LRDs (m=535) was 3.4%, and hyposp. was 5.1%. Since the rate was high for hypospadias I looked at clomiphene use among the sample control series — 11 exposed of (255) compared to 85 exposed of 3741 other controls. Very interesting! Please call if this is confusing

Regards, Martha

(617) 734−6006

5 cats.   5 cats.
MAT AGE & INTERVIEW YEAR
≤20 20-29 30-39   76 − 91
                 ≥3 yr. Cancer

EXHIBIT 16

Ovulation induction and risk of neural tube defects

Martha M Werler, Carol Louik, Samuel Shapiro, Allen A Mitchell

The relation between use of ovulation-inducing drugs and risk of neural tube defects (NTDs) was studied in a case-control surveillance programme. The frequency of any use of such drugs during the 6 months before the last menstrual period or during pregnancy was 3·6% for 1034 mothers of infants and fetuses with NTDs (cases) and 2·6% for 4081 mothers of those with other major congenital malformations (controls) (relative risk 1·1, 95% CI 0·8–1·7). Relative risks for clomiphene and for hormones were 0·8 (0·5–1·3) and 1·5 (0·7–3·4), respectively. These data suggest that use of ovulation-inducing drugs before conception does not increase the risk of NTDs.

Lancet 1994; 344: 445–46

Use of ovulation-inducing medications has increased,[1] and questions have been raised about teratogenic risk, especially for neural tube defects (NTDs).[2-6] One contribution uses data collected as part of a case-control surveillance programme of birth defects.

The Slone Epidemiology Unit Birth Defects Study (ongoing since 1976) identifies fetuses and infants affected with major malformations at prenatal diagnostic clinics and maternity and tertiary-care hospitals in the metropolitan areas of Boston, Philadelphia, and Toronto (and Iowa in 1983–85). Interviews were done in person within 6 months of delivery. Women who reported use of ovulation-inducing drugs at any time during the 6 months before the last menstrual period or during pregnancy were asked about specific drugs. Such drugs included clomiphene, follicle-stimulating and luteinizing hormones (FSH+LH), and human chorionic gonadotropin (HCG), and bromocriptine.

Cases were 1034 subjects with NTDs (776 with spina bifida, 135 with anencephaly, and 123 with encephalocele), after exclusion of subjects with syndromes or genetic disorders. Cases represent an 80% participation for physicians and mothers. Subjects with other malformations (except defects of central nervous system, eye, or bowel) were used as potential controls. To counter-balance any potential drug-related risk, the use of ovulation-inducing drugs for the largest subgroups (n>600): inguinal hernia, cleft lip with or without cleft palate, ventricular septal defect, chromosomal anomalies, pyloric stenosis, and hypospadias. Maternal age and interview-year-adjusted frequencies ranged from 2·3% to 5·1% (2·6% for the group overall). For efficiency, controls were matched by frequency to cases by five categories each of maternal age and interview year. The control/case ratio was 4:1, except two categories had fewer cases because of smaller pools of controls. The final control pool was 4081 infants/fetuses (mothers). Case and control mothers were compared for the use of any and specific ovulation-inducing drugs. Relative risks (odds ratios) were estimated by unconditional logistic regression. Terms were included for maternal age, interview year, geographic area, birth status, gravidity, maternal education, planned pregnancy, and daily use of folic-acid-containing vitamin supplements around conception. Multivariate models for specific ovulation-inducing drugs included terms for each of the drugs.

The frequency of use of an ovulation-inducing drug was 3·6% for case mothers and 2·6% for control mothers (table). For timing of use relative to last menstrual period (data not shown), relative risk estimates ranged from 1·3 for exposure during the first lunar month before use was reported.

Drug	Cases (%)	Controls (%)	Relative risk (95% CI)
Any	31 (3·0)	113 (2·8)	1·1 (0·8–1·7)
Clomiphene	22 (2·1)	95 (2·4)	0·8 (0·5–1·3)
FSH + LH and/or HCG	11 (1·1)	31 (0·8)	1·5 (0·7–3·4)
Hormones	4 (0·4)	16 (0·4)	

Table: Use of ovulation-inducing drugs among mothers of 1034 case-defined cases and 4081 malformed controls

during 4–6 months before last menstrual period to 0·9 for exposure during the first lunar month. Only 1 case mother and 12 control mothers reported use during the second lunar month; no later use was reported. Clomiphene was used by the mothers of 2·1% of cases and 2·4% of controls. For timing of use (data not shown), relative risk estimates ranged from 1·0 for exposure 4–6 months before last menstrual period to 0·6 for exposure during the first lunar month. Overall, 1·1% of cases and 0·8% controls were exposed to FSH + LH and/or HCG. Only 0·4% of case and 0·2% of control mothers used bromocriptine.

Subgroup analyses were limited to clomiphene because of small numbers exposed to hormones and bromocriptine. For the 776 cases of spina bifida, 17 (2·2%) mothers used clomiphene (relative risk 0·8, 95% CI, 0·5–1·5). 5 cases with anencephaly and no cases with encephalocele were exposed. Among the NTD cases, 839 subjects were considered to be isolated (they had no associated defects other than sequelae of the NTD); 15 (1·8%) were exposed (relative risk 0·6, 0·3–1·2). Of the 636 isolated cases of spina bifida, 12 (1·9%) mothers used clomiphene (relative risk 0·7, 0·3–1·3). The mixed subgroup of cases with associated defects was too small to examine separately.

We found no increase in risk of NTDs for overall use of ovulation-inducing drugs; less than a doubling in risk was ruled out with 95% confidence. For clomiphene, the most commonly used agent, an even smaller increase was ruled out. We also observed no associations for all spina bifida, isolated NTDs, isolated spina bifida, and when timing of exposure was considered. For FSH + LH and/or HCG, the risk for NTDs was slightly increased, but not statistically so. Although bromocriptine use was more common among cases, there were too few exposed subjects to provide stable risk-estimates.

Selection bias was unlikely for several reasons. Subject ascertainment was probably not related to subfertility treatments, especially because controls were also malformed. Participation rates were similar for cases and controls. The controls included a wide range of defects, so the exposure frequency of each defect would have little influence on that of the overall group. For the largest control subgroup, exposure to ovulation-inducing drugs differed only slightly. Also, when each subgroup was separately excluded, relative risks ranged from 1·1 to 1·2. Anencephaly cases may have been under-ascertained during the study's early years, but our findings were consistent for spina bifida and NTDs overall.

Interviews were conducted up to 22 months after the exposure period of interest, but our findings are unlikely to have been affected by incomplete reporting because subjects were specifically asked about drug treatment for infertility and clomiphene in particular. Also, the experience of subfertility and its treatment tends to be emotional, and unlikely to be forgotten.

Although control for effects of several factors revealed little or no confounding, we cannot rule out confounding by other factors, such as indication for treatment. For certain types of subfertility, pregnancy may occur only with treatment, and clomiphene and the hormones studied have no indications other than subfertility. In an observational study, it is not possible to separate the effects of subfertility from those of its treatment.

Concern about a relation between use of ovulation-inducing drugs and NTDs was raised in case reports during the 1970s.[7] Subsequent findings from birth-defect registry[2,3,6] case-control,[4,7] and cohort studies have estimated risks ranging from 0 to 9·3. Before the latest studies[6-8] were unstable, each with less than 5 exposed cases. Of the larger investigations, our risk-estimate — based on an apparent near-field ascertainment, and two case-control studies[4,7] found no increased risk.

In the largest study to date, our findings for use of ovulation-inducing drugs and, specifically for clomiphene, were reassuring. Estimates approximated unity with narrow confidence intervals. For other drugs, we were unable to rule out increases in NTD risk; the data were sparse and these drugs require further study.

We thank Theresa Gillman, Dawn Pellusso, Sally Perkins, Jean Shimelo, Diane Gallagher, Annamaria Durkin, and Mary Tanwhisa for their help. We also thank all the participating families and the institutions that gave access to their patients. Major support was provided by NICHD grant R01–HD25697 and Maternal and Child Health Resources Development grant MCJ-250560; additional support was provided by Medical Marvell Dow.

References

1 Glazener AM, Aten S, Eskin BA. Ovulation induction with clomiphene and its role in human reproduction. J Reprod Med 1990; 35: 175–78.

2 Harlap S. Ovulation induction and congenital malformations. Lancet 1976; ii: 961.

3 Czeizel E, Wind R. Ovulation induction and neural tube defects. Lancet 1989; ii: 1251.

4 Mills LJ, Simpson JL, Rhoads GG, et al. Risk of spinal tube defects in relation to maternal fertility and fertility drug use. Lancet 1990; 336: 103–04.

5 Robert E, Francannet C, et al. Ovulation induction and neural tube defects: a registry study. Reprod Toxicol 1991; 5: 83–84.

6 Milli F, Khoury Mj, Lo X. Association between clomiphene citrate use and the risk of birth defects. Am J Epidemiol 1991; 134: 744 (abstract).

7 Fritz S, Kerr C. Ovulation stimulation and defects of neural tube? Lancet 1994; 343: 415.

8 Shapiro S, Siegel S. Possible relationship between clomiphene and neural tube defects. J Pediatr 1978; 93: 152.

Slone Epidemiology Unit, Boston University School of Public Health, 1371 Beacon Street, Brookline, MA 02146, USA (M M Werler MSc, C Louik MPH, S Shapiro MB, A A Mitchell MD)

Correspondence to: Dr Martha M Werler

EXHIBIT 17

HALF-LIFE TABLE OF CLOMIPHENE CITRATE

Cycle Day	Day 5	Day 6	Day 7	Day 8	Day 9	Total
5	100 mg.					100 mg.
6	90 mg.	100 mg.				190 mg.
7	80 mg.	90 mg.	100 mg.			270 mg.
8	70 mg.	80 mg.	90 mg.	100 mg.		340 mg.
9	60 mg.	70 mg.	80 mg.	90 mg.	100 mg.	400 mg.
10	50 mg.	60 mg.	70 mg.	80 mg.	90 mg.	350 mg.
11	45 mg.	50 mg.	60 mg.	70 mg.	80 mg.	305 mg.
12	40 mg.	45 mg.	50 mg.	60 mg.	70 mg.	265 mg.
13	35 mg.	40 mg.	45 mg.	50 mg.	60 mg.	230 mg.
14/1 *	30 mg.	35 mg.	40 mg.	45 mg.	50 mg.	200 mg.
15/2	25 mg.	30 mg.	35 mg.	40 mg.	45 mg.	175 mg.
16/3	22.5 mg.	25 mg.	30 mg.	35 mg.	40 mg.	152.5 mg.
17/4	20.0 mg.	22.5 mg.	25.0 mg.	30.0 mg.	35.0 mg.	132.5 mg.
18/5	17.5 mg.	20.0 mg.	22.5 mg.	25.0 mg.	30.0 mg.	115.0 mg.
19/6	15.0 mg.	17.5 mg.	20.0 mg.	22.5 mg.	25.0 mg.	100.0 mg.
20/7	12.5 mg.	15.0 mg.	17.5 mg.	20.0 mg.	22.5 mg.	87.5 mg.
21/8	11.3 mg.	12.5 mg.	15.0 mg.	17.5 mg.	20.0 mg.	76.3 mg.
22/9	10.0 mg.	11.3 mg.	12.5 mg.	15.0 mg.	17.5 mg.	66.3 mg.
23/10	8.8 mg.	10.0 mg.	11.3 mg.	12.5 mg.	15.0 mg.	57.6 mg.
24/11 **	7.5 mg.	8.8 mg.	10.0 mg.	11.3 mg.	12.5 mg.	50.1 mg.
25/12	6.3 mg.	7.5 mg.	8.8 mg.	10.0 mg.	11.3 mg.	43.9 mg.
26/13	5.6 mg.	6.3 mg.	7.5 mg.	8.8 mg.	10.0 mg.	38.2 mg.
27/14	5.0 mg.	5.6 mg.	6.3 mg.	7.5 mg.	8.8 mg.	33.2 mg.
28/15	4.4 mg.	5.0 mg.	5.6 mg.	6.3 mg.	7.5 mg.	28.8 mg.
29/16	3.8 mg.	4.4 mg.	5.0 mg.	5.6 mg.	6.3 mg.	25.1 mg.
30/17	3.1 mg.	3.8 mg.	4.4 mg.	5.0 mg.	5.6 mg.	21.9 mg.
1/18 ***	2.8 mg.	3.1 mg.	3.8 mg.	4.4 mg.	5.0 mg.	19.1 mg.

* Conception; ** Teratogenic Susceptibility; *** Organogenesis/Neural Groove Forms

EXHIBIT 18

512

www.ingramcontent.com/pod-product-compliance
Lightning Source LLC
Chambersburg PA
CBHW032047020426
42335CB00011B/218